ATLAS OF THE

ATLAS OF THE CANINE BRAIN

Authored by
O. S. Adrianov and T. A. Mering

Translated by
E. Ignatieff

Edited by
Kenneth E. Domino and Edward F. Domino

NPP Books
http://www.nppbooks.com

NPP Books, 15 Sunset Road, Arlington, Massachusetts, 02474, USA
Copyright 2010 by NPP Books

Printed in the United States of America.

Second Edition

International Book Standard Number (ISBN): 978-0-916182-17-5 (Softcover)

First Edition ISBN: 978-0-916182-01-4)

Translated and published in English with the permission of the authors, the Medical Publishing House, and the All-Union Society International Hooks, USSR.

Library of Congress Catalog Card No. 64-63010.
Supported in part by Grant NB-04713-01 United States Public Health Service.

ИНСТИТУТ МОЗГА АМН СССР

О. С. АДРИАНОВ, Т. А. МЕРИНГ

АТЛАС
МОЗГА СОБАКИ

ГОСУДАРСТВЕННОЕ ИЗДАТЕЛЬСТВО МЕДИЦИНСКОЙ ЛИТЕРАТУРЫ

Москва — 1959 — Медгиз

Cover of Atlas of the Canine Brain published in 1959

ATLAS OF THE CANINE BRAIN

By

O. S. ADRIANOV and T. A. MERING
Brain Institute, Academy of Medical Sciences, USSR

Translated by
E. Ignatieff
Department of Slavic Languages
University of Michigan
Ann Arbor

Edited by
E. F. Domino
Department of Pharmacology
University of Michigan
Ann Arbor

Published originally in Russian as a Government Publication of Medical Literature
Moscow - 1959 - Medgiz

Cover of Atlas of the Canine Brain published in 1964

EDITORS' REMARKS, SECOND EDITION

The first English edition of this book, Atlas of the Canine Brain, was published in 1964. Currently, this book is not generally available. Hence, the present second edition was composed and re-edited to meet current printing standards.

The changes to this book include: typesetting using LaTeX; updating the Table of Contents, Bibliography, Symbols, and Index; reordering and renumbering figures and text; correcting errata; rewording chapter and section titles; and, italicization of Latin terms.

Publication of this revised book has been made possible with the help of Zarina Memon. Her efforts in scanning the original Russian and English books, and the editing of the figures using Adobe Photoshop, were invaluable.

K.E. Domino & E.F. Domino
March 12, 2010
Arlington, Massachusetts, U.S.A.

EDITOR'S REMARKS, FIRST EDITION

Translation of information from one language to another inevitably loses some of the flavor of the original. This book is no exception. We have tried to retain the style of authors Adrianov and Mering as much as possible consistent with understandable English. It is our belief that this atlas of the canine brain offers data and a point of view which so far have been unavailable to Western scientists. The increasing use of the dog in experimental neurology, physiology and pharmacology makes this atlas especially important. It is a valuable adjunct to other atlases of the dog brain now available in English.

Publication of this atlas has been made possible by Mrs. Edith Price who helped in the translation, Mrs. Ruth Good for editorial assistance, and Mrs. Ellen Howard for typing the manuscript. Mrs. Edith Ignatieff, our translator, deserves a special debt of gratitude for the many long hours required to make this book a reality. Translation errors in the scientific aspects of this book are the editor's. It is hoped that there are not too many.

E.F. Domino
January, 1964
Ann Arbor, Michigan

ABSTRACT

The Atlas of the Canine Brain offers a systematic and detailed analysis of the structure, connections, and functional peculiarities of various parts of the canine central nervous system, from the spinal cord through the cerebral cortex. The cytoarchitectural areas in the cerebral cortex, shown in a new map devised by the authors, are based on the principles of I.P. Pavlov's teaching on analyzers.

The exact information on the topography of various areas will permit the experimenter to destroy a selected portion of the brain without materially disturbing the other parts.

The reader of the atlas will become acquainted with structural details not by means of schematic drawings, but primarily through photographs of specimens prepared in the laboratories of cytoarchitecture of the Brain Institute of the Academy of Medical Sciences, USSR.

The atlas provides a bibliography compiled according to the various sections of the central nervous system, in conformity with the text.

The atlas is meant for a wide circle of practical and scientific workers: physicians, biologists, and veterinarians.

Professor E.P. Kononova
Scientific Consultant – Head of the Laboratory of Cytoarchitecture of the Brain Institute AMN USSR
The photographs were made in the Photolaboratory of the Brain Institute AMN USSR, by A.A. Kudriashov

PREFACE

One of the most widely used subjects for experimental neuroanatomical studies is the dog. This makes it necessary to have detailed and systematic information on the central nervous system of this animal. However, in the literature on this subject there are no studies that delineate the macro- and microscopic structure of all sections of the spinal cord and cerebral cortex of the dog. There are many reports containing data on the brain of the rabbit and of the cat (Winkler and Potter [65, 66]; Papez [59]), the horse (Ellenberger and Baum [20]), man and animals (Kononova [38]). Some studies include a minute description of the structure of only one portion of the canine central nervous system (Klempin [737]; Filimonov [713, 715]; Rioch, 1929 [*Editors' note: The Rioch reference cannot be found in the bibliography.*]; Gurevich and Bykhovskaya [725]; Rose [778] and others).

The present atlas gives a systematic description of the macro- and micro-anatomic structure of the canine spinal cord, brainstem, and cerebral hemispheres. The atlas is divided into three chapters.

The first chapter sets forth in detail the macroscopic structure of the spinal cord, the brainstem, and the subcortical formations. There is also a detailed analysis of a great number of serial sections made through the entire brain and the spinal cord. The original photomicrographs of the spinal cord and the brainstem shown in the atlas have been enlarged so as to make it possible to inspect the entire area of the sections and to expose with precision the various nuclear groups and conducting tracts of the canine brain.

The second chapter contains a description of sulci and gyri of the hemispheres of the dog's brain. The cytoarchitecture of various regions and areas of the cerebral cortex is described minutely. Comparatively little research has been devoted to this subject (Betz [980]; Campbell [704] and others). Widest attention has been given to the investigations and maps compiled by Klempin [737] and Gurevich and Bykhovskaya [725]. These studies do contain interesting material; however, supplemental data and certain corrections are required. The data on the boundaries of some sections and areas of the cortex are rather ambiguous, and there are no photomicrographs of the cellular structure of many areas.

The present atlas includes photomicrographs of all sections of the cortex and a map of the cytoarchitectural areas of the neocortex, based on extensive material. The materials of Filimonova were used for the description of the areas of the paleocortex, the archiocortex, and the intermediate cortex.

In their studies of the cellular structure of the cortex, the authors proceeded from Pavlov's viewpoint with respect to the end stations of various analyzers. The cortex is divided (where this is possible) into regions corresponding to the analyzers.

The third chapter, written by Leontovich and Mering gives details on the topography of subcortical nuclei and their projection upon the cranium. Photographs of a series of sections through the cranium and the brain are presented, as well as the projections of the cerebral hemispheres, basic sulci, and subcortical formations on the surface of the cranium. Also, calculations of the location of the most important subcortical formations are included. A similar report on the canine does not exist in the literature.

The material in this atlas greatly enriches our concepts of the structure of the dog's central nervous system.

The uniqueness of this atlas of the canine brain lies in the fact that its authors are not only morphologists, but are also qualified physiologists, which enhances considerably the value of their complex morpho-physiological work.

The atlas will be indispensable to a wide circle of scientific workers: physicians, morphologists, physiologists, and biologists who are studying problems of experimental medicine and biology and whose subject is primarily the dog.

Professor S.A. Sarkisov,
Active Member of the Academy of Medical Sciences USSR

CONTENTS

EDITORS' REMARKS, SECOND EDITION   vii

EDITOR'S REMARKS, FIRST EDITION   viii

ABSTRACT   ix

PREFACE   x

CONTENTS   xi

THE STRUCTURE OF THE SPINAL CORD, BRAINSTEM, AND SUBCORTICAL NUCLEI   1

General Characteristics 1

The Spinal Cord (*Medulla Spinalis*) (Fig. 2, 3, 4, 8, 9, 10) 1

Ascending (Centripetal) Tracts of the Spinal Cord 5

     Goll's Fasciculus and Burdach's Fasciculus (*Fasciculus Golli et Fasciculus Burdachi*) 5

     Straight or Dorsal Cerebellospinal Flechsig's Tract (*Fasciculus spinocerebellaris dorsalis, fscd*) 5

     The Decussated or Ventral Spinocerebellar Tract of Govers (*Fasciculus spinocerebellaris ventralis, fscv* 5

     Cerebrothalamic Tract (*Fasciculus spinothalamicus, fsth*) 7

Descending (Centrifugal) Tracts of the Spinal Cord 7

     Corticospinal or pyramidal tract (*Fasciculus corticospinalis s. pyramidalis, py*) 7

     Rubrospinal Tract or Monakov's Fasciculus (*Fasciculus rubrospinalis, frs*) 7

     Tectospinal or Predorsal Tract (*Fasciculus tectospinalis s. praedorsalis, fts*) 8

     Posterior Longitudinal Fasciculus (*Fasciculus longitudinalis posterior s. medians, flp*) 8

     Vestibulospinal Tract or Lowental's Fasciculus (*Fasciculus vestibulospinalis Lowentali*) 8

     Reticulospinal Tract (*Fasciculus reticulospinalis*) 8

The Brainstem 9

     The Medulla Oblongata (*medulla oblongata, mo*) and the pons Varolii (*pons Varolii, pV*) (Figs. 5,
         6, 11-27) 9

     The Cerebellum (Fig. 7) 15

     The Midbrain (mesencephalon) (Fig. 5, 6, 26-31) 18

     The Diencephalon (Fig. 6, 31-41) 19

     The Epithalamic Region 21

     The Hypothalamic Region 21

     The central ganglia, the lateral ventricles, and the commissures of the terminal brain (Fig. 5, 35-43) . 23

A Section through the Upper Part of the Cervical Spinal Cord (Fig. 8) 26

A Section at the Level Where the Spinal Cord Changes into the Medulla Oblongata, on a Level with the
     Decussation of the Fibers of the Pyramidal Tract (Section 10, Fig. 11) 30

A Section at the Level of the Lowest Portion of the Medulla Oblongata (Section 40, Fig. 12) 32

A Section at the Level of the Inferior Olivary Body of the Medulla Oblongata (Section 120, Fig. 13) 34

A Section through the Caudal Part of the Nucleus of the Hypoglossal Nerve (Section 200, Fig. 14) 36

A Section at the Level of the Opening of the Central Canal into the Cavity of the IV Ventricle (Section
     240, Fig. 15) 38

A Section through the Central Nucleus of the Reticular Formation (section 280, Fig. 16) 40

A Section at the Level of the Upper Part of the Inferior Olive (*oi*) (Section 360, Fig. 17) 42

A Section at the Level of the Emergence of the Nucleus of the Facial Nerve (Section 400, Fig. 18) 44

A Section of the Level of the Maximal Development of the Nucleus of the Facial Nerve (Section 490, Fig.
     19) 46

A Section at the Level of the Appearance of the Nuclei of the Auditory Nerve and the Beginning of the
     Superior Olive (Section 550, Fig. 20) 48

A Section through the Nucleus of the Abducent Nerve (Section 590, Fig. 21) 50

A Section on the Level of the Emergence of the Superior Cerebellar Peduncles (Section 650, Fig. 22) . . . 52

A Section through the Pons Varolii at the Level of the Appearance of the Motor Nucleus of the Trigeminal
     Nerve (Section 700, Fig. 23) 54

A Section through the pons Varolii, somewhat more Anterior (Section 760, Fig. 24) 56
A Section at the Level of the Maximal Development of the Pons' Nuclei and Fibers (Section 820, Fig. 25)   58
A Section at the Level of the Maximum Development of the Posterior Corpus Bigeminum (Which in the
    Dog Reaches Considerable Dimensions, Section 950, Fig. 26) 60
A Section through the Midbrain on the Level with the Corinissure of the Posterior Corpus Bigeminum
    (Section 990, Fig. 27) 62
A Section through the Midbrain at the Level of the Nuclei of the Trochlear Nerve (Section 1020, Fig. 28) . 64
A Section through the Midbrain at the Level of the Emergence of the Anterior Corpus Bigemini (Section
    1040, Fig. 29) 66
A Section through the Midbrain at the Level of the Emergence of the Red Nuclei (Section 1090, Fig. 30) .   68
A Section through the Mesencephalon at the Level of the Greatest Development of the Nuclei of the
    Oculomotor Nerve and the Red Nucleus (Section 1120, Fig. 31) 70
A Section at the Level of the Maximal Development of the Medial and Lateral Geniculate Bodies (Section
    1200, Fig. 32) 72
A Section at the Level of the Opening of the Cavity of the Sylvian Aqueduct into the *III* Ventricle (Section
    1260, Fig. 33) 74
A Section at the Level of the Maximal Development of the Mammillary Bodies (Section 1300, Fig. 34) . .   76
A Section slightly Anterior to the Previous One, at the Level of the Maximal Development of Corpus Luysi
    (Section 1330, Fig. 35) 78
A Section at the Level of the Infundibulum (Section 1380, Fig. 36) 80
A Section at the Level of the Maximal Development of the Central Lateral Nucleus of the Optic Thalamus
    (Section 1420, Fig. 37) 82
A Section at the Level of the Emergence of the Caudate Nucleus (Section 1460, Fig. 38) 84
A Section at the Level of the Optic Chiasm (Section 1490, Fig. 39) 86
A Section through the Optic Gniasm, slightly to the Front of the Previous Section (Section 1520, Fig. 40)   88
A Section at the Level of the Anterior Commissure (Section 1580, Fig. 41) 90
A Section at the Level of the Emergence of the Mass of the Septum Pellucidum (Section 1620, Fig. 42) .   92
A Section at the level of the Maximum Size of the Head of the Caudate Nucleus (Section 1820, Fig. 43) .   94

THE STRUCTURE OF THE CANINE CEREBRAL CORTEX   **97**

The Sulci and Gyri of the Cerebrum 97
The Sulci of the Lateral Surface of the Hemisphere (Fig. 44, 45) 97
The Sulci of the Medial Surface of the Hemisphere (Fig. 46) 100
The Sulci of the Lower Surface of the Hemisphere (Fig. 46) 101
The Cerebral Gyri (Fig. 47-48) 101
The Cellular Structure of the Cerebral Cortex (Fig. 49-51) 104
The Occipital Region (*Regio Occipitalis*) (Fig. 52-56) 111
The Parietal Region (*Regio Parietalis*) (Fig. 57, 58) 112
The Temporal Region (*Regio Temporalis*) (Fig. 59-66) 112
The Insular Region (*Regio Insularis*) (Fig. 67-72) 113
The Postcoronal Region (*Regio Postcoronalis*) (Fig. 73-80) 113
Area Pc_4 (*Area Postcoronalis Quarta*) (Fig. 76, 77) 114
Precoronal Region (*Regio Praecoronalis*) (Fig. 81-83) 114
The Frontal Region (*Regio Frontalis*) (Fig. 84-89) 115
Limbic Area (*Regio Limbica*) (Fig. 90-93) 115
Area O_1 (*Area Occipitalis Prima*) (Fig. 52) 118
Area O_2 (*Area Occipitalis Secunda*) (Fig. 53, 54) 120
Area *OP* (*Area Occipto Parietalis*) (Fig. 55, 56) 123
Area *P* (*Area Parietalis*) (Fig. 57, 58) 126
Area T_1 (*Area Temporalis Prima*) (Fig. 59) 130
Area T_2 (*Area Temporalis Secunda*) (Fig. 60) 132
Area T_3 (*Area Temporalis Tertia*) (Fig. 61) 134
Area T_4 (*Area Temporalis Quarta*) (Fig. 62, 63) 136
Transition of Cortical Areas from Temporal into the Entorhinal Region (*TE_1* and *TE_2*) (Fig. 64-66) 140
Area TE_1 (*Area Temporoentorhinalis Prima*) (Fig. 65) 142
Area TE_2 (*Area Temporoentorhinalis Secunda*) (Fig. 66) 144
Area I_1 (*Area Insularis Prima*) (Fig. 67) 146

Area I₂ (*Area Insularis Secunda*) (Fig. 68) 148
Area PI₁ (*Area Parainsularis Prima*) (Fig. 69) 150
Area PI₂ (*Area Parainsularis Secunda*) (Fig. 70) 152
Area Pc₁ (*Area Postcoronalis Prima*) (Fig. 73) 156
Area Pc₂ (*Area Postcoronalis Secunda*) (Fig. 74) 158
Area Pc₃ (*Area Postcoronalis Tertia*) (Fig. 75) 160
Subarea Pcˢ₄ (*Subarea Postcoronalis Quarta Superior*) (Fig. 76) 162
Subarea Pcⁱ₄ (*Subarea Postcoronalis Quarta Inferior*) (Fig. 77) 164
Area TPc (*Area Temporopostcoronalis*) (Fig. 78) 166
Area Prc₁ (*Area Praecoronalis Prima*) (Fig. 81) 170
Area Prc₂ (*Area Praecoronalis Secunda*) (Fig. 82) 172
Subarea Prc₂-L₂ (*Subarea Praecoronalis Limbica*) (Fig. 83) 174
Area F₁ (*Area Frontalis Prima*) (Fig. 84) 176
Area F₂ (*Area Frontalis Secunda*) (Fig. 85) 178
Area F₃ (*Area Frontalis Tertia*) (Fig. 86) 180
Area F₄ (*Area Frontalis Quarta*) (Fig. 87, 88) 182
Subarea F-L₂ (*Subarea Fronto-Limbica*) (Fig. 89) 186
Area L₁ (*Area Limbica Prima*) (Fig. 90) 188
Area L₂ (*Area Limbica Secunda*) (Fig. 91) 190
Area Pt₁ (*Area Peritectalis Prima*) and *Pt₂* (*Area Peritectalis Secunda*) (Fig. 92) 192
Area Pt₃ (*Area Peritectalis Tertia*) (Fig. 93) 194
The Paleocortex, Archicortex, and Intermediate Cortexi (*Paleocortex, Archicortex Et Cortex Intermedius*) . 197

THE TOPOLOGY OF THE SUBCORTICAL FORMATIONS AND THEIR PROJECTION UPON THE CRANIUM   **205**

BIBLIOGRAPHY   **243**
Research concerning all areas of the central nervous system 243
The Spinal Cord 246
The Medulla Oblongata, Pons Varolii and the Mesencephalon 250
The Cerebellum 258
The Midbrain 261
Subcortical Nuclei 266
Cerebral Cortex 269
Occipital Region (Optic Analysor) 274
Temporal Region (Auditory Analysor) 277
Postcoronal Area (Cutaneous Analysor) 280
Precoronal Region (Motor Analyser) 281
Frontal Region 284
Parietal, Limbic Regions, Archicortex, Paleocortex and Intermediate Cortex and Other Cortical Regions . . 286

SYMBOLS   **289**

INDEX   **295**

THE STRUCTURE OF THE SPINAL CORD, BRAINSTEM, AND SUBCORTICAL NUCLEI

General Characteristics

There are numerous reports in the literature on the structure of the spinal cord, brainstem, and subcortical nuclei in the carnivores. The subject has been dealt with in great detail in the atlas of Winkler and Potter [66], the handbook of Papez [59], and the works of Ingram, Hannett, and Ranson [531], Monnier [53, 54], and Rexed [150], in which there are drawings of serial sections of the cat's brain and photomicrographs of separate cellular groups. A description of the macroscopic structure of the canine brain is given in the handbooks of Flatau and Jacobsohn [23], Ellenberger and Baum [19, 20]. Extensive material on the macro- and microstructure of the human and animal brainstem can be found in the atlas compiled by E.P. Kononova [38]; however, the number of photomicrographs of serial sections of the canine brain is not adequate. In the studies by Langley [41], Bekhterev [1, 192], Lewandovski [46], Neiding [573], Rioch [588, 587], Papez [578] and others, there are descriptions of diverse areas or portions of the central nervous system of the dog.

In the investigations mentioned above there are a number of discrepancies particularly in the data on the structure of the optic thalamus. The information on the conducting tracts of the spinal cord and cerebrum of the dog is incomplete.

In writing this chapter, a great many publications concerning the structure and function of the various parts of the central nervous system were consulted. There is a description of original photomicrographs of sections of the spinal cord and cerebrum, stained according to Nissl's method. The brain was treated in a manner used by the Brain Institute (Kononova [738]). After the cranium was opened, the brain was fixed in formalin for 3 to 5 days and then photographed, the photographs showing all sulci; after further induration, the brain was dehydrated in alcohol of increasing strength, then embedded in paraffin. After that, serial sections were prepared and stained with cresyl violet. The thickness of each section was 20 μ, or approximately 40 sections to 1 mm.

Fig. 1 shows a photograph of the canine brain, with lines indicating the position of the sections represented in Chapter 1 of the atlas. As seen in this figure, the distance between the sections is usually from 1 to 1.5 mm.

The Spinal Cord (*Medulla Spinalis*) (Fig. 2, 3, 4, 8, 9, 10)

The canine spinal cord has the shape of a long cylinder and reaches a length of 38 cm (Fig. 2).

The spinal cord is constructed on a segmental principle and is subdivided into segments; 8 cervical, 13 thoracic, 7 lumbar, 3 sacral, and 5 to 6 coccygeal (Fig. 3). Each segment has corresponding pairs of ventral (anterior) and dorsal (posterior) roots. Thus, from each side extend 8 pairs of cervical roots, 13 pairs of thoracic, 7 pairs of lumbar, 3 pairs of sacral, and 5 to 6 pairs of coccygeal roots. The canine spinal cord, as is the case in other mammals, lengthwise does not completely fill the vertebral canal in which it is encased. For this reason, only the more central cervical roots extend from the spinal cord in a horizontal direction. The remaining roots extend at an angle, which become more pointed in the posterior regions of the spinal cord. The lower lumbar, sacral, and coccygeal roots lie completely vertical, and form the so-called horse tail (*cauda equina*). The posterior segments of the spinal cord form the conus medullaris, which in the canine, is located on the same level as lumbar vertebrae VI to VII.

The cervical and lumbar swellings of the spinal cord correspond to the beginning of those roots which innervate the upper and lower extremities.

On the ventral surface of the spinal cord, along the midline, lies the anterior medial fissure (*fissura mediana anterior, fma*). The dorsal surface of the spinal cord is separated in the middle by a shallow posterior median, or longitudinal fissure (*sulcus medianus posterior, smp*). Lateral to the anterior median fissure, on each side, lie anterior lateral fissures (*sulci laterales anterior, sla*). On both sides of the posterior longitudinal fissure are the posterior lateral fissures (*sulci laterales posterior, slp*).

Every segment of the spinal cord, composed of two symmetrical halves, consists of gray matter (nerve cells) surrounded by white substance (nerve axons). In general, the shape of the gray matter resembles a butterfly. This shape varies from one area to another in the spinal cord; however, it can always be discerned in the anterior and posterior horns. The anterior horns are composed mainly of large neural cells of polyangular shape, which send their

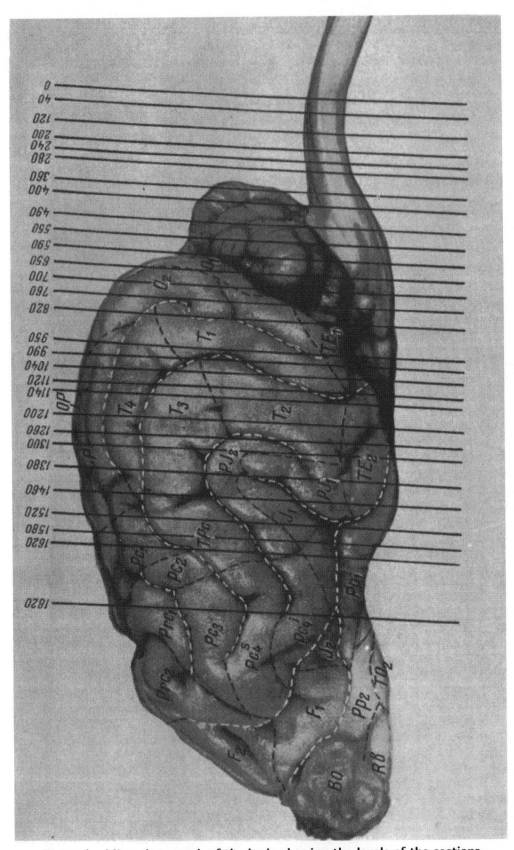

Figure 1 - Microphotograph of the brain showing the levels of the sections

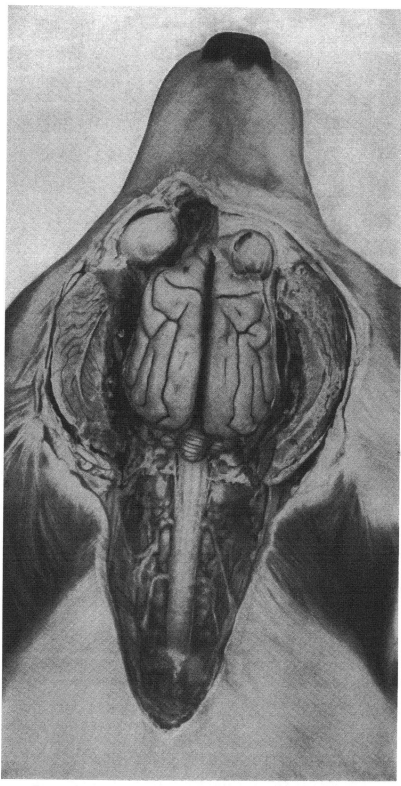

Figure 2 – The cerebrum and the spinal cord of the dog.
Photograph made from a preparation of the Brain Institute.

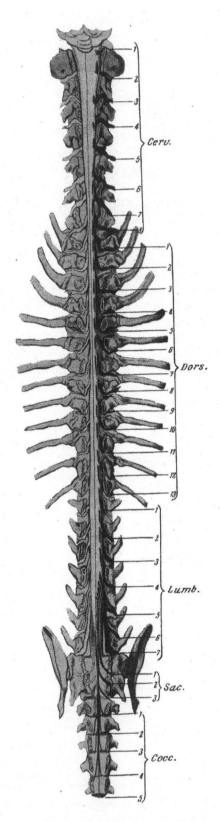

Figure 3 – The spinal column with an open spinal canal (after Flatau)

axons in the form of the anterior roots to the periphery, to the skeletal muscles of the trunk and extremities. The posterior horns consist of sensory neural cells.

In the thoracic segments of the spinal cord, there can be observed also lateral horns, situated between the anterior and posterior horns. The lateral horns are amaller in the lumbar area, and in the cervical area, they merge with the very massive anterior horns.

The lateral horns contain groups of cells which form Jacobsohn's external sympathetic nucleus (*nucleus sympaticus lateralis Jacobsohni*). From these cells extend preganglionic sympathetic fibers toward the sympathetic ganglia. The latter are, as we know, outside the spinal cord.

Lateral to the base of the posterior horns is a reticular process (*processus s. formatio reticularis, ret*) formed by seams of gray and white matter.

In the sacral part of the spinal cord is the so-called sacral portion of the vegetative neural system. It consists of cells that send preganglionic fibers of the parasympathetic system to the parasympathetic ganglia.

In the center of the gray matter lies the central canal which has an oval or circular shape (*canalis centralis, cc*), which continues in the brain and connects to the ventricles.

The white matter of the spinal cord is divided into columns: anterior, lateral, and posterior, which are penetrated by systems of short and long centripetal (ascending) and centrifugal (descending) neural fibers (Fig. 4.)

The major portion of this section is devoted to a description of the conducting tracts of the spinal cord of carnivores Yacubovich [174]; Lebedev [117]; Schifferdecker [156]; Lenhossek [118]; Bekhterev [78]; Goltzinger [101]; Vorotynskiy [172]; Troshin [166]; Amassian [69] Getz [97]; Glees [99]; Verhaart [169, 170]; Maffre [125] and others).

We are providing a short description of the conducting tracts, so that the reader may later obtain a more precise concept of the topography and the functions of various cellular groups of the spinal cord, described and illustrated in the series of figures.

Ascending (Centripetal) Tracts of the Spinal Cord

The peripheral neuron of the centripetal tracts is represented by the cells of the cerebrospinal or intervertebral ganglion (*gangl. spinale s. intervertebrale*), located on the outside of the spinal canal, in the intervertebral foramen. The peripheral processes of these cells, in the shape of diverse receptor endings, begin in the skin, the muscles, fascias, and internal organs. The central processes of the cells of the cerebrospinal ganglia, in the form of the posterior roots, enter the spinal cord and separate into different portions according to length and direction; the longest fibers go from the posterior root into the posterior column of the spinal cord, forming Goll's fasciculus and Burdach's fasciculus. The shorter fibers end at the

cells of the anterior horns, as the afferent part of the simplest or direct reflex arc, consisting of only two neurons, the sensory and motor. There is also an indirect reflex arc, which consists of a sensory, internuncial, and motor neuron. The shortest fibers of the neural cells of the cerebrospinal ganglia end at the cells of the posterior horns and Clark's column.

Goll's Fasciculus and Burdach's Fasciculus (*Fasciculus Golli et Fasciculus Burdachi*)

In the posterior column of each half of the spinal cord, lateral from the longitudinal fissure, lie Goll's fasciculus gracilis (*fasciculus s. funiculus gracilis Golli, fg*) and Burdach's fasciculus cuneatus (*fasciculus s. funiculus cuneatus Burdachi, fc*). Goll's fasciculus extends the entire length of the spinal cord and carries the impulses from the hind legs. Goll's and Burdach's fasciculi end in the medulla oblongata in the nuclei corresponding to those of the gracilis funiculus (*nucleus funiculi gracilis, ng*) and the cuneiform funiculus (*nucleus funiculi cuneati, nc*). The axons of these nuclei extend toward the midline as the internal fibers (*fibrae arcuatae internae, ari*) and form a decussation (*decussatio lemniscorum, dlm*), and as the medial lemnisaus (*lemniscus medians, lm*) they ascend to the nuclei of the optic thalamus.

There are indications that there is a connection between the medial lemniscus and the reticular formation (Jacobson [266]). The nuclear cells of the optic thalamus send out fibers through the posterior portion of the internal capsule, to the sensory as well as the motor cortex of the analyzors. The above system serves mainly for conduction of impulses of epicritical sense (deep and kinesthetic) and represents one of the main conductive systems of the motor and cutaneous analyzors. Some of the fibers of Goll's and Burdach's nuclei enter in the shape of external posterior acriform fibers (*fibrae arcuatae externae posteriores, arep*) into the restiform bodies (*corpus (corpora) restiforme, rest*) and reach the vermis cerebelli through the cerebellar peduncle.

Straight or Dorsal Cerebellospinal Flechsig's Tract (*Fasciculus spinocerebellaris dorsalis, fscd*)

The fibers of the cells of the intervertebral ganglia end at the cells of Clark's column; the axons of the latter ascend within the lateral column on the ipsilateral side of the spinal cord, occupying its external posterior section. The fasciculus keeps the same position in the rear area of the medulla oblongata. Out of the medulla oblongata the fibers of the dorsal spinocerebellar tract, as a component of the restiform body, enter into the cerebellum and end in the cells of the cortex of the vermis cerebellum, mainly in the lobulus centralis and partly in the culmen (Grundfest and Campbell [103]).

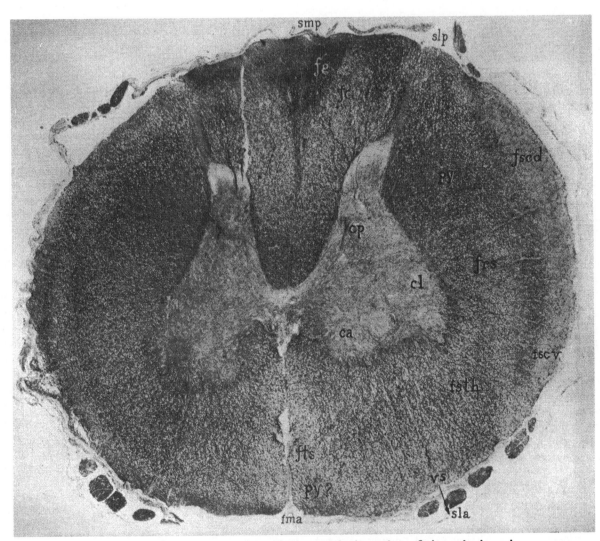

Figure 4 – Cross section through the cervical portion of the spinal cord

The Decussated or Ventral Spinocerebellar Tract of Govers (*Fasciculus spinocerebellaris ventralis, fscv*)

The fibers of the cells of the intervertebral ganglia end at the column cells of the posterior horn; the axons of the latter extend to the opposite side through the commissura anterior alba, and ascend within the anteroexternal section of the lateral column of the spinal cord, through the medulla oblongata to the pons Varolii. Gower's tract rounds the upper cerebellar peduncles, enters into the anterior cerebellar vellum, where it decussates and ends in the cortex of the vermis and the adjacent areas of the cerebellar hemisphere.

The above tracts conduct the impulses from the receptors of proprioception to the cerebellum; i.e., they are included in the system of reflex coordination of movements, and play an important part in the activity of the kinetic analysor.

Cerebrothalamic Tract (*Fasciculus spinothalamicus, fsth*)

The fibers of the cells of the intervertebral ganglia enter the posterior roots and end at the cells of the posterior horns. The axons of these cells cross into the lateral column of the opposite side and end at the cells of the lateral nucleus of the optic thalamus. The cerebrothalamic tract extends the length of the spinal cord and the medulla oblongata toward the medial side of Gower's tract, but is located in the pons Varolii between the fibers of the medial and the lateral lemniscus. This tract conducts the impulses of pain, temperature and, partly, tactile sensitivity. In other words, it is one of the main systems of the cutaneous analysor.

Side by side with the tracts discussed above, there also exist other ascending conductive systems, the course of which has not been sufficiently investigated: the dorsotactile tract (*fasciculus spinotactalis*), which begins in the cells of the gray matter of the spinal cord, crosses through the commissura alba into the lateral column of the spinal cord of the opposite side and ends in the cells of the lamina quadrigemina; the spinoolivary tract (*fasciculus spinoolivarius*), which ends in the olivary body of the medulla oblongata. Brodal, Walberg, and Blackstad [85] pointed out that the fibers of this tract pass through the anterior (ventral) column, and partly the lateral column of the spinal cord; most of these fibers decussate on the level of the cervical sections of the spinal cord and end mostly in the ventrolateral parts of the dorsal and medial supplementary olivary body. These authors are of the opinion that a great number of impulses from the spinal cord, by way of this tract and the olivocerebellar connections, go to the anterior lobe of the vermis, some of them to the pyramis and a few to the uvula and nucleus fastigii. Grundfest and Garter [104] assume that this anatomically isolated tract is polysynaptic. Di Bia-

gio and Grundfest [90], Krieger and Grundfest [109] are of the opinion that the synapse of this tract occurs on a level with the second cervical vertebra in a special lateral nucleus of the spinal cord. The above authors point out the functional similarity of the spinoolivary and the dorsal spinocerebellar tract.

Insufficiently investigated also are the spinoreticular tract (*fasciculus spinoreticularis*) leading toward the cellular formation of the brainstem, and the spinopontine tract fibers leading to the nuclei of the pons. These surround the pyramidal tracts (Walberg and Brodal [811]).

Descending (Centrifugal) Tracts of the Spinal Cord

Corticospinal or pyramidal tract (*Fasciculus corticospinalis s. pyramidalis, py*)

This tract begins primarily in the cells of the motor area and partly in the sensory area; it descends through the posterior part of the base of the cerebellar peduncle and enters the base of the pons Varolii and the medulla oblongata. On the borderline between the medulla oblongata and the spinal cord, most of the fibers of the pyramidal tract cross to the opposite side, forming a decussation of the pyramids (*decussatio pyramidum, dpy*), and descend within the posterior section of the lateral column of the spinal cord to the cells of the anterior horns. Half of the fibers of this fasciculus end in the cervical area and only a few reach the sacral area. Until now, data on the existence of a direct or non-decussated pyramidal tract, in the case of the Carnivora, have been contradictory. Bekhterev [192], Lewandowsky [46], Lassek [116], Lance [111], Chiarugi, Rossi, and Zanchetti [87] deny the existence of such a tract, while Romanov [350], Papez [142], Brodal and Walbert [84], Brodal and Kaada [82] affirm the presence of the tract in the anterior column on the ipsilateral side of the spinal cord. The pyramidal tract, as it descends, sends collaterals to the motor nuclei of the brainstem, in particular to the trigeminal, facial, glossopharyngeal, and hypoglossal nerves, to the nuclei of the vestibular nerves, and to the cells of the reticular formation.

In recent years, reports have been published on the formation of a pyramidal tract, apart from the sensorimotor area, in the temporal and occipital areas of the cat's cerebral cortex, and on the existence of ascending fibers in the cat's pyramidal tract (Brodal and Walberg [84]; Brodal and Kaada [82]).

The pyramidal tract conducts the impulses from the cortical end of the motor analysor to the muscular apparatus. It is therefore one of the important tracts which mediate the motor reactions of the animal.

Rubrospinal Tract or Monakov's Fasciculus (*Fasciculus rubrospinalis, frs*)

The tract begins in the macrocellular part of the red nucleus. Below this site of origin, the tract immediately decussates (Forel's decussation - *decussatio Foreli, dF*) and continues in the region of the brainstem tegmentum, descending in the lateral column to the lowest levels of the spinal cord.

The rubrospinal tract lies above and lateral to the pyramidal tract. This tract is considerably developed in the subprimates and plays a vital part in the conduction of impulses from the red nucleus, and through the latter also impulses from the cerebellum, in the regulation of the contractile (contracting) muscle tone (Magnus [296]; Rademaker [771] and others).

Tectospinal or Predorsal Tract (*Fasciculus tectospinalis s. praedorsalis, fts*)

The fibers of this tract begin primarily in the cells of the anterior corpus bigeminum (stratum griseum profundum), continue in a ventromedial direction, completely decussate along the midline (Meynert's fountain-shaped decussation-*decussatio Meynerti, dM*) and pass near the midline ventrally in the posterior longitudinal fasciculus.

In the spinal cord, the tract descends within the anterior column, close to the anterior medial fissure, and ends at the cells of the anterior horns.

Posterior Longitudinal Fasciculus (*Fasciculus longitudinalis posterior s. medians, flp*)

The majority of authors are of the opinion that the posterior longitudinal fasciculus is formed by ascending and descending fiber systems. There is some question, however, as to where the fibers of this fasciculus begin.

It was determined that the beginning of the descending system of fibers of this fasciculus is represented by the cells of Cajal's interstitial nucleus (Muskens [316]; van Gehuchten [386]; Klosovskiy [279] and others). However, there are indications that the formation of the descending fibers of the posterior longitudinal fasciculus also occurs in Darkshevich's nucleus (Bekhterev [192]; Lewandovsky [46]; Blumenau [3]; and others). In the brainstem, the descending fasciculus goes straight down to the base of the Sylvian aqueduct and the fourth ventricle; in the spinal cord, it lies in the anterior column, close to the anterior medial fissure.

The ascending fibers of the posterior longitudinal fasciculus consist of two systems that begin in the vestibular nuclei of the brainstem. Through the lateral part goes a direct, non-decussated, vestibulo-mesencephalic system that begins in Bekhterev's nucleus and ends in the nuclei of the oculomotor and trochlear nerves. Through the medial part passes a decussated, vestibulo-mesencephalic system that begins in the cells of the triangular nucleus (dorsal nucleus of Schwalbe) and also ends in the nuclei

of the oculomotor and trochlear nerves (van Gehuchten [386]; Muskens [316]; Gray [257]; Rasmussen [343]; Klosovskiy [279] and others).

According to Muskens, and also to Buchanan [216], Deiter's nucleus sends out fibers into the ascending decussated part of the posterior longitudinal fasciculus where these fibers end in the nuclei of the oculomotor, trochlear, and abducent nerves.

According to some authors, the posterior longitudinal fasciculus regulates the associated movements of both eyeballs, takes part in the combined work of the vestibular and oculomotor apparatus, and plays an important part in the mechanism of vestibular nystagmus.

Vestibulospinal Tract or Lowental's Fasciculus (*Fasciculus vestibulospinalis Lowentali*)

The tract begins, for the most part, in the cells of the vestibular nuclei; according to some authors, it begins in the cells of Deiter's nucleus. It descends as a whole, not decussating, within the outer portion of the lateral column, on the borderline between the lateral and anterior column of the spinal cord, and ends at the cells of the anterior horns.

The topography of other centripetal tracts, in the case of the dog, has not been investigated adequately. This includes: the olivospinal tract, the Bekhterev-Gelweg fasciculus (*fasciculus olivospinalis Bekhterevi-Wegwegi*), leading from the cells of the inferior olivary body to the upper parts of the spinal cord. It occupies the periphery of the anterolateral column of the spinal cord; the thalamospinal tract (*fasciculus thalamospinalis*), proceeds from the cells of the optic thalamus in the lateral column of the spinal cord.

Reticulospinal Tract (*Fasciculus reticulospinalis*)

The tract begins in the cells of the reticular formation of the brainstem and descends to the first lumbar segment of the spinal cord (Verhaart [169]), with three (Papez [142]) or two (Niemer and Magoun [137]) large systems of diffusely located fibers: the medial reticulospinal tract, going through the anterior column of the spinal cord, and the lateral reticulospinal tract in the lateral column of the spinal cord.

Thus the spinal cord consists of an apparatus which regulates the spinal cord's own functions, and of a long conducting apparatus (of projective conducting tracts), which carries the stimulation from the receptors to the cerebrum and, conversely, from the cerebrum to the muscles. The actual functions of the canine spinal cord include the innervation of all skeletal muscles of the body and the extremities, which are responsible for simple reflex motor reactions, for instance: the flexor and extensor, the tendinous, and several other reflexes. The spinal cord makes possible the reflex regulation of the activity of the internal organs. The spinal cord is also responsible for the operation of reflexes from the urinary bladder and the rectum, the majority of vascular reflexes, the reflex regulation of heat exchange, and the metabolism of most tissues. Consequently, the spinal cord is responsible for the realization of many simple unconditioned reflex actions of a somatic and vegetative type (Goltz and Ewald [100]; Sherrington et al. [158]; Rademaker [771]; Popov [147]; Tower [165]; Asratian [72, 73]; Gambarian [96] and others). The part played by the spinal cord in conditioned reflexes has been investigated (Novikova and Khanutina [138]; Gambarian [96]; Barsegian [75]; Urgandzhian [168] and others).

The Brainstem

The brainstem is located between the spinal cord and the hemispheres of the cerebrum (Figs. 5 and 6). The brainstem is subdivided into the *medulla oblongata (mo)*, the *pons Varolii (pV)*, the cerebellum (*cer*), the mesencephalon and the diencephalon.

The Medulla Oblongata (*medulla oblongata, mo*) and the pons Varolii (*pons Varolii, pV*) (Figs. 5, 6, 11-27)

The medulla (Figs. 5, 6), the immediate continuation of the spinal cord, appears in the shape of a coniform body which becomes narrower toward the back. The ventral surface of the medulla is divided into two symmetrical halves by the sagittal fissure (*sulcus sagittalis s. fissura mediana anterior, fma*). Along the sides of the fissure extend two pyramids (*pyramis, py*), which narrow toward the back and gradually disappear in the decussation of the pyramids (*decussatio pyramidum, dpy*). On the outside, the pyramids are almost entirely separated by the anterior lateral sulcus (*sulcus lateralis anterior, sla*) from the olivary bodies (*olivae, o*). The latter are represented by long, narrow protractions, bounded in the back by the posterior lateral sulcus (*sulcus lateralis posterior, slp*). On the average, the width of these bodies is 1-2 mm.

The posterolateral border of the medulla is formed by restiform bodies (*corpora restiformia, rest*).

Laterally from the anterior segment of the pyramids, perpendicular to the latter, are clearly seen the fibers of the trapezoid body. The greater part of the dog's trapezoid body, in contrast to the primates, is not covered by the fibers of the pons, because of their insufficient development in the carnivores.

In connection with this, some authors refer the above mentioned area of the spinal cord in carnivores to the medulla, others to the pons Varolii.

Anterior to the fibers of the trapezoid body are the transverse fibers of the pons Varolii, making its surface uneven, as if crenated. The pons Varolii is the continuation of the medulla. Through the middle of the pons

passes a slightly raised, basal or longitudinal sulcus (*sulcus basilaris s. sulcus longitudinalis, sln*, Fig. 5), which frequently does not reach the posterior border of the pons. Laterally, the pons narrows and becomes the cerebellar peduncles (*crura cerebelli ad pontem s. crura pontis, s. pedunculi cerebelli medius, pcm*).

The dorsal surface of the medulla is divided in the middle by the posterior medial sulcus (*sulcus medianus posterior, smp*, Fig. 6). On both sides of the fissure lie Goll's funiculus (*funiculus gracilis, fg*), which swells here into the shape of a callus (clava). On the outside of the *funiculus gracilis* passes Burdach's cuneiform funiculus (*funiculus cuneatus, fc*). The funiculi are separated by the posterior intermediate sulcus (*sulcus intermedius posterior, sip*). The lateral surface of the medulla is crossed by the posterior lateral sulcus (*sulcus lateralis posterior, slp*), which is the continuation of the same sulcus of the spinal cord. Alongside the latter lies the descending root of the trigeminal nerve (*radix descendens nervi trigemini, rVd*), intersected in the upper regions by the external arciform fibers (*firbae arcuatae externae, are*).

On the dorsal surface (Fig. 6) of the medulla lies a rhomboid fossa (*fossa rhomboidea*), representing the floor of the fourth ventricle. The posterior part of this pit belongs to the medulla; however, its anterior part belongs to the pons Varolii. The posterolateral section of the rhomboid fossa is bordered by the restiform bodies, and its anterior part by the anterior or upper cerebellar peduncles (*pedunculi cerebelli superiores, pcs*). The rhomboid fossa is divided into two symmetrical halves by a medial sulcus (*sulcus medianus fossae rhomboideae, smfr*). On both sides of the latter, there is a small round eminence (*eminentia tares, et*), which is bordered, from the side, by the lateral sulcus of the rhomboid fossa (*sulcus lateralis fossae rhomboideae, slfr*), and which corresponds to the genu of the facial nerve. The medial part of the posterior triangle of the rhomboid fossa is called calamus scriptorius (*calamus scriptorius, cal*) and corresponds to the location of the nuclei of the hypoglossal nerve (*trigonum hypoglossi*). Slightly lateral is the dorsal nucleus of the vagus nerve, or ala cinerea. The lateral part of the rhomboid fossa occupies the auditory area (*area acustica, aa*), corresponding to the location of the nuclei of the vestibular nerve. Into the cavity of the fourth ventricle, in its ventrolateral part, enters the *area postrema (ap)*, which is related in innervation to glands or vessels (Brizzee and Borison [203]; Brizzee and Neal [204]; Clemente and van Breemen [227]).

From the medulla and the pons Varolii extend roots of nerves of the craniocerebral type, beginning in the corresponding nuclei.

From the anterolateral fissure extend the roots of the hypoglossal nerve (*nervus hypoglossus, XII*). Its fibers begin in a macrocellular nucleus. The intracerebral root extends in a ventral direction, lateral from the inferior olivary body and appears on the surface of the medulla as a multitude of roots. The nerve leaves the cranium through

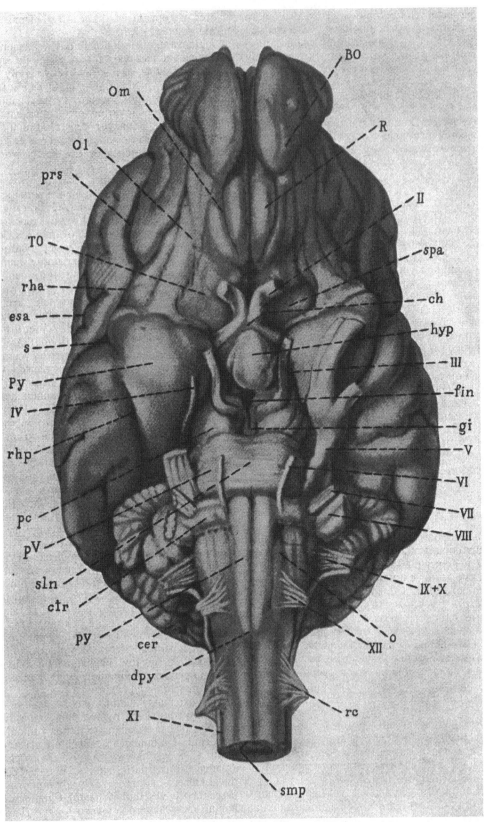

Figure 5 – The base of the cerebrum

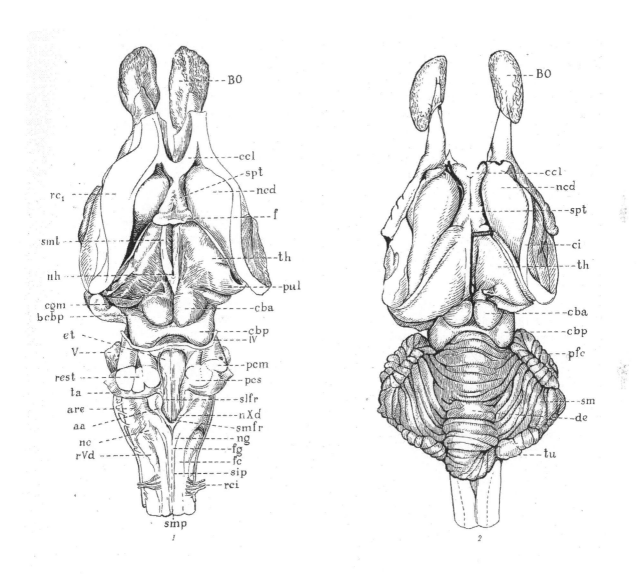

Figure 6 – Illustrations 1 and 2 depict the dorsal surface of the brainstem (after Papez)

the *canalis nervus hypoglossi* in the occipital bone and innervates the muscles of the tongue.

From the posterolateral fissure of the medulla extend the roots of the accessory, vagus, and glossopharyngeal nerves.

The accessory nerve (*nervus accessorius Willisii, XI*) is a motor nerve, formed by upper and lower roots.

The upper root begins in the cells of the dorsal nucleus of the accessory nerve (*nucleus dorsalis nervus accessorii, nXId*) anastomosing with the vagus nerves and leaves the medulla alongside of it. The lower, or spinal root, begins in the cells of the ventral nucleus of the accessory nerve (*nucleus ventralis nervus accessorii, nXIv*), located in the anterior horns of the upper cervical segments of the spinal cord. Leaving the spinal cord, these roots extend into the fissures formed by anterior and posterior spinal roots of the first pair of cervical nerves. Upon entering into the cerebrum through the foramen occipital magnum, the spinal root of the accessory nerve joins its upper root. The accessory nerve leaves the cranium through the jugular foramen (*foramen jugulare*) and innervates the muscles of the brachial plexus.

The vagus and glossopharyngeal nerves (*nervus vagus, X et nervus glossopharyngeus, IX*), of mixed origin, have common nuclei, located in the medulla. The nerves leave the lateral surface of the medulla in the form of numerous thin roots.

The fibers of the sensory part of the vagus nerve begin in the cells of the jugular and nodose ganglia. The fibers of the sensory part of the glossopharyngeal nerve begin in the cells of the superius and petrosal ganglia. The nerve processes originating in these cells divide into two branches, peripheral and central. Some of the fibers, extending toward the center, end in the sensory nucleus (*nucleus sensibilis*). Other central fibers - forming the solitary fasciculus (*tractus s. fasciculus solitarius, fsl*) - proceed in a downward direction and end in the concomitant nucleus of the solitary fasciculus (*nucleus tractus solitarius, nsl*). The solitary fasciculus contains mainly gustatory fibers; in recent years, data have become available on the relation of the nucleus of the solitary fasciculus to breathing. In the sensory and solitary nuclei begins the central sensory neuron, which, together with the medial lemniscus, extends toward the optic thalamus, and from there to the cortex.

The motor parts of the nerves under consideration begin primarily in the ventral nucleus of the *nucleus ambiguus (nXa)*. In addition, some of the motor fibers of the vagus originate in the dorsal nucleus of this nerve (*nucleus dorsalis n. vagi s. ala cinerea, nXd*).

The motor fibers of the vagus nerve innervate striated as well as smooth musculature of the pharynx, larynx, esophagus, stomach, the small and large intestines, trachea, bronchi, liver, and myocardium. The sensory fibers of the vagus nerve appear in the same organs, which are innervated by the motor fibers of this nerve. The vagus nerve forms a plexus (on the lungs, the esophagus, and

the heart). Some of its fibers, together with the fibers of the sympathetic nerve, extend toward the spleen, the pancreas, the adrenal glands, and the kidneys.

The motor part of the glossopharyngeal nerve innervates the muscles of the pharynx. The sensory fibers of the nerve appear in the posterior third of the tongue and in the pharynx. The fibers which innervate the salivary glands begin in the cells of the dorsal nucleus.

The facial nerve (*n. facialis, VII*) is a mixed nerve, with motor, sensory, and secretory fibers. The sensory fibers begin at the bipolar cells of the peripheral ganglion (*gangl. geniculi*). The central processes of the cells of this ganglion form the intermediate nerve (*n. intermedius*), enter into the medulla together with the motor part of the facial nerve, and reach the solitary fasciculus. The peripheral processes of the cells of the *gangl. geniculi* pass through as the chorda tympani into the lingual nerve (*n. lingualis*), a branch of the trigeminal nerve, and receive the gustatory stimuli from the anterior parts of the tongue. Through the chorda tympani also pass secretory fibers for the sublingual and submaxillary glands. The fibers of the motor portion begin in the cells of the nucleus of the facial nerve (*nucleus n. facialis, n VII*), located in the ventral parts of the medulla. The intracerebral root of the facial nerve rises upwards, makes a loop around the nucleus of the abducent nerve, and leaves the cerebrum on a level with the anterior part of the medulla. After leaving the cranium through the foramen stylomastoideum, the facial nerve innervates all of the most important facial muscles of the canine head.

The auditory nerve (*n. acusticus s.n. statoacusticus, VIII*) is formed by two roots or subnerves: *n. vestibularis* and *nervus cochlearis*. In the former are inherent the functions of conducting vestibular sensation, and in the latter conduction of acoustic sensation. Both nerves form the peripheral part of the vestibular and auditory analyzors, respectively.

The vestibular nerve (*nervus vestibularis, rVIIIv*) begins in the cells of the vestibulary ganglion (*gangl. vestibulare s. gangl. Scarpe*), located at the bottom of the meatus acusticus internus. The peripheral fibers of these cells extend toward the ampules of the semicircular canals (*canalis semicircularis*) and to the saccules (*utriculus et sacculus*). The vestibular nerve, after entering the brainstem as a compact fasciculus, turns around the dorsal surface of the descending root of the trigeminal nerve, and then divides into an ascending and a descending part.

The descending branch can be traced up to the external nucleus of the cuneiform fasciculus, or Burdach's nucleus, or Monakov's or Bekhterev's (*nucleus externus funiculi cuneati, nce, s. nucleus Burdachi s. Monakowi s. Bechterewi*); on its way, it sends collaterals to the triangular nucleus, or the dorsal nucleus of Schwalbe (*nucleus triangularis, ntr. s. nucleus dorsalis Schwalbe*), and to the nucleus of the descending root of the vestibular nerve (*nucleus radicis descendentis vestibularis, ndv*). It has not been determined whether the fibers of the descending root end in Deiter's nucleus or in the giant cell nucleus (*nucleus Deitersi, nD, s. nucleus magnocellularis*). The ascending branch of the vestibular nerve ends in the angular nucleus, or Bekhterev's nucleus (*nucleus angularis, s. nucleus Bekhterewi, nB*, and in the nuclei and cortex of the *vermis cerebelli*.

The connections of the vestibular nuclei are complicated and varied. As was pointed out before, in Bekhterev's nuclei, in the triangular nucleus and possibly in Deiter's nucleus, originate the ascending system of the fibers of the posterior longitudinal fasciculus, connecting the vestibular nuclei with the nuclei of the trochlear, abducent, and oculomotor nerves. A considerable number of fibers of the vestibular nuclei (Bekhterev's, Deiter's nuclei and the triangular nucleus) extend toward the cerebellum through the medial part of the inferior peduncle of the cerebellum within the vestibulocerebellar tract (*tractus s. fasciculus vestibulocerebellaris, fvc*). As mentioned before, the vestibular tract begins in Deiter's nucleus. There are indications of decussated connections of vestibular nuclei, leading to the nuclei of the optic thalamus.

Details as to how vestibular functions are represented in the cortex are still rather vague. According to some authors, these functions are represented in the posterior part of the suprasylvian gyrus (Bunichi [1103]; Bremer [697]; Dell and Bonvallet [896]), and according to others, in the anterior part of the suprasylvian and ectosylvian gyri (Andersson and Gernandt [1094]; Mickle and Ades [1125]; Ruwaldt and Snider [1136]).

The peripheral part of the auditory analysor - the cochlear nerve (*nervus cochlearis, rVIIIc*) - originates in the inner ear from the spiral ganglion of the cochlea. Through the internal auditory foramen of the temporal bone, the cochlear nerve enters into the cranial cavity, and, becoming a part of the brain substance, ends in two nuclei: in the ventral nucleus (*nucleus ventralis n. cochlae, nVIIIcv*) and in the *tuberculum acusticum* (*tac*). The cell axons of the ventral nucleus form the trapezoid body and end in the superior olivary body as well as in the nuclei of the trapezoid body, on both the ipsilateral and contralateral sides. The superior olivary complex reached a considerable development in the case of the dog. It consists of a medial part of the superior olive (*oliva superior medians, osm*) and of a lateral part (*oliva superior lateralis, osl*). From the cells of the superior olive and the nuclei of the trapezoid body, fibers extend within the lateral lemniscus and end in the nuclei of the lateral lemniscus (*nuclei lemniscus lateralis, nll*), in the posterior corpus bigeminum (*corpus bigeminum posterius, cbp*), and in the medial geniculate body (*corpus geniculatum mediale, cgm*). The posterior corpus bigeminum is connected, by the brachium (*brachium corporis bigemini posterioris, bcbp*), with the medial geniculate body. From the medial geniculate body begins the central neuron of the auditory tract, the auditory radiation, which passes through the sublenticular part of the internal cap-

sule and ends in the cortex of the temporal area in the nucleus of the auditory analysor. There are indications of the existence of numerous collaterals from the cells of the superior olive and the nucleus of the lateral lemniscus to the reticular formation (Rasmussen [346]; Stotler [370]).

The abducent nerve (*nervus abducens, VI*) is a motor nerve. It begins in the cells of the nucleus (*nVI*), located beneath the floor of the *IV* ventricle. The intracerebral root of the abducent nerve leaves the brain between the posterior edge of the trapezoid body and the pyramid. The nerve innervates the lateral rectus muscle of the eyeball.

On a level with the posterior parts of the pons Varolii emerges the very large root of the trigeminal nerve.

The trigeminal nerve (*nervus trigeminum, V*) is a mixed sensory-motor nerve. The sensory root (*portio major*) is thicker than the motor root (*portio minor*).

The fibers of the sensory root begin in the cells of Gasser's ganglion (*gangl. Gasseri*). The peripheral processes of the cells of this ganglion form three branches, *n. ophthalmicus, n. maxillaris*, and *n. mandibularis*; all of them innervating the conjunctiva of the eyeballs, the mucous membranes of the nose and mouth cavities, the teeth, and the skin of the muzzle. The central processes of the cells of Gasser's ganglion enter into the pons, some of them ending in the sensory nucleus of the trigeminal nerve (*nucleus sensibilis nervi trigemini, nVs*), and a larger number forming the descending, or spinal, root of the trigeminal nerve (*radix descendens, s. spinalis n. trigemini, rVd*) which ends in the nucleus of the spinal root of the trigeminal nerve (*nucleus radicis descendentis n. trigemini, nVd*). The spinal root of the trigeminal nerve crosses immediately into the gelatinous Roland's spinal cord substance, which forms the apex of the posterior horns.

The axons of the cells of the sensory nucleus and of the gelatinous Roland's substance cross to the opposite side, and rise within the medial lemniscus to the cells of the ventral nucleus of the optic thalamus. The cells of the latter send their fibers to the sensory area of the cortex.

The motor root begins in the motor nucleus of the trigeminal nerve (*nucleus motorius, nervus trigemini, nVm*) located in the tegmentum of the pons Varolii. Its fibers extend in a thin root from the pons, continue together with the sensory part of the trigeminal nerve and, within its third branch (ramus s.n. mandibularis), proceed toward the masticatory musculature.

There is some question about the nucleus of the trigeminal nerve, located in the midbrain, on both sides of the central gray substance of the sylvian aqueduct. This nucleus is called the nucleus of the mesencephalic root of the trigeminal nerve (*nucleus radicis mesencephalicus s. nucleus radicis ascendentis, n. trigemini nVa*). A majority of authors consider it a motor nucleus and assume that from its ventricular cells extends a mesencephalic root (*radicis mesencephalicus n. trigemini*), which adjoins the motor root. Other authors think that this is a sensory nucleus which receives, through the mesencephalic root, proprioceptive impulses from the masticatory muscles.

In the ventral portion of the medulla, lateral to the pyramids, lies the inferior olivary complex, which is divided into the basal olive (*olive inferior, oi*), and the supplemental olive (*oliva inferior accessoria ventralis, oiv*).

One of the systems connected with the inferior olivary body is the central tract of Bekhterev's tegmentum (*fasciculus centralis tegmenti, fct, s. tractus thalamorubro olivaris*), which begins in the cells of the optic thalamus and red nucleus, and ends at the cells of the inferior olive of the medulla.

According to Ogawa [323], the central tract of the dog's and cat's tegmentum is poorly developed; better developed is the so-called medial tract of the tegmentum. Both tracts of the tegmentum, medial as well as central, originate in the nuclei of the field of Forel, Darkshevich and Cajal and in the rostral parts of the medial accessory and basal olive. The central tract of the tegmentum lies lateral to the medial tract.

Bürgi [219] assumes that there exist not one but several central fasciculi of the tegmentum, which have a different beginning and ending.

It is assumed that the extrapyramidal system is connected with the cerebellum by the fibers which extend from the basal ganglia and the red nucleus to the inferior olive (Snider and Barnard [365]; Walberg [391]).

The inferior olive also receives impulses from the spinal cord and passes them on to the cerebellum through the spino-olivo-cerebellar system of fibers (Lisitsa [292] and others). The connections of the inferior olive indicate its importance in the operation of motor functions.

In the lateral area of the medulla lies the lateral nucleus of the medulla (*nucleus lateralis medullae oblongatae, s. nucleus lateralis reticularis, nlt*), well developed in the canine.

Due to the fact that there is a connection between the spinal cord and the lateral nucleus, and between the latter and the cerebellum, the lateral nucleus seems to be a station between the spinal cord, the brainstem, and the cerebellum, all of which are possibly crossed by exteroceptive tactile impulses (Brodal [207]; Walberg [389] and others).

The pons is divided into the base and tegmentum. In the canine, as compared with primates, the base of the pons is rather poorly developed. Through the base of the pons pass the fibers of the pyramidal tract, surrounded by the pons' own nuclei (*nuclei proprii pontis, npp*), which extend in a transverse direction and are subdivided into a superficial (*sts*), a complex (*stratum complexum, stc*), and a deep (*stratum profundum pontis, stp*) layer.

The central areas of the medulla and of the pons varolii are occupied by a well developed reticular formation (*formatio reticularis, ret*). As to its topography, the reticular formation is not clearly separated from the other nuclear formations and the main conducting systems of

the brainstem. The cellular formations which enter into the reticular formation are numerous. According to the size of the cells they can be divided, essentially, into two groups: a medial group containing small, medium, and very large cells, and a lateral group consisting mainly of small cells. In the medial group of the reticular formation, in the dog, the central nucleus of the reticular formation (*nucleus centralis formatio reticularis, ncr*) and the gigantocellular nucleus (*nucleus gigantocellularis, ngc*), the central nucleus of the tegmentum (*nucleus centralis tegmenti, nct*), the caudal nucleus of the pons (*nucleus pontis caudalis, npc*) and the oral nucleus of the pons (*nucleus pontis oralis, npo*), are all distinctly isolated.

The cells of the reticular formation at different levels of the brainstem receive collaterals and fibers from the conductive systems of the majority of analysors, from the motor and sensory nuclei of the brainstem, from the pyramidal tract, from the cells of the cerebellum, the optic thalamus, the cerebral cortex, etc.

In recent times, the attention of many investigators (Magoun [299] Scheibel [359]; Jasper [534]; Moruzzi [314]; Narikashvili [569, 570]; Anokhin [688] and others) has been drawn to the study of the structure, connections, and functions of the reticular formation of the brainstem. In Mislayskiy's (1885) and Bekhterev's [1] time there already existed data on the relationship between the cells of the reticular formation and the respiratory and vasomotor centers, and there also was information available on the basis of the anatomical structure of the reticular formation.

One assumes, at present, that the diverse parts of the reticular formation have their functional peculiarities. Stimulation of the ventromedial part of the reticular formation of the medulla, according to Magoun [298] leads to an inhibition of motor reactions; on the other hand, stimulation of the reticular formation of other areas of the brainstem results in an intensification of the motor effect. Many foreign investigators acknowledge the activating influence of the reticular system on the cortex, and for this reason, the above mentioned system has been given the name of "the ascending activating system" of the brainstem.

One should not assume, however, that it is only the reticular formation that keeps the cortex in a state of vigilance. The first and basic source giving rise to activity in the cortex are the stimuli of the environment, which are sent as impulses into the brain along specific tracts of the analyzors. Some of these impulses switch to the cells of the reticular formation, which sends a supplemental flow of impulses to the cortex of the brain. An important point in explaining the activating influences of the reticular formation is its close connection with the hypothalamus and the vegetative nervous system of the organism (Bonvallet et al., [497], and others), which sustains the tonus in the cortex of the brain.

Through the medulla and the pons Varolii passes the basic mass of the most important conducting systems described above, connecting various parts of the brain and the spinal cord.

The base of the medulla and the pons Varolii is taken up by the pyramidal tract. Above the latter, in the tegmentum, closer to the raphe (*raphe, r*) pass the tectospinal tract and the posterior longitudinal fasciculus - the central tract of the tegmentum. The medial lemniscus, located in the tegmentum, on the borderline between the latter and the base of the pons, gradually moves away from the centerline and settles directly above the pyramids.

Through the lateral parts of the medulla and the pons Varolii extends the rubrospinal tract. In the lower regions lies the spinothalamic tract, and lateral to it the lateral lemniscus.

The above-mentioned receptor and motor formations and their connections permit the medulla and the pons Varolii to realize numerous, very important unconditioned reflexes of a somatic as well as of vegetative character. Only when the medulla is healthy and functioning normally can there be a realization of reflex regulation of cardiac activity, breathing, digestion, and the act of swallowing. Here also are represented the centers of sympathetic neural regulation - the center of sweating, and the vasomotor center.

The complex systems of the trigeminal, facial, abducent, sublingual, and glossopharyngeal nerves are responsible for the realization of the protective oculomotor reflexes, the movement of the musculature of the jaw, the tongue and the pharynx. The presence of the four nuclei of the vestibular nerve, and the extensively developed system of connections with the spinal cord and the cerebellum permit the medulla to play an important part in the preservation of the reflex regulation of the tonus of the musculature (the realization of position reflexes, of labyrinthine tonic reflexes). Of great importance for the coordination of movements and the preservation of tonus are the systems of the spinocerebellar fibers, extending through the medulla, as well as the systems of Goll's and Burdach's tracts with their nuclei - *nuclei gracilis et cuneatus*, located in the medulla.

The formation of the auditory analysor is highly developed in the canine medulla and pons Varolii.

The Cerebellum (Fig. 7)

The cerebellum is the dorsal part of the rhombencephalon and is partly covered by the large hemispheres. In the works of older authors, the cerebellum in Carnivora as well as other Mammalia was divided into a middle part - the vermis or body of the cerebellum (vermis or corpus cerebelli) and the hemispheres of the cerebellum (*hemisphaerium cerebelli*). The surface of the cerebellum is covered with parallel sulci which have in the vermis a transverse direction, and in the hemispheres an ellipsoidal direction. Phylogenically, the oldest systems of the cerebellum are the vermis, *flocculus (fl)*, and *paraflocculus*

(*pfl*), all unified under the concept of old cerebellum - palaeocerabellum. The hemispheres of the cerebellum appear phylogenically as a more recent formation, called the neocerebellum. The development of the cerebellar hemispheres is connected with the development of the cerebral hemispheres. In the canine, the cerebellar hemispheres are much more weakly developed than in the primates.

It should be mentioned, however, that the division of the cerebellum into vermis and hemispheres is rather provisional, as comparative anatomical data show. More thorough is the subdivision of the vermis, as well as the hemispheres, into lobes: anterior, central, and posterior.

The subdivision of the cerebellum, in this work, is based mainly on the work of Ingvar [434].

The anterior lobe (*lobus anterior*) is separated from the central primary fissure (*fissura prima, fpr*) and is subdivided into the *lingula (li)*, the central lobule (*lobulus centralis, lc*), the *culmen (cu)* and the anterior part, weakly developed in the Carnivora, of the tetragonal lobule (*lobulus quadrangularis, lqd*). The wings of the central lobule (*ala*) clearly defined in primates, are absent in the canine.

The central lobe (*lobus medius*) lies between the primary fissure (*fpr*) and the prepyramidal sulcus (*sulcus praepyramidalis, spp*). To it belongs the declive (*de*), the tuber (*tub*), the posterior larger part of the quadrangular lobule (*lqd*), the ansiform or semilunar lobe (*lobulus ansiformis s. lobulus semilunaris, lsm*) and the paramedian lobule (*lobulus paramedianus, lmp*), or the tonsil (*tonsilla*). Some authors distinguish in the lobulus semilunaris an upper and a lower lobule (lobulus semilunaris superior et lobulus samilunaris inferior), called also crus (*crus primum et crus secundum lobuli ansiformis*).

The posterior lobe (*lobus posterior*) consists of the pyramid (*pyr*), the uvula (*uv*), the nodule (*nodulus, nod*), the flocculus (*fl*) and the paraflocculus (*pfl*).

The above classification differs little from the subdivision of the cerebellum in the work of Volk [807], who distinguished the lobus anterior, lobus simplex, and lobus complicatus.

The *fissura paramediana (fpm)* clearly separates the vermis from the hemispheres of the cerebellum on its lower and posterior surface, while on the anterosuperior surface of the cerebellum the borderline is not clearly defined.

In the literature, the vermis of the cerebellum is often subdivided into a superior and an inferior vermis. To the former belong the lingula, lobulus centralis, culmen and declive, and to the latter the tuber, pyramid, uvula, and nodule.

The cerebellum consists of gray and white matter. The gray matter forms the cerebellar cortex and four subcortical nuclei. In the cortex of the cerebellum, there can be distinguished three basic cellular layers:

1. The exterior, or molecular layer (*stratum molceulare*), containing few cells and consisting predominantly

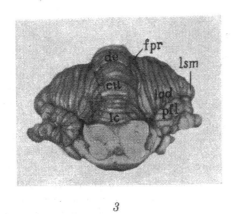

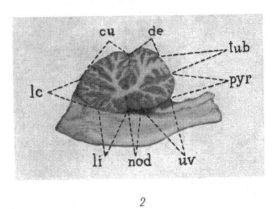

1

2

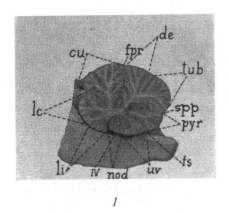

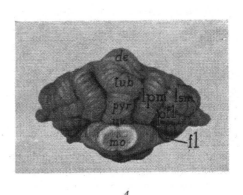

3

4

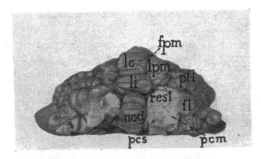

5

Figure 7 – Photographs 1 – 5 depict different views of the cerebellum

of fibers. In the superior part of the layer lie small superficial stellate cells; in the inferior part lie basketlike or deep stellate cells.

2. The ganglionic layer (*stratum ganglionare*), consists of the large cells of Purkinje. The axons of the latter are directed toward the nuclei of the cerebellum, and the dendrites rise toward the molecular layer.

3. The granular layer (*stratum granulosum*) is the deepest, consisting of numerous granular or the so-called claw-like cells, and of sparsely distributed large stellate cells - Golgi's cells.

The nuclear formations, located deep in the white matter of the cerebellum, are represented by the fastigial nucleus (*nucleus fastigii s. tecti, s. nucleus medians, nfs*), the dentate nucleus (*nucleus dentatus, s. nucleus lateralis, ndn*), the nucleus globosus (*nucleus globosus, ngb*), and the emboliform nucleus (*nucleus emboliformis, neb*). Frequently the two last nuclei are called, in the case of the Carnivora, *nucleus interpositus*.

The cerebellum is connected to the brainstem with three pairs of peduncles: the anterior, or superior peduncles (*pedunculi conjunctiva s. superior, s. pedunculi cerebelli ad corpora quadrigemina, pcs*) with the midbrain, the middle peduncles (*pedunculi medius s. pedunculi cerebelli ad pontem, pcm*) - with the pons Varolii, and the posterior or inferior peduncles (*pedunculi inferior s. pedunculi cerebelli ad medullam oblongatum, pci*) with the medulla oblongata. The superficial part of the posterior peduncle is formed by the corpus restiforme, which consists of the cerebellospinal tract of Flechsig, the tracts from Goll's and Burdach's nuclei, and also the phylogenetic new system of connections - the olivocerebellar tract (*fibrae olivocerebellares, foc*). Some of the studies show the exact topographical relations of the diverse areas of the olivary body to definite zones of the cerebellum, and the presence of efferent cerebello-olivary connections (*fibrae cerebello-olivares*).

The medial part of the posterior peduncle (*corpus juxta restiforme*) is formed by vestibulocerebellar fibers. To the efferent tracts, passing through the posterior peduncle, belong the tracts from the fastigial nucleus to Deiter's and Bekhterev's nuclei and the cells of the reticular formation.

The medial peduncles of the cerebellum contain fibers that begin at the nuclei at the base of the pons and, decussating along the midline, extend into the cerebellum (cerebellopontile fibers). The corticopontine fibers (*fibrae cortico-pontines*) which carry impulses from the cortex to the pons terminate, as we know, in the nuclei at the base of the pons. The system of the middle cerebellar peduncles sends these impulses to the cerebellum. According to Brodal and Jansen [211], all parts of the cerebellar cortex of the cat (except, perhaps, nodulus and flocculus) receive fibers from both the same side of the pons and, in part, from the opposite side.

There are indications of the existence, in the middle peduncles, of not only cerebellopetaline, but also of cere-

bellofugaline fibers (Besta [411]).

The anterior (superior) cerebellar peduncles are formed mainly by efferent fibers, which begin in the dentate and partly fastigial nuclei, and end, after a decussation (Vernekink's decussation), in the cells of the red nucleus and the ventral group in the nuclei of the optic thalamus. Impulses coming from the cerebellum can be transmitted through the red nucleus to the cerebrum and through the rubrospinal tract to the spinal cord.

Fibers were recently discovered extending from the cells of the red nuclei within the superior peduncles of the cerebellum, mainly to the dentate nucleus of the latter (Brodal and Gogstad [210]). Thus, within the superior peduncles of the cerebellum takes place a bilateral transmission of impulses between the red nucleus and the cerebellum.

Through the anterior peduncles of the cerebellum also passes the decussated spinocerebellar tract of Govers. A number of authors describe the unciform tract of the cerebellum (*fasciculus uncinatus*), which, according to Probst's [461] description, begins at the fastigial nucleus of the cerebellum, giving fibers mainly to Bekhterev's and the triangular nuclei, then to Deiter's and Roller's nuclei, and descends into the spinal cord. Mussen [455] points out, that from the unciform tract extend collaterals toward the nucleus of the abducent nerve, to the superior olive, etc.

The ascending and descending, straight and decussated reticulocerebellar connections, in the case of the cat, have been described in great detail.

There exist numerous connections between the various parts of the cerebellum. The system of various connections permit the cerebellum to realize an important role in the regulation of muscle tone, of proprioceptive tendinous reflexes and sensations from the skin. The extensive connections between the cerebellum and the vestibular nuclei give evidence of its participation in maintaining the equilibrium of the body. Important, although not sufficiently investigated as to their functions in the subprimates, are the connections between the cerebral cortex and the cerebellum (*fibrae cortico-pontino-cerebellares*), and the optic thalamus and the cerebellum. The latter are achieved through the central tract of the tegmentum (*fasciculus thalamo-rubro-olivaris, fct*) and further through the olivocerebellar fibers (*foc*).

There are data on the somatotopical representation of diverse functions in the brain. Thus, for instance, in the cortex of the lingula of the vermis of the cat's cerebellum, there is a representation of the tail, in the central part of the culmen the hind legs and the eyes, in the caudal part of the culmen and the lobulus simplex the front legs, thoracic area, and head and the neck, in the tuber of the vermis the head, neck, eyes, and ears. The vestibular function is widely represented all along the vermis (Larsell [444]; Chambers and Sprague [422]).

According to Snider and Stowell [470], the front and hind legs of the cat have their representation in both lobuli paramediani. The auditory zone is represented in the lobulus simplex, tuber, culmen, and pyramid by the internal part of the crus primum, lobulus paramedianus. The visual zone partly overlaps the auditory and frequently coincides with the latter. Larsell [444], Bürgi [420], Dow [425], on the basis of the study of the afferent connections of the cerebellum, divided the cerebellum into three basic zones (the vestibulary, spinal and cortico-pontile-cerebellar projections).

In the works of Jansen and Brodal [435] and Chambers and Sprague [422] the concept was put forward of the localization of the functions in the zonal longitudinal direction, based upon the studies of the efferent connections between the cerebellar cortex and its nuclei. The first internal or medial zone (the cortex of the vermis and the nucleus fastigii) realizes the control of posture, locomotion and the equilibrium of the body. The second paravermal zone (the cortex of the cerebellum around the vermis and the nucleus interpositus) controls the reflexes of the body posture and the individual movements of the extremities of the same name. The third lateral zone (the cortex of the hemispheres and of the nucleus dentatus) has to do with delicate coordinated movements without the regulation of postural reflexes.

In cats and dogs, the removal of the cerebellum leads to a change of activity in respect to conditioned reflexes, as well as to a considerable increase in the stimulating process and a marked weakening of the inhibiting process (Karamian [439]). In dogs with different types of nervous systems, the influence of the cerebellum on the activity of the cortex is not uniform (Lifshitz [446]).

The important role of the cerebellum as an adaptational tropic center, regulating the functional condition of somatic and vegetative reflexes, has been proved (Luciani [447]; Bekhterev [2]; Orbeli [456, 457]; Asratian [408]; Popov [460]; Aleksanian [406]; Pines and Zelikin [459]; Karamian [439] and others).

The Midbrain (mesencephalon) (Fig. 5, 6, 26-31)

The midbrain lies between the rhombencephalon and the diencephalon. On the dorsal side, the midbrain is formed by the lamina quadrigemina (*lamina quadric gemina*), composing the tectum of the midbrain (*tectum*), and on the ventral side by the cerebral peduncles (*pedunculi cerebri, pc*). In turn, the cerebral peduncles are divided into the tegmentum and the base (*pes pedunculi, pp*). Between the cerebral peduncles is located the interpeduncular fossa (*fossa interpeduncularis, fin*), the bottom of which is formed by the posterior perforated substance (*substantia perforata posterior*). On the dorsal side, into the midbrain enter the superior peduncles of the cerebellum (*pedunculi cerebelli superior, pcs*); between them lies the anterior cerebral vellum (*vellum medullare anterius, vma*). The lamina quadrigemina are located above the sylvian aqueduct (*aquaeductus Sylvii, aS*) - the cavity of

the midbrain which connects the fourth and third cerebral ventricles.

The lamina quadrigemina is formed by the posterior tubercles, or posterior corpus bigeminum (*corpus bigeminum posterius, cbp*), and by the anterior tubercles or anterior corpus bigeminum (*corpus bigeminum anterius, cba*). The corpus quadrigeminum is well developed in the canine.

The posterior corpus bigeminum represents a nucleus formation which receives some of the fibers of the lateral lemniscus. The tubercles of the posterior corpus bigeminum are connected with each other by the commissure of the posterior corpus bigeminum (*commissura corporis bigemini posterioris, ccbp*).

From the posterior corpus bigeminum extends the brachium of the posterior corpus bigeminum (*brachium corporis bigemini posterioris, bcbp*), through which passes the basic mass of fibers to the medial geniculate body (*corpus geniculatum mediale, cgm*). The posterior corpus bigeminum is connected with the unconditioned reflex orienting auditory reactions, entering into the system of the auditory analysor. There are indications of a connection of the posterior corpus bigeminum and the red nucleus [*fasciculus colliculorubralis* (Klosovskiy [280])] to the anterior corpus bigeminum.

The anterior corpus bigeminum represents a complicated formation, consisting of a number of layers of alternating gray and white matter. Through the uppermost or zonal stratum (*stratum zonale, sz*) and the optic layer (*stratum opticum, so*) pass some of the fibers of the optic tract, which end in the superficial gray layer (*stratum grisum superficiale, sgs*) located between the zonal and the optic layers. Below lies the medial gray layer (*stratum griseum medium, sgm*), from the cells of which extend fibers into the deeper layer of the corpus bigeminum, and the fibers from the cortex end near the cells. The medial layer of the white matter (*stratum album medium, sam*) receives collaterals from the medial and the lateral lemniscus and the fibers of the spinotectal tract. In the deep gray layer (*stratum griseum profundum, sgp*) begin the fibers of the tectospinal tract and also, according to some reports, the fibers which enter the reticular formation. The deep layer of the white matter (*stratum album profundum, sap*) receives fibers from various layers of the anterior corpus bigeminum. The anterior corpus bigeminum, having to do with the system of the optic analysor, takes part in the realization of complicated unconditioned reflex optic reactions (through the system of oculomotor nerves and the posteriorlongitudinal tract). In the conjunctive activity of the eyes and the connection of the optic with the vestibulary functions, an important role, aside from the posterior longitudinal tract, is played by the predorsal or tectospinal tract, beginning in the superior corpus bigeminum.

Taking into account the connections of the upper corpus bigeminum with the lower corpus bigeminum, the medial and lateral lemniscus, and the reticular formation, it stands to reason that the upper corpus bigeminum takes part in the activity of not only the visual analysor but others also.

The sylvian aqueduct is surrounded by the central gray matter. Immediately ventrally lies Darkshevich's nucleus (*nucleus Darkschewitschi, nDr*) and the interstitial nucleus of Cajal (*nucleus interstitialis Cajali, nC*), in which originate the fibers of the posterior longitudinal fasciculus. According to the investigations of Peche and also of Klosovskiy, Kosmarskaya and Afanasyeve (1951) Darkshevich's nucleus represents a formation of the vegetative nervous system. Below the nuclei of Darkshevich and Cajal lie the nuclei of the trochlear and oculomotor nerves.

The trochlear nerve (*nervus trochlearis, IV*) is a motor nerve; it begins in the nucleus located ventrally from the central gray substance on a level with the posterior corpus bigeminum. It is the only nerve emerging from the dorsal surface of the brainstem. The trochlear nerve decussates in the anterior cerebral vellum and innervates the upper oblique eye muscle.

The oculomotor nerve (*n. oculomotorius, III*) is a motor nerve; it originates in the corresponding nuclei, which lie ventrally from sylvian's aqueduct. These are: the paired principal, or macrocellular motor nucleus, the paired microcellular motor nucleus of Edinger-Westphal, and the unpaired, or central nucleus of Perlia. The nerve leaves the cerebral peduncle in the form of several small stems on the same level with the interpendiculnr fossa, and innervates the muscles of the eyeball (except for the lateral rectus and the superior oblique). The vegetative fibers, contained in the system of this nerve (beginning in the nuclei of Edinger-Westphal and Perna) innervate the smooth muscle, which causes constriction of the pupil (*m. sphincter pupillae*) and of the eyelash muscle (*m. ciliaris*).

Dorsally from the sylvian aqueduct, on the same level with the foremost sections of the anterior corpus bigeminum, can be observed the posterior commissure of the brain (*commissura posterior, cmp*) and alongside it the nucleus of the posterior commissure (*nucleus commissura posterioris, nap*).

This nucleus receives some of the fibers of the optic tract and sends fibers into the posterior commissure. In addition, fibers from the nuclei of the oculomotor nerve enter into the posterior commissure, the medial lemniscus, the anterior corpus bigeminum, the optic thalamus, the subthalamus, and the cells of the reticular formation. Some of the fibers of the commissure end in the interstitial nucleus of Cajal and in Darkshevich's nucleus.

In the tegmentum of the cerebral peduncle is the red nucleus (*nucleus ruber, nr*), which is well developed in the dog. It can be subdivided into a posterior macrocellular area, older phylogenetically, in which originate the fibers of the rubrospinal tract, and into the anterior microcellular area, the newer part, connected with the cerebrum. In Carnivora, the macrocellular part of the red nucleus is better developed. The fibers of the anterior cerebellar peduncle (*pedunculum cerebelli superior, pcs*) terminate

in the red nucleus, as do the fibers coming from the optic thalamus and the globus pallidus. On the borderline between the tegmentum and the base of the midbrain lies the black substance of Soemmering (*substantia nigra Soemmeringi, sn*). In contrast to the substantia nigra in man the cells of the substantia nigra of the canine brain lack melanin pigment. There are data on the existence of direct connections of the substantia nigra with the pallidum (Kimmel [275]) and with the cerebral cortex (Sager [356]).

To the base of the cerebral peduncle (*pes pedunculi, pp*) extends the corticobulbar tract and the pyramidal tract; to the exterior of the latter, the temporal and occipitopontile tracts; and medially the frontopontile tract. Between the peduncles is the interpeduncular ganglion (*gangl. interpedunculare, gi*), reaching large dimensions in the dog. It is connected with the frenulum of the midbrain and has to do with olfactory functions.

The midbrain plays a rather important part in many complicated unconditioned reactions and in the correct realization of most important tonic reflexes (*contractile tonus*). The separation of the midbrain from the rhombencephalon causes a sharp intensification of the tonus of the extensor muscles, as well as of the so-called decerebrate or extensor rigidity. In the origination of the latter, together with the red nucleus (Magnus [296]; Rademaker [341]), an important part is played by other connections of the midbrain and the fibers of the pyramidal tract (Mussen [455]; Ingram and Ransom [265]; Burkenko and Klosovskiy [222], and others).

The Diencephalon (Fig. 6, 31-41)

The diencephalon forms the anterior portion of the brainstem. The diencephalon is subdivided into: (1) the optic thalamus (*thalamus opticus, th*), consisting of several groups of nuclei; (2) the epithalamus (*epithalamus*) into which enter medullary striae (striae medullares thalami, or *stria medullaris thalami, smt*), the frenulum (*habenula s. nucleus habenulae, nh*) and the epiphysis (*glandula pinealis s. epiphysis*); (3) the subthalamic region (*regio subthalamica s. subthalamus*), enclosing Luysi's nucleus (*corpus Luysi, cL*), the *zona incerta* (*zin*), the fields H_1 and H_2 of Forel (*campus et H_2 Foreli, H_1, H_2*) and others; (4) the hypothalamus or the hypothalamic region (*hypothalamus, s. regio hypothalamica*) which is composed of mammillary bodies (*corpora mamillaria, cml, cmm*), the gray tuber (*tuber cinereum, tc*), the *infundibulum* (*in*), the posterior part of the hypophysis (*hypophysis, hyp*) and a number of other nuclei; (5) the metathalamus, to which belong the geniculate bodies (*corpus (corpora) geniculata laterale, cgl et mediale, cgm*).

The optic thalamus represents a paired formation, divided by the cavity of the third ventricle (*ventriculus tertius, vIII*), into which opens the sylvian aqueduct. The third ventricle has the appearance of a vertical fissure, divided into two halves by the gray commissure (commissura grisea media s. commissura mollis, cm) which connects both optic thalami. The roof of the third ventricle is a vascular lamina (tela chloroidea), which forms the vascular plexus of the ventricle. The lateral surface of the ventricle is formed by the medial surface of the optic thalamus; the posterior wall is formed by the posterior commissure and its nuclei; the bottom is formed by the hypothalamus. The anterior wall of the ventricle is formed by a thin lamina (lamina terminalis), which adjoins, at its upper end, the anterior commissure of the hemispheres (commissura anterior, can), and at the lower end the upper border of the chiasm. The superior regions of the anterior wall of this ventricle are composed of the columns of the fornix (columnae fornicis).

The optic thalamus represents in itself a voluminous cellular mass, located on the internal surface of the hemisphere under the corpus callosum and the fornix. A narrow marginal stria (stria terminalis, st) separates the optic thalamus from the caudate nucleus. Microscopic investigations reveal that the optic thalamus is of very complex construction and is subdivided into a series of nuclei. The topography and the classification of the nuclei of the optic thalamus have been elucidated in a rather contradictory manner (Monakov [564]; Neiding [573]; Papez [59]; Rioch [588]; Ingram, Hannet and Ranson [531]; Kononova [38]). According to the majority of the authors, the thalamus in the dog consists of: (1) the anterior group of nuclei, (2) the medial group, (3) nuclei of the central line, (4) the lateral group, (5) the ventral group of nuclei. The nuclei or groups of nuclei are separated from each other by laminae of white matter (laminae medullares). The classification of the nuclei of the optic thalamus, as followed in this atlas, is based on the works of Rioch [588]. The anterior group of nuclei of the optic thalamus occupies the tuberculum anterium and the foremost pole of the optic thalamus. It is formed by three nuclei: the anterodorsal nucleus (nucleus anterodorsalis, and), and the anteroventral nucleus (nucleus anteroventralis, anv) and the anteromedial nucleus (nucleus anteromedialis, anm). The anterior group of nuclei receives a larger number of fibers from the mammillary bodies through the mamillothalamic fasciculus of Vicq d'Azyr (fasciculus mamillothalamicus s. fasciculus Vicq d'Azyr, fmt) which points to the relationship of these nuclei to the olfactory analysor. In addition, according to some published reports, the anterior group is connected with the striatum (Papez [59]; Rioch [588]) and with the cerebral cortex, predominantly with the cortex of the limbic region of the hemispheres (Waller and Barris [614]; Rose and Woolsey [1132], and others).

The internal or medial group of nuclei lie along the entire length of the optic thalamus in its medial part. According to Rioch, this group is formed by 10 nuclei; among them should be mentioned, first of all, the medial dorsal nucleus (nucleus medians dorsalis, md), the parafascicular nucleus (nucleus parafascicularis, prf), the central lateral nucleus (nucleus centralis lateralis, cnl), the paracentral nucleus (nucleus paracentralis, pcn), the nucleus sub-

medium (smd), the paratenial nucleus (nucleus paratae-nialis, pt), the nucleus of the habenulo-peduncular tract (nucleus tractus habenulopeduncularis, hp). The central medial nucleus of Luysi (centrum medianum Luysi, cmd), quite pronounced in the primates, can barely be discerned in the dog, especially in Nissl preparations.

The medial group of nuclei have vast connections with the periventricular system of the midbrain, the gray substance surrounding the sylvian aqueduct, and the reticular formation of the mesencephalon (Rioch [588]). Other reports have given data on the connections with the striatum, the paleocortex and the cortex of the frontal region (through the anterior peduncle of the thalamic radiation) (Papez [59]; Droogleever-Fortuyn and Steffens [513]; Auer [490], and others).

The nuclei of the midline are situated between the two optic thalami. Among them can be distinguished the rhomboid nucleus (nucleus rhomboidalis, rhm), the central medial nucleus (nucleus centralis medialis, cnm), the reunial nucleus (nucleus reuniens thalami, reu), the anterior and posterior paraventricular nuclei (nuclei paraventriculares anterior, pra, et posterior, prp), the commissurial nuclei (nucleus interparataenialis, nucleus interanterodorsalis, nucleus interanteromedialis, iam, nucleus intermediodorsalis, imd). Except for the nucleus centralis medians, these nuclei are insignificant in size, and are comparatively poorly differentiated in the dog.

The lateral group of nuclei is represented by the following formations: (a) the lateral nucleus (nucleus lateralis), which is subdivided into an anterior, posterior, and intermediate part (pars anterior, lta, pars posterior, ltp, and pars intermedia, lti); (b) the pulvinar nucleus (pul); (c) the reticular nucleus (nucleus reticularis, nret); (d) the posterior nucleus (nucleus posterior, post); (e) the pretectal area (area praetectalis, prt); (f) the marginal nucleus (nucleus limitans, lmt); (g) nucleus supragenicu-latus, scg.

Some of the fibers of the spinothalamic tract terminate in the lateral nucleus. This tract sends a system of fibers of the thalamocortical radiation into the postcoronal and parietal regions, into the area of the cutaneous analysor, i.e., the area that receives tactile stimuli from the trunk and extremities.

The cells of the pulvinar receive some of the fibers of the optic tract and send axons to the occipital region of the large hemispheres within the optic radiation.

The posterior nucleus is located in the topographic vicinity of the pulvinar, lateral, and medial geniculate bodies, and is connected with them. According to a number of authors, this fact may point to a relationship between this nucleus and the visual and auditory analyzors. However, the ending of some of the fibers of the medial lemniscus in the posterior nucleus points to a functional importance of another kind (Rioch [588]).

The ventral nuclear group is represented by the ventral nucleus (nucleus ventralis), which is subdivided into four parts: the anterior (pars anterior nucleus ventralis, vna), the medial (*pars medians nucleus ventralis, vnm*), the external (*pars externa nucleus ventralis, vne*), and the arciform (*pars arcuata nucleus ventralis, vnar*). At the present time, the medial, the external and the arciform parts are usually known under the name of posterior ventralis nucleus - nucleus ventralis posterior (Clark [507] and others). The ventral nucleus receives the basic part of the fibers of the spinothalamic tract, the fibers from the cerebellum through its superior peduncle, the larger part of the fibers of the medial lemniscus (Rioch [588]), and a considerable number of fibers of the trigeminal nerve (Papez [59]; Magoun and McKinley [557]). Information is available on the topographical distribution of the tactile sensibility in the ventral nucleus (Dusser de Barenne and Sager [514]; Mountcastle and Henneman [568]; Robiner [589]; Getz [97]; Rose [591]; Gaze and Gordon [517], and others). The ventral nucleus sends fibers through the superior peduncle of the thalamic radiation, evidently to the motor radiation, but also to the somesthetic region of the cortex.

All nuclei of the optic thalamus are connected with specific regions of the cortex through the peduncles of the optic thalamus, forming the radiation of the optic thalamus (*radiatio thalami optici*).

The optic thalamus is thus the most important formation, correlating the diverse afferent signals coming out of the spinal cord and the medulla, the pons Varolii and the midbrain, and in turn passing on various impulses to the cerebral cortex, the striatum, and the areas lying below.

All of the most important types of the exteroceptive sensibility (with the possible exception of hearing), and also of interoceptive (kinesthetic) sensibility, are analyzed and synthesized in the nuclei of the optic thalamus.

In recent years, many investigators (Magoun [556]; Jasper [534]; Nauta and Whitlock [572], and others) have brought to attention the so called nonspecific or diffuse thalamic nuclei of the optic thalamus. To these belong the reticular nucleus of the optic thalamus, the nuclei of the midline and the intralaminar nuclei. The intralaminar nuclei comprise centrum medianum Luysi, nucleus centralis medialis, nucleus centralis lateralis, and nucleus paracentralis. According to some authors, the following also belong to the diffuse thalamic nuclei: nucleus submedius, nucleus parafascicularis, a part of nucleus anteromedialis, nucleus ventromedialis, and the lower part of nucleus medialis dorsalis. However, the relationship of some of the above mentioned nuclei to the nonspecific formations of the optic thalamus is rather dubious.

Together with the cells of the reticular formation of the lower lying regions of the brainstem, these areas are regarded as nonspecific systems of the brainstem, exerting an activating influence on the cerebral cortex.

Poorly investigated and debatable is the question of the connection of the nonspecific nuclei of the optic thalamus with the cerebral cortex. Nauta and Whitlock have shown, in the cat, that the nuclei of the midline and the intralaminar nuclei are connected with the phylo-

genetically old part of the cortex - the prepyriformal, the infralimbical, and the cortex of the limbic region. A small number of fibers end in the marginal stria of the neocortex, near the formation of the paleocortex. Noted also are the cross connections of the limbic and infralimbic cortex with the nonspecific nuclei of the optic thalamus. Jasper considers that all sensory, frontal, motor, and parietal areas and the structures of the so called olfactory brain belong to the cortical regions which receive nonspecific projective fibers. Connections of the diffuse nuclei of the optic thalamus with the projective parts of the cortex have also been pointed out by Nashold, Hanbery and Olszewsky [571], Auer [490] and others.

It is assumed that connections with the cortex can be realized through a system of specific nuclei of the optic thalamus, or else through a reticular nucleus, or a striatal system. We have recently observed direct connections of the majority of intralaminar and other "nonspecific" thalamic nuclei with the frontal, motor, and somesthetic regions of the cortex, which is in conformity with the electrophysiological investigations of a more or less local projection of these nuclei on the cerebral cortex.

It has been found that fibers from the lower lying formations of the brainstem, particularly the medial ansa and the spinothalamic tract, terminate in the nonspecific nuclei of the optic thalamus.

The Epithalamic Region

An important formation of this region in the dog, located upward from the medial nucleus of the optic thalamus, is the nucleus of the frenulum (*nucleus habenulae, nh*), which consists of a lateral macrocellular (*nhl*) and a medial microcellular (*nhm*) nucleus. The frenulum enters the system of the olfactory analysor, receiving the fibers of the olfactory-frenular tract (*tractus olfactohabenularis s. stria medullaris thalami, smt*). Through the frenulum pass impulses to the interpeduncular ganglion in the midbrain via the decussated olfacto-peduncular tract (*tractus habenulo-peduncularis s. fasciculus retroflexus Maynerti, frM*).

Immediately below the optic thalamus lies the subthalamic region, consisting of seams of white and gray matter. To the white matter of the subthalamic region belong: field H_1 of Forel, or the thalamic fasciculus (*fasciculus thalamicus, H_1*) and field H_2 of Forel, or the lenticular fasciculus (*fasciculus lecticularis, H_2*. The above mentioned fasciculi are important conductive tracts, connecting the periventricular nuclei and Luysi's body with the striopallidal system. Between fields H_1 and H_2 of Forel are accumulations of cells designated as the zona incerta (*zin*). Below field H_2 of Forel is the corpus of Luysi (*corpus hypothalamicus s. corpus Luysi, cL*).

The Hypothalamic Region

This lies at the bottom of the third ventricle between the

chiasm of the optic nerves and the posterior pole of the mammillary bodies. This area comprises, in the dog, about 20 nuclei and can be subdivided into a medial and a lateral zone, or a medial and lateral hypothalamus. It is rather difficult to establish a borderline between the majority of nuclei.

The medial part of the anterior section of the hypothalamus is occupied by the anterior hypothalamic nucleus (*nucleus hypothalamicus anterior, hpa*). The lateral part of the anterior hypothalamic region forms the lateral hypothalamic area (*area hypothalamica lateralis, hpl*), which extends back to the anterior section of the mammillary bodies.

Medial to the anterior hypothalmic nucleus, near the cavity of the third ventricle, lie the small *nucleus filiformis anterior* (*fa*) and *nucleus filiformis principalis* (*fp*). Above the chiasm, more medially, lies the diffuse supraoptic nucleus (*nucleus supraopticus diffusus, nsp*), and lateral to the latter the tangential nucleus (*nucleus tangentialis, tg*).

The caudal areas of the anterior hypothalamic nucleus merge into the large medial hypothalamic nucleus, in which there can be distinguished a dorsal part (*nucleus hypothalamicus dorsomedialis, hpmd*) and a ventral part (*nucleus hypothalamicus ventromedialis, hpmv*).

Toward the rear lies the posterior hypothalamic nucleus (*nucleus hypothalamicus posterior, hpp*), the *tuber cinereum* (*tc*), changing into the *infundibulum* (*in*), which ends with the hypophysis cerebri (*hypophysis, hyp*). To the hypothalamus belongs the upper third of the hypophysis cerebri, while the remaining part constitutes the endocrine gland. The posterior parts of the hypothalamic region are formed by the mammillary bodies, separated from each other by a longitudinal fissure. In the mammillary bodies can be found a lateral and medial part (*nuclei corporae mamillares lateralis, cml, et medialis, cmm*).

Above the mammillary bodies lies a small supramammillary nucleus (*nucleus supramammillaris, scm*). Around the cavity of the third ventricle lie the periventricular masses of the thalamus and the hypothalamus (*per*).

The connections of the hypothalamic region are numerous and multiple. In the cells of the mammillary bodies end the fibers of the columna fornicis which constitute the projective system of the olfactory analysor. To the afferent fibers of the mammillary bodies belong also the peduncles of the mammillary bodies (*pedunculi corporae mamillariae, pm*), which begin in the cells of the tegmentum of the pons Varolii. From the cells of the mammillary bodies extend fibers toward the tegmentum of the pons Varolii (*fasciculus mamillotegmentalis, s. fasciculus Guddeni*) and to the anterior nucleus of the optic thalamus (*fasciculus mamillothalamicus s. fasciculus Vicq d'Azyr*), and through the latter to the cerebral cortex. There are indications of an immediate connection of the hypothalamic region with the cerebral cortex, particularly with the cortex of the limbic and orbital areas of the hemisphere. The connection with the cortex of the limbic area (ac-

cording to Clark and Meyer [509]) is possibly achieved within the limits of a specific functional circle, from the mammillary bodies through the anterior nucleus of the optic thalamus, the limbic cortex, the hippocampus, the fornix, and back to the mammillary bodies.

The hypothalamic region is one of the important areas taking part in the regulation of activity of the vegetative nervous system. According to some authors, stimulation of the posterior part of the hypothalamic region excites the sympathetic nervous system, while stimulation of the anterior part excites the parasympathetic system (Clark, Beattie, Riddock and Dott [508]).

In recent years, investigators have pointed out the functional differences between the lateral and medial hypothalamic areas. Stimulation of the lateral hypothalamus is accompanied by a considerable increase of alimentary excitability (Anand and Dua [487]). Kogan [546] considers the lateral hypothalamus a part of the nutritive subcortical center.

The hypothalamic area is closely connected with the glandular part of the hypophysis, and by means of the latter exerts an influence on water and salt metabolism. The hypothalamus also has an influence on carbohydrate, protein, and lipid metabolism.

The nuclear formations also belong to the diencephalon – the lateral and medial geniculate bodies, located lateral and posterior to the optic thalamus. These form the so-called posterior thalamus. The first formation constitutes the nearest subcortex of the optic analysor and the second, the auditory analysor.

The lateral geniculate body (cgl) has a complicated lamellar structure and is the terminal point for most of the fibers of the optic tract. The only craniocerebral nerve of the diencephalon is the optic nerve (nervus opticus, II), which forms the peripheral part of the optic analysor. The fibers of the optic nerve are formed by the axons of the ganglion cells of the retina of the eye. The optic nerve enters through the optic foramen (foramen opticum) into the cavity of the cranium and, extending toward the midline, forms with the nerve of the same name of the opposite side a partial chiasma (chiasma opticorum, ch). Approximately three fourths of the fibers of the optic nerves are decussated. These together with the non-decussated fibers form the optic tract (tractus opticus, to). The fibers of the tract end in the lateral geniculate body, the pulvinar of the optic thalamus, partly in the superior corpus bigeminum. The superior corpus bigeminum is connected with the lateral geniculate body (through the anterior arm of the corpus bigeminum) and with the optic thalamus. From the cells of the lateral geniculate body and the pulvinar of the optic thalamus begin the fibers of the powerful central optic tract – the optic radiation (radiation optica), which passes through the reticular part of the interior capsule and ends in the area of the optic analysor.

Below and slightly to the rear of the lateral geniculate body lies the medial geniculate body (cgm), which is subdivided into a macrocellular and a microcellular part. As described above, numerous fibers of the lateral lemniscus and the brachia o fthe lower corpus bigeminum end in the medial geniculate body. From the medial geniculate body extends the auditory radiation, which passes within the sublenticular part of the internal capsule to the cortex of the temporal region.

The central ganglia, the lateral ventricles, and the commissures of the terminal brain (Fig. 5, 35-43)

The central or basal ganglia lie in the depth of the hemispheres of the cerebrum and are subdivided into three basic nuclei: (1) the caudate nucleus (nucleus caudatus, ncd), (2) the lenticular nucleus (nucleus lenticularis), (3) the amygdale (amygdale, am).

The caudate nucleus is a massive cellular accumulation forming the external and in part the lower wall of the lateral ventricle. It is divided into the capitellum (caput nuclei caudate), the body (corpus), and the tail (cauda). The latter is poorly developed in the dog. On the outside, the caudate nucleus borders on the anterior limb of the internal capsule (*capsula interna, ci*), which separates it from the lenticular nucleus, which in turn represents a cellular formation of a triangular shape.

The lenticular nucleus is subdivided into two cellular formations: the *putamen* (*put*) and the globus pallidus consisting of the external (*pallidum externum, pe*) and the internal (*pallidum internum, pi*) parts.

Laterally the lenticular nucleus is separated from the *claustrum* (*cls*) by the external capsule (*capsula externa, ce*). In the anterior sections, the putamen unites immediately with the capitellum of the caudate nucleus. The striopallidal system should be considered in connection with the caudate and lenticular nuclei. The caudate nucleus and the putamen belong to the phylogenetically more recent formations (neostriatum or striatum), while the globus pallidus constitutes a phylogenetically more ancient formation (palaeostriatum or pallidum).

The striopallidal system (striopallidum) is characterized by its wealth of connections with other formations of the cerebrum. The striopallidum is connected by the optic thalamus with the cerebral cortex and, first and foremost, with the frontal and the precoronal regions.

The existence of direct fibers from the cortex of the large hemispheres to the pallidum has been firmly established. The majority of investigators have definitely settled the question as to the direct connections of the cerebral cortex with the caudate body. The pallidum, and especially the striatum, receive numerous connections from the optic thalamus. There is evidence that direct tracts from the nuclei of Goll and Burdach enter into the pallidum. The pallidum sends a great number of efferent fibers to the optic thalamus, to the substantia nigra, to the subthalamic and the hypothalamic formations, and to several other formations of the brainstem.

The connections of the pallidum with the red nucleus (the pallidorubral tract) deserve special attention, for through these are directed impulses which regulate motor functions and tonic reactions.

Many authors have traced the direct tracts from the striatum to the nuclei of the brainstem and to the substantia nigra.

The striopallidal system is the most important part of the extrapyramidal system. In a tight complex with the cerebral cortex and the nuclear formations of the brainstem, the striopallidum participates in the coordination of the complicated, stereotype unconditioned reflex movements which constitute the basis of the activity of the motor analysor (Shaikevich [665]; Bekhterev [2]; Liddel and Philipps [649]; Mettler [652] and others).

It is assumed that the striopallidum is included in the realization of instinctive reactions which belong, as is well known, to the category of the most complex unconditioned reflexes (Ivanov-Smolenskiy [30]; Rozhanskiy [781, 61]; Vasilyev [612]; Shumilina [1072]; Lagutina and Rozhanskiy [551]). The participation of the striopallidum in the region of a series of vegetative processes has also been established. The above mentioned numerous connections of the striopallidum with other areas of the cerebrum point to its complex functions.

Recently, Klosovkiy and Volzhina [641] have come to the conclusion that bilateral removal of the caudate nuclei is accompanied by an abrupt disturbance in conditioned reflex activity. These authors negate the vegetative functions ascribed to the caudate nucleus and emphasize the functional connection of these formations with basic instincts.

To the subcortical ganglia belongs also the amygdaloid nucleus, or almond, located in the anterior part of the pyriform gyrus (*gyrus piriformis, Pi*) ventrally from the capsule. The amygdala is formed by numerous accumulations of nerve cells, which are subdivided into a series of nuclei, poorly separated from the cortical lamina of the periamygdalar region, located ventrally and belonging to the paleocortex. The amygdala is connected through afferent fibers with the olfactory tubercle and with the septum pellucidum through the stria terminalis (st) and presumably can be referred to the system of the olfactory analysor.

In each hemisphere, toward the medial side of the central ganglia lie the cavities of the lateral ventricle.

The lateral ventricle begins slightly to the front of the corpus callosum, extends backward and downward and consists of the anterior horn (*cornu anterior*), the central part (*pars centralis*), the lower horn (*cornu interius*), and the posterior horn (*cornu postrius*).

The anterior horn, which has the form of a fissure, borders on adjacent structures as follows: in front and above, on the white matter of the frontal lobe and on the fibers of the corpus callosum; from within, on the mass of the septum pellucidum (*massa septi pellucidi, spf*); from the outside and partly from underneath, on the caudate body (*nucleus caudatus, ncd*). In the posterior end of the anterior horn, approximately where the columns of the fornix (*columnae fornicis*) border on the septum pellucidum, is Monroe's foramen (*foramen Monroi, fM*), which connects the lateral ventricle with the superior part of the third ventricle.

The central part is limited from above by the fibers of the corpus callosum and the epithelial lamina of the vascular plexus (*plexus chorioideus*), and from below by the fimbria and Ammon's horn. In the posterior sections, the central part widens, and toward the back changes into the posterior horn, and downward into the inferior horn.

The inferior horn, in the shape of a narrow, fissure-like cavity, descends in an arched way, downward and toward the front, up to the top of the pyriform gyrus. From below and from within, the inferior horn is bounded by Ammon's horn (*cornu Ammonis*), by the fimbria and the vascular plexus (*plexus choroideus)* from above by the tapetum.

The posterior horn is the continuation of the central part of the lateral ventricle. From below and from the outside it is covered by the tapetum and is lined with the ependyma of the ventricle.

The cerebrum is divided by a longitudinal fissure (*fissura longitudinalis cerebri, flc*) into two hemispheres, which are connected in the middle by a commissure of white matter - the corpus callosum (*corpus callosum, ccl*).

The corpus callosum consists of the genu (*gen*), the stem (*truncus, trn*), and the torulus (*splenium, spn*). The central, largest part of the corpus callosum forms the stem, which curves toward the front and forms the genu. Below, the genu tapers off into the rostrum. Toward the back, the stem of the corpus callosum thickens and changes into the torulus. The fibers of the corpus callosum penetrate into the mass of the cerebral hemispheres and form the corona of the corpus callosum (*corona corporis callosi*). The fibers of the anterior part of the corpus callosum are directed toward the frontal region, forming the anterior forceps (*forceps anterior*); the fibers of the posterior part, going in the direction of the occipital and the temporal areas, form the posterior forceps (*forceps posterior*).

Underneath the corpus callosum lies the *fornix* (*f*), through which pass the projective fibers from the region of the archicortex toward the mammillary bodies, and the commissural fibers of the archicortex. The fornix is formed by two arches, joined together in the central part. In the anterior portion, the fornix is divided into the columns of the fornix (*columnae fornicis*) which pass through the hypothalamus and end in the cells of the mammillary bodies. The posterior section of the fornix is formed by the crura fornicis, which changes into the fimbria which is solidly connected with the dentate fascia. The crura fornicis are joined together by the transverse fibers, which form the commissure of the fornix, or the lyre of David (*commissura fornicis*) which connects the cortex of Ammon's horn of both hemispheres.

Between the corpus callosum and the columns of the fornix lies the thin lamina, named the mass of the septum pellucidum (*massa septi pellucidi, spt*) between the leaves of which is a closed cavity (*cavum septi pellucidi*). The third commissure of the cerebrum is the anterior commissure (*commissura anterior, can*) which connects, predominantly, the structures of the archicortex.

Ventral to the anterior portion of the optic thalamus, between the anterior commissure and the chiasm of the optic nerves, lies the preoptic area (*area praeoptica, hpr*), which is subdivided into medial and lateral parts. The medial part is occupied by the medial preoptic area (*area praeoptica medialis, hprm*) and the nucleus of the anterior commissure (*nucleus interstitialis commissurae anterioris, nca*, s. "bed nucleus" - Rioch, 1929 [*Editors' note: The Rioch reference cannot be found in the bibliography.*] and others).

The lateral part of this zone is represented by the lateral preoptic area (*area praeoptica lateralis, hprl*).

A Section through the Upper Part of the Cervical Spinal Cord (Fig. 8)

The gray and white matter of the spinal cord stand out clearly in the preparation.

The central canal (*canalis centralis, cc*) extends through the center of the gray matter. It is lined from within by the ependyma and surrounded by the central gelatinous substance (*substantia gelatinosa centralis*). Above it lies the posterior gray commissure (*commissura grisea posterior, cpg*), below it lie the anterior gray and white commissures (*commissurae anteriores grisea, cag, et alba, caa*). The gray matter consists of massive anterior horns (*corna anteriores, ca*) and posterior horns (*corna posteriores, cp*).

The posterior horn consists of three parts: the cells of the posterior horn (*nuclei cornu posterioris*), the gelatinous substance (*substantia gelatinosa Rolandi, sgR*), and the marginal zone lying more posteriorly (*zona marginalis, zm*). The latter structures unite into the apex of the posterior horn (*apex cornu posterioris*), which does not reach the periphery of the spinal cord. Between the apex and the periphery lies a small area of the white matter - the marginal zone of Lissauer. The posterior and anterior horns are connected with thin lamina of gray matter which, together with the white matter, make up the reticular formation (*formatio reticularis, ret*).

The anterior horn consists predominantly of large triangular cells which can be distinguished as lateral (*lb*), ventral (*v*), medial (*m*), and central (*c*) groups.

The white matter of the spinal cord is formed by the anterior (*columnae anteriores, cla*), lateral (*columnae laterales, cll*), and posterior (*columnae posteriores, clp*) columns, divided by the anterior median fissure (*fissura mediana anterior, fma, s. sulcus medianus anterior, sma*), the anterior lateral fissure (*sulcus lateralis anterior, sla*), the posterior lateral fissure (*sulcus lateralis posterior, slp*), and the posterior median or longitudinal fissure (*sulcus medianus posterior, smp*).

The tracts extending within these columns are described in the text and are labeled in Fig. 4.

As pointed out above, the form of the gray matter in different sections of the spinal cord is variable. Thus, the lateral horns are best developed (*cornu lateralis, cl*) in the thoracic portion (Fig. 9, ill. 1). In the cervical portion, they merge with the massive anterior horns (Fig. 8). In the lumbar area (Fig. 9, illustration 2), the anterior horns correspond in size approximately to the posterior horns. The amount of white matter of the spinal cord varies in different areas. It decreases considerably in the sacral and the coccygeal portions of the spinal cord (Fig. 10).

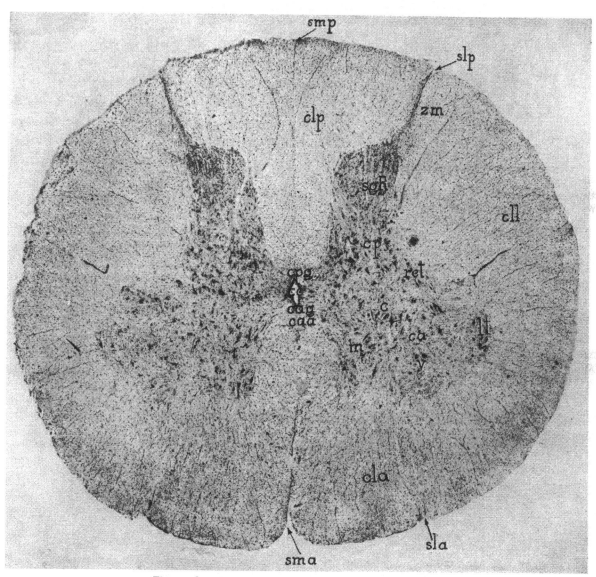

Figure 8 – The cervical portion of the spinal cord

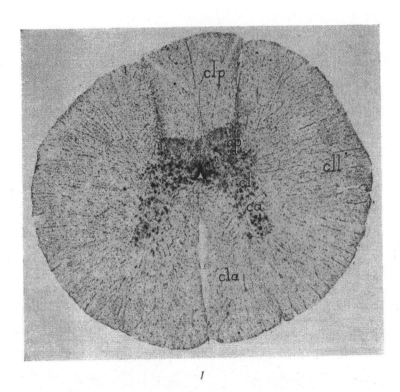

1

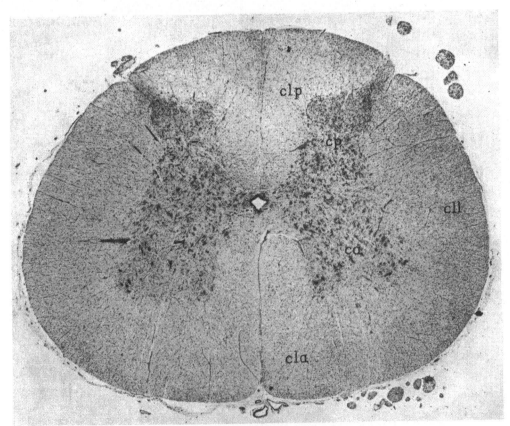

Figure 9 – Illustration 1: The thoracic portion of the spinal cord;
Illustration 2: The lumbar portion of the spinal cord.

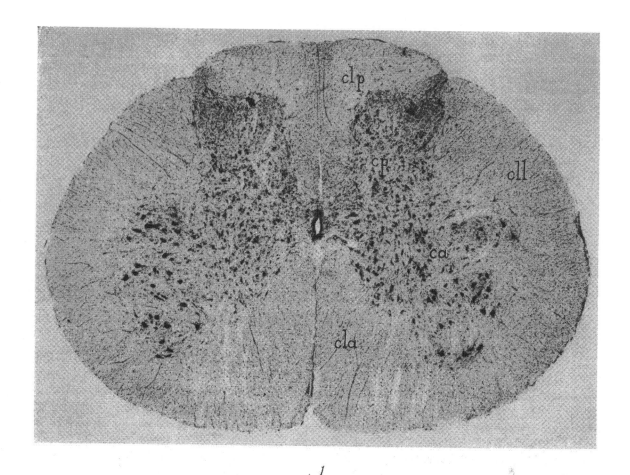

1

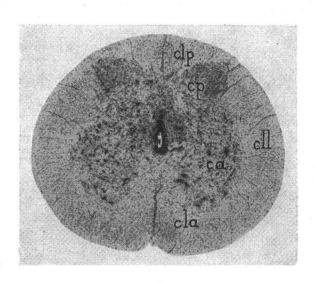

2

**Figure 10 – Illustration 1: the sacral portion of the spinal cord;
Illustration 2: The coccygeal portion of the spinal cord**

A Section at the Level Where the Spinal Cord Changes into the Medulla Oblongata, on a Level with the Decussation of the Fibers of the Pyramidal Tract (Section 10, Fig. 11)

The gray matter still keeps its configuration and is subdivided into the anterior and posterior horns. The anterior horns begin to isolate themselves from the posterior horns by the fibers of the pyramidal tract. The central canal (*cc*) is displaced more dorsally. By the side of the latter lies the dorsal nucleus of the accessory nerve (*nucleus dorsalis nervus accessorii, nXId*).

Emerging above the central canal are the nuclei of the gracilis (delicate) fasciculus (*nucleus funiculi gracilis, ng*) and the cuneiform fasciculus (nucleus funiculi cuneati, nc), with their fibers (*funiculus gracilis, fg, et funiculus cuneatus, fc*). There is a considerable increase of the gelatinous substance of Rolando (*sgR*) in the posterior horn. Ventral to the central canal is the decussation of the fibers of the pyramidal tract (*decussatio pyramidum, dpy*); the anterior horns lie laterally and here one can distinguish the ventral nucleus of the accessory nerve (*nucleus ventralis nervus accessorii, nXIv*) and the nucleus of the first pair of cervical nerves (*nucleus nervus cervicalis I, nc$_1$*). Between the anterior and posterior horns lies the reticular formation (*ret*).

Lateral to the decussation of the pyramidal tract pass the fibers of the posterior longitudinal fasciculus (*fasciculus longitudinalis posterior, flp*) and the tectospinal tract (*fasciculus tectospinalis, fts*). In the lateral area of the section lie, from the bottom up: the spinothalamic tract (*fasciculus spinothalamicus, fsth*), the ventral spinocerebellar tract of Cowers (*fasciculus spinocerebellaris ventralis Gowersi, fscv*), the dorsal spinocerebellar tract of Flechsig (*fasciculus spinocerebellaris dorsalis Flechsigi, fscd*), and the rubrospinal tract (*fasciculus rubrospinalis, frs*).

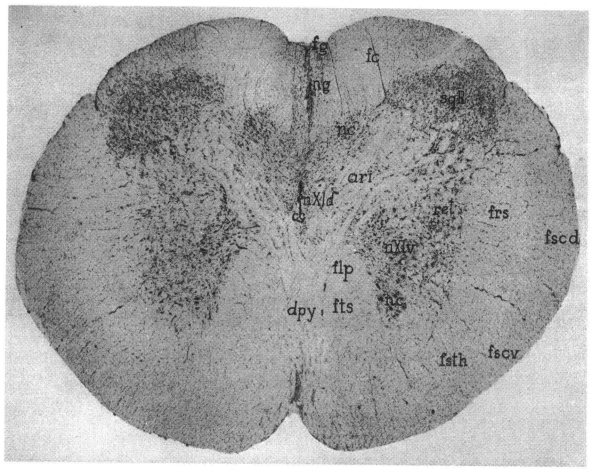

Figure 11 – Section 10

A Section at the Level of the Lowest Portion of the Medulla Oblongata (Section 40, Fig. 12)

The cavity of the central canal (*cc*) is displaced in a dorsal direction. The gray matter begins to lose its characteristic butterfly shape, becoming separated into discrete nuclei. At the side of the central canal lies the dorsal nucleus of the vagus nerve (*nucleus dorsalis nervus vagus, xXd*). Dorsal to the canal can be seen the cuneiform (*fc*) and the gracilis (*fg*) funiculi with their nuclei (*nc, ng*), which increase in size; more laterally is seen the gelatinous substance of Rolando (*sgR*) with the descending root of the trigeminal nerve (*radix descendens n. trigemini, rVd*).

Lateral to the central canal lie the internal arcuate fibers (*fibrae arcuatae internae, ari*), which ventrally decussate along the midline (*decussatio lemniscorum medialium, dlm*). Lateral to the decussation pass the fibers of the posterior longitudinal fasciculus (*flp*) and the tectospinal tracts (*fts*), and extending downward are the fibers of the pyramidal tract (*fasciculus pyramidalis, py*). The anterior horns of the gray matter (*ca*) are smaller; within them can be distinguished the nucleus of the first pair of cervical nerves (C_1 or nC_1). In the lateral parts of the section emerges the lateral nucleus of the medulla oblongata (*nucleus lateralis, nlt*); below it pass the spinothalamic (*fsth*) and the ventral spinocerebellar (*fscv*) tracts, and above are the dorsal spinocerebellar (*fscd*) and the rubrospinal (*frs*) tracts.

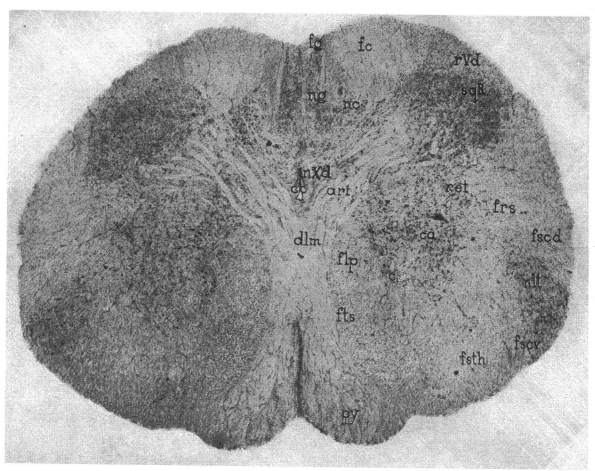

Figure 12 – Section 40

A Section at the Level of the Inferior Olivary Body of the Medulla Oblongata (Section 120, Fig. 13)

Alongside the central canal (*cc*) is the dorsal nucleus of the vagus nerve (*nXd*); above can be seen the small cells of the nucleus of the solitary fasciculus (*nucleus tractus solitarius, nsl*).   Above the central canal lie the nuclei of the cuneiform and the *gracilis funiculi* (*nc, ng*).   From the latter extend the internal arciform fibers (*ari*), forming a decussation (*dlm*) immediately below the central canal.   Among the decussating fibers lie the fibers of the posterior longitudinal fasciculus (*flp*).   In a more ventral direction lies the tectospinal tract (*fts*) and the massive pyramidal tract (*py*).   Lateral to the pyramidal tract emerges the inferior olive (*oliva inferior, oi*).   The photograph shows the olivocerebellar fibers (*fibrae olivocerebellares, foc*) coming from the olive.   The anterior horns of the spinal cord are already missing.   The reticular formation (*ret*) with its nuclei is increased in size.   The lateral nucleus (*nlt*) is considerably developed.   Between the olive and the lateral nucleus lie the spinothalamic (*fsth*) and the ventral spinocerebellar (*fscv*) tracts.   The dorsal spinocerebellar tract (*fscd*) is pushed in a more dorsal direction.   The rubrospinal tract (*frs*) is more medial.

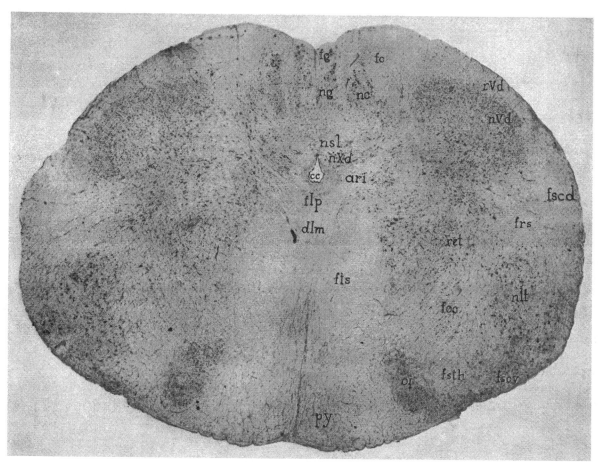

Figure 13 — Section 120

A Section through the Caudal Part of the Nucleus of the Hypoglossal Nerve (Section 200, Fig. 14)

The cavity of the central canal (*cc*) is even more dislodged in a dorsal direction. Lateral to the central canal lies the massive nucleus of the hypoglossal nerve (*nucleus hypoglossi, nXII*) and above it can be seen the dorsal nucleus of the vagus nerve (*nXd*) and the nucleus of the solitary fasciculus (*nsl*).

The nuclei of the gracilis (*ng*) and cuneiform (*nc*) fasciculi with the fibers (*fg, fc*) lie in the dorsal area of the section. Laterally appears the external nucleus of the cuneiform fasciculus, or the nucleus of Burdach, or of Monakov, or of Bekhterev (*nucleus externus funiculi cuneati s. nucleus Burdach, s. Monakowi, s. Bechterewi, nce*). Lateral to this nucleus lies the descending root of the trigeminal nerve (*rVd*) and its nucleus (*nVd*). Above the latter pass the posterior exterior arcuate fibers (*fibrae arcuatae externae posteriores, arep*). Below the central canal can be seen the raphe (*raphe, r*), on both sides of which lie the fibers of the posterior longitudinal fasciculus (*flp*), the tectospinal tract (*fts*), the medial lemniscus (*lemniscus medians, lm*), and the pyramid (*py*). Lateral to the pyramids lies the complex of the inferior olive (*oi*). At the cells of the olive, originate the olivocerebellar fibers (*foc*) which are clearly visible in the section. Above the medial lemniscus and the olive pass the fibers of the root of the hypoglossal nerve (*rXII*), extending in a ventral direction. The reticular formation (*ret*) with its nuclei is considerably developed, as is the lateral nucleus (*nlt*). The spinothalamic (*fsth*), ventral spinocerebellar (*fscv*), dorsal spinocerebellar (*fscd*), and rubrospinal (*frs*) tracts retain their previous positions.

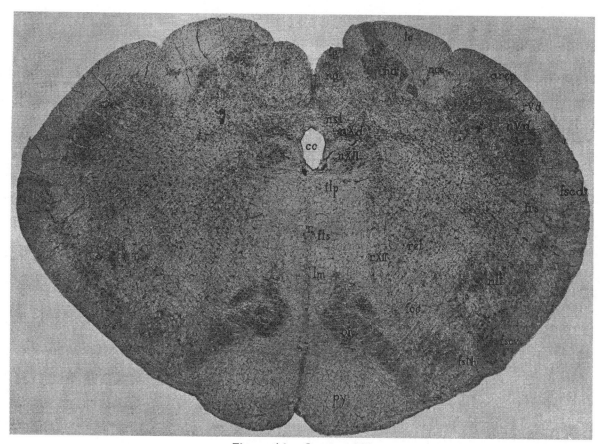

Figure 14 – Section 200

A Section at the Level of the Opening of the Central Canal into the Cavity of the IV Ventricle (Section 240, Fig. 15)

The floor of the IV ventricle is formed by the calamus scriptorius (*calamus scriptorius, cal*) and the *ala cinerea*. From the side the *area postrema* (*ap*) enters into the cavity of the ventricle. The roof of the ventricle is formed by the posterior medullary velum (*velum medullare posterius, vmp*). The nucleus of the hypoglossal nerve (*nXIII*), which can become quite large lies on both sides of the ventricle. Above it can be seen the *nucleus intercalatus* (*nin*), the dorsal nucleus of the vagus nerve (*nXd*), and the nucleus of the solitary fasciculus (*nsl*). The nuclei of the gracilis and cuneiform fasciculi (*ng, nc*) decrease noticeably in size. From them extend the posterior exterior arciform fibers (*arep*), which go into the restiform body (*corpus restiforme, rest*). The fibers of the restiform body are grouped around the exterior nucleus of the *cuneiform fasciculus* (*nce*).

On both sides of the commissure (*raphe, r*) lie the posterior longitudinal fasciculus (*flp*) and the tectospinal tract (*fts*); further down lie the medial lemniscus (*lm*) and the pyramids (*py*). Here the complex of the inferior olive reaches considerable dimensions; one can distinguish the main olive (*oi*), the dorsal accessory olive (*oliva inferior accessoria dorsalis, oid*), and the ventral accessory olive (*oliva inferior accessoria ventralis, oiv*).

From the medial sections of the olive extend the olivocerebellar fibers (*foc*), crossing through the raphe (*r*) to the opposite side; from the lateral sections of the olive the olivocerebellar fibers rise toward the restiform body (*rest*) on the same side.

Above and lateral to the olives lies the well developed reticular formation (*ret*) with its nuclei. Its lateral portions surround the motor nucleus of the vagus nerve (*nucleus motorius n. vagi s. nucleus ambiguus, nXa*). The lateral nucleus (*nlt*) is much smaller in size; below it can be seen the spinothalamic (*fsth*) and ventral spinocerebellar tracts (*fscv*). Still more externally lies the descending root of the trigeminal nerve (*rVd*), its nucleus (*nVd*), the rubrospinal tract (*frs*) and the external arciform anterior fibers (*fibrae arcuatae externae anteriores, area*), representing the continuation of Flechsig's fasciculus.

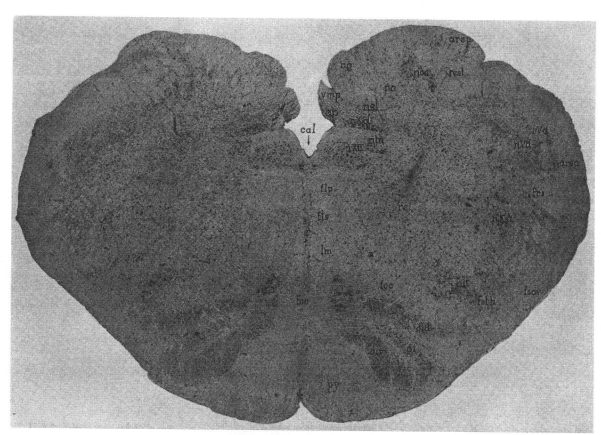

Figure 15 – Section 240

A Section through the Central Nucleus of the Reticular Formation (section 280, Fig. 16)

The cavity of the IV ventricle (ventriculus quartus, vIV) gradually widens. On the top, it is bounded by the posterior medullary vellum (*velum medullare posterius, vmp*) and a few cells of the *area postrema* (*ap*). Below the floor of the IV ventricle, on both sides of the raphe (*raphe, r*), lies the nucleus of the hypoglossal nerve (nXII); lateral to it is nucleus intercalates (*nin*), below it is Roller's nucleus (*nucleus sublingualis, nR*), and slightly above is the dorsal nucleus of the vagus nerve (*nXd*). Next to the nucleus of the vagus nerve can be seen the solitary fasciculus (*tractus s. fasciculus solitarius, fsl*) and its nucleus (*nucleus tractus solitarius, nsl*). The external nucleus of the *cuneiform fasciculus* (*nce*) reaches considerable dimensions.

Below the IV ventricle and near the midline lie the fibers of the posterior longitudinal fasciculus (*flp*) and the tectospinal tracts (*fts*). In a still more ventral direction lie the medial lemniscus (*lm*) and the fibers of the pyramidal tract (*py*). More laterally can be seen the complex of the inferior olive (*oi*) with the olivocerebellar fibers (*foc*) extending from it. Above and exterior to the olive lies the reticular formation (*ret*) with its nuclei, among which can be distinguished the central nucleus of the reticular formation (*nucleus centralis formation reticularis, ncr*). The outer areas of the section are taken up by the motor nucleus of the vagus nerve (*nXa*), the lateral nucleus (*nlt*), and the spinothalamic tract (*fsth*), all of which are decreasing in size. As before, the descending root of the trigeminal nerve (*rVd*) and its nucleus (*nVd*) can be seen clearly. Below is the rubrospinal tract (*frs*). In the outermost portions of the section lie the ventral spinocerebellar tract (*fscv*) and the restiform body (*corpus restiforme, rest*), and entering the latter, the external anterior arciform fibers (*fibrae arcuatae externae anteriores, area*).

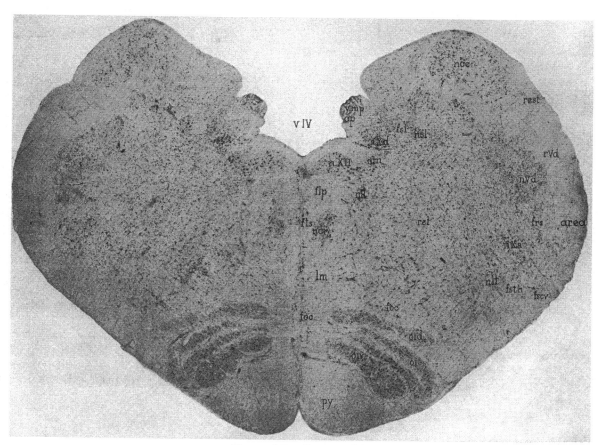

Figure 16 – Section 280

A Section at the Level of the Upper Part of the Inferior Olive (*oi*) (Section 360, Fig. 17)

The cavity of the *IV* ventricle (*vIV*) is wide open. Below the *IV* ventricle, on both sides of the raphe (*r*), can be seen: the posterior longitudinal fasciculus (*flp*), the nucleus of the hypoglossal nerve (*nXII*) with its descending root (*rXII*), Roller's nucleus (*nucleus sublingualis, nR*), *nucleus intercalatus* (*nin*), and the dorsal nucleus of the vagus nerve (*nXd*). Above the dorsal nucleus lies the triangular nucleus, or the internal vestibular nucleus of Schwalbe (*nucleus triangularis s. nucleus vestibularis, medians Schwalbe, ntr*). Immediately lateral to the dorsal nucleus of the vagus nerve lies the solitary fasciculus (*fsl*) and its nucleus (*nsl*). Below the posterior longitudinal fasciculus can be seen the tectospinal tract (*fts*) and the medial lemniscus (*lm*), and among its fibers lie large cells - the gigantocellular nucleus of the reticular formation (*nucleus gigantocellularis formatio reticularis, ngc*). Again, the lateral microcellular portion of the reticular formation (*ret*) is seen to be well developed. On both sides of the anterior central fissure lie two pyramids (*py*); dorsally from them can be seen the much smaller inferior olive (*oi*). Between the olives, along the midline, is the arciform nucleus of the medulla oblongata (*nucleus arcuatus medullae oblongatae, narc*), in which originate the external arciform anterior fibers. The motor nucleus of the vagus nerve (*nXa*) is clearly defined. Below it lie the spinothalamic (*fsth*) and the ventral spinocerebellar (*fscv*) tracts; above it are the rubrospinal tract (*frs*), the descending root of the trigeminal nerve (*rVd*) and its nucleus (*nVd*), the external nucleus of the cuneiform fasciculus (*nce*), and the restiform body (*rest*) with the external arciform anterior fibers (*area*) entering into it (see the left side of the figure).

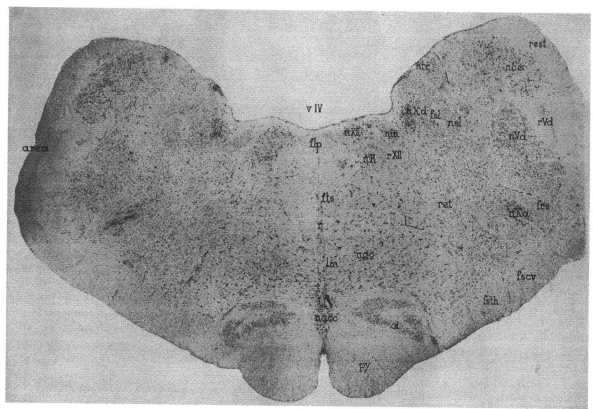

Figure 17 – Section 360

A Section at the Level of the Emergence of the Nucleus of the Facial Nerve (Section 400, Fig. 18)

At this level, the cavity of the *IV* ventricle (*vIV*) is still wider. At its bottom, on both sides of the raphe (*r*), is the nucleus of the sublingual nerve (*nXII*), Roller's nucleus (*nR*), and the dorsal nucleus of the vagus nerve (nXd). To the exterior of the latter are the solitary fasciculus (*fsl*) and its nucleus (*nsl*), the triangular nucleus of the vestibulary nerve (*ntr*), the descending root of the vestibular nerve (*radix descendens nervi vestibularis, rdv*) and its nucleus (*nucleus radicis descendentis nervus vestibularis, ndv*). Still more lateral appears Deiter's nucleus, or the external vestibular nucleus (*nucleus Deitersi s. nucleus vestibularis lateralis, nD*), formed by large cells. The external nucleus of the cuneiform fasciculus (*nce*) is smaller. Laterally from this nucleus lies the restiform body (*rest*) with its external arciform anterior fibers (*area*) entering into it (see the left half of the figure).

Below the floor of the *IV* ventricle can be seen the posterior longitudinal fasciculus (*flp*), the tectospinal tract (*fts*), and the medial lemniscus (*lm*). The pyramids (py) lie in the form of compact fasciculi on both sides of the anterior central fissure. In the midline, above from the pyramids, lies the arciform nucleus (*narc*). The reticular formation (*ret*) is tremendously developed and occupies a large area. Among its cells can be distinguished the gigantocellular nucleus (*ngc*). In the inferolateral parts of the section emerges the nucleus of the facial nerve (*nucleus n. facialis, nVII*). Below it are the fibers of the spinothalamic (*fsth*) and the ventral spinocerebellar (*fscv*) tracts, and laterally and above lie the rubrospinal tract (*frs*) and the descending root of the trigeminal nerve (*rVd*) and its nucleus (*nVd*), which is gradually growing smaller.

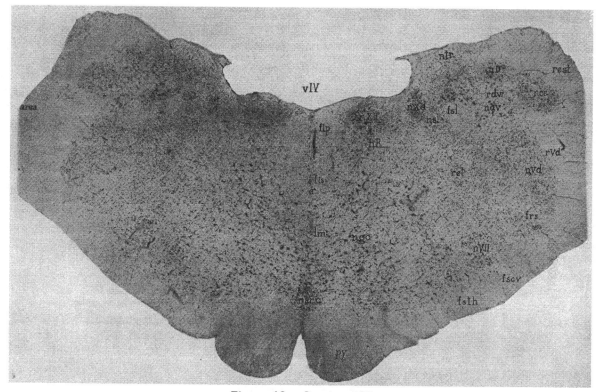

Figure 18 – Section 400

A Section of the Level of the Maximal Development of the Nucleus of the Facial Nerve (Section 490, Fig. 19)

At the bottom of the *IV* ventricle (*vIV*), on both sides of the raphe (*r*), passes the posterior longitudinal fasciculus (*flp*). Lateral to it lie the nucleus of Roller (*nR*), the triangular nucleus (*ntr*), Deiter's nucleus (*nD*), and the external nucleus of the cuneiform fasciculus (*nce*), which is considerably smaller in size.

Below the posterior longitudinal fasciculus (*flp*) lie the tectospinal tract (*fts*) and the medial lemniscus (*lm*). The ventral parts of the section are occupied by the compact fasciculus of the pyramids (*py*).

The reticular formation (*ret*), as before, takes up a considerable area; in it can be clearly distinguished the gigantocellular nucleus (*ngc*).

In the external parts of the Section can be seen the nucleus of the facial nerve (*nVII*), the spinothalamic (*fsth*), ventral spinocerebellar (*fscv*), and rubrospinal (*frs*) tracts, the powerfully developed descending root of the trigeminal nerve (*rVd*) and its nucleus (*nVd*), as well as the restiform body (*rest*), which is growing larger.

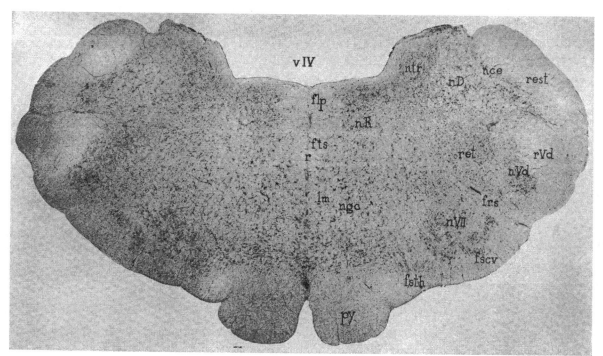

Figure 19 – Section 490

A Section at the Level of the Appearance of the Nuclei of the Auditory Nerve and the Beginning of the Superior Olive (Section 550, Fig. 20)

Below the *IV* ventricle (*vIV*), on both sides of the raphe (*r*), lie the posterior longitudinal fasciculus (*flp*) and the genu of the facial nerve (*genu n. facialis, gVII*). Near the latter structure are the triangular nucleus of the vestibular nerve (*ntr*) and Deiter's nucleus (*nD*), and below it the tectospinal tract (*fts*).

In the ventral portion of the section are the medial lemniscus (*lm*), the cells of the superior olive (*oliva superior, os*) emerging in this location, and the well isolated compact fasciculi of the pyramids (*py*). Among the fibers of medial lemniscus, and lateral to it, one can see the cells of the reticular formation (*ret, ngc*).

The nucleus of the facial nerve (*nVII*) is much smaller in size. To the exterior of these structures lie the fibers of the spinothalamic (*fsth*), the rubrospinal (*frs*) tracts, the descending root of the trigeminal nerve (*rVd*) and its nucleus (*nVd*), and above this the restiform body (*rest*). The lateral parts of the section are occupied by the cochlear branch of the auditory nerve (*ramus cochlearis n. acustici, rVIIIc*) and its two nuclei: the dorsal nucleus, or auditory tubercle (*nucleus dorsalis ramus cochlearis s. tuberculum acusticum, tac*) and the ventral nucleus (*nucleus ventralis, nVIIIcv*). It can be clearly seen how the fibers of the trapezoid body (*corpus trapezoides, ctr*) extend from the ventral nucleus; some of these end in the superior olive on the ipsilateral side, but most of them pass to the opposite side, immediately above the pyramids and ending in the olive of the contralateral side. From the auditory tubercle extend the *striae acusticae* (*sa*), which cross the raphe and enter the lateral lemniscus. Between the descending root of the trigeminal nerve and the restiform body is the vestibular portion of the auditory nerve (*ramus vestibularis, n. acustici, rVIIIv*).

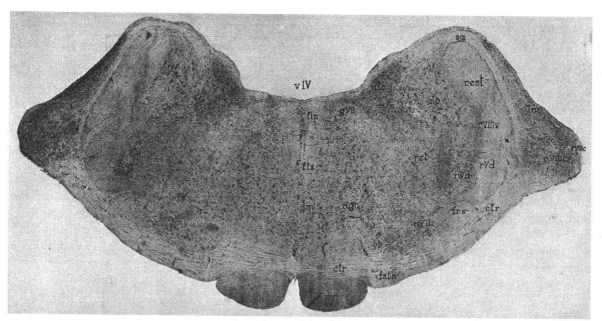

Figure 20 – Section 550

A Section through the Nucleus of the Abducent Nerve (Section 590, Fig. 21)

In the figure can be seen the closed cavity of the *IV* ventricle (*vIV*). At the bottom of the ventricle, on both sides of the raphe (*r*), lies the posterior longitudinal fasciculus (*flp*). Lateral to it can be seen the genu of the facial nerve (*gVIII*), the triangular nucleus (ntr), and Deiter's nucleus (*nD*). Above the latter lies Bekhterev's nucleus (*n. angularis, s.n. Bekhterewi, nB*). The figure clearly shows how the vestibulocerebellar fibers (*fibrae vestibule-cerebellares, fvc*) extend from these nuclei toward the cerebellum.

Above the cavity of the *IV* ventricle are the nuclei of the cerebellum - the fastigial nucleus (*nucleus fastigii, nfs*), the globular nucleus (*nucleus globesus, ngb*), the dentate nucleus (*nucleus dentatus, ndn*), and the *nucleus emboliformis* (*neb*). Below the ventricle can be seen the nucleus of the abducent nerve (*nucleus nervi abducentis, nVI*) and its descending roots (*radix n. abducentis, rVI*) extending in the direction of the base of the pons, the tectospinal tract (*fts*), the medial lemniscus (*lm*), and the compact fasciculi of the pyramids (*py*), immediately exterior to which can be seen the spinothalamic tract (*fsth*). The central and lateral parts of the section are occupied by the reticular formation (*ret, ngc*), by the well developed complex of the superior olive, containing the superior (*oliva superior lateralis, osl*) and the medial (*oliva superior medians, osm*) olives, and the fibers of the lateral lemniscus (*lemniscus lateralis, ll*); somewhat above lie the rubrospinal tract (*frs*), the descending root of the trigeminal nerve (*rVd*) and its nucleus (*nVd*). External to the latter lie the auditory tubercle (*tac*) and the ventral nucleus of the auditory nerve (*nVIIIcv*), from where originate the fibers of the trapezoid body (*ctr*), ending in the olives on the same and opposite side. Between the restiform body (*rest*) and the descending root of the trigeminal nerve lie the fibers of the vestibular nerve (*rVIIIv*).

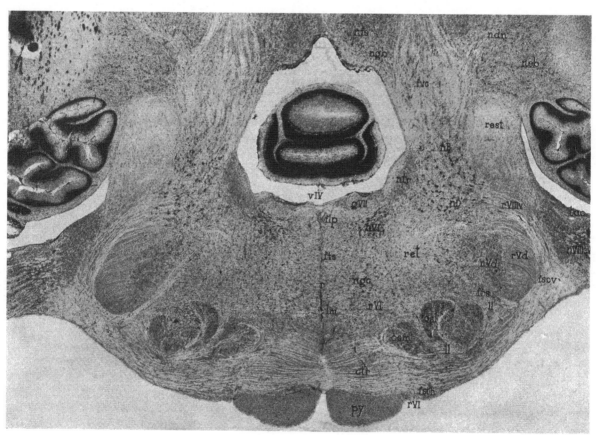

Figure 21 – Section 590

A Section on the Level of the Emergence of the Superior Cerebellar Peduncles (Section 650, Fig. 22)

The lobule of the cerebellum penetrates into the cavity of the *IV* ventricle. Below the ventricle lie the posterior longitudinal fasciculus (*flp*), the genu of the facial nerve (*gVII*) and the central tract of the tegmentum (*fasciculus-thalamorubro-olivaris s. fasciculus centralis tegmenti, fct*).

In this section, one can trace the fibers of the facial nerve (*rVII*), which proceed in a central direction between the nucleus of the descending root of the trigeminal nerve and the superior olive. Outside the genu of the facial nerve is the nucleus of Bekhterev (*nB*) with the vestibulocerebellar (*fvc*) fibers and Deiteris nucleus (*nD*) extending from it. Dorsolateral to the cavity of the ventricle pass the superior cerebellar peduncles (*pedunculi superior s. pedunculi cerebelli ad corpora quadrigemina, pcs*). Above and to either side of them lie the fastigial (*nfs*) and dentate (*ndn*) cerebellar nuclei. Still more lateral are the inferior cerebellar peduncles (*pedunculi inferior s. pedunculi cerebelli ad medullam oblongatum, pci*) with their fibers and the medial cerebellar peduncles (*pedunculi medius s. pedunculi cerebelli ad pontem, pcm*) extending from them.

Below the *IV* ventricle lie the posterior longitudinal fasciculus (*flp*), the tectospinal tract (*fts*), the medial lemniscus (*lm*), the decussation of the fibers of the trapezoid body (*ctr*), and the pyramids (*py*), lateral to which pass the fibers of the spinothalamic tract (*fsth*).

In the reticular formation (*ret*) originates the caudal nucleus of the pons (*nucleus pontis caudalis, npc*). The ventrolateral portions of the section show the complex of the superior olive (*osm, osl*) with the fibers of the lateral lemniscus (*ll*) extending from it. Above the latter are the fibers of the rubrospinal tract (*frs*), the descending root of the trigeminal nerve (*rVd*) and its nucleus (*nVd*). The most lateral area of the section is occupied by the central nucleus of the auditory nerve (*nVIIIcv*) with the fibers of the trapezoid body (*ctr*) extending from it. Between the central nucleus and the descending lemniscus (*rVd*) lies the vestibular branch of the auditory nerve (*rVIIIv*).

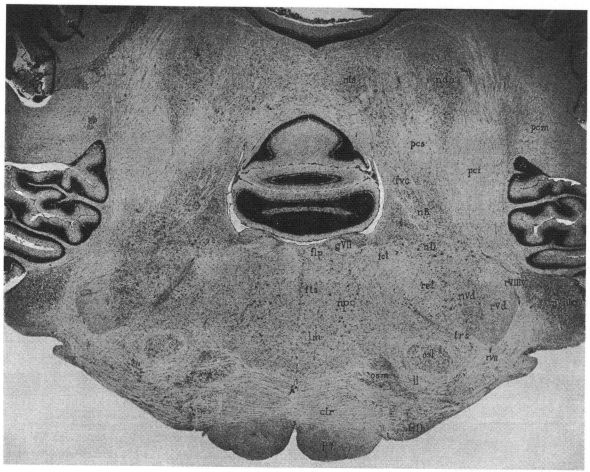

Figure 22 – Section 650

A Section through the Pons Varolii at the Level of the Appearance of the Motor Nucleus of the Trigeminal Nerve (Section 700, Fig. 23)

The cerebellar lobule penetrates into the cavity of the *IV* ventricle. At the bottom of the ventricle lies the posterior longitudinal fasciculus (*flp*), and lateral to it the central tract of the tegmentum (*fct*) and the angular nucleus of Bekhterev (*nB*); more dorsally lie the cerebellar peduncles: superior (*pcs*), medial (*pcm*), and inferior (*pci*).

The pons is divided into the base (*basis pontis*) and the tegmentum (*tegmentum pontis*). In the tegmentum is the tectospinal tract (*fts*), the medial lemniscus (*lm*), the reticular formation (*ret*) with the caudal nucleus of the pons (*npc*), the fibers of the trapezoid body (*ctr*), and the superior olive (*os*), which is now smaller in size. In the outer sections of the preparation can be seen: the macrocellular motor nucleus of the trigeminal nerve (*nucleus motorius n. trigemini, rVm*), the sensory nucleus of the trigeminal nerve (*nucleus sensorius nervi trigemini, nVs*), the descending root of the trigeminal nerve (*rVd*), the fibers of the well developed lateral lemniscus (*ll*), the spinothalamic tract (*fsth*), the massive intracerebral root of the trigeminal nerve (*radix nervi trigemini, rV*), coming out of the cerebrum, and the rubrospinal tract (*frs*).

Within the base of the pons pass the fibers of the pyramidal tract (*py*), surrounded by the pons' own nuclei (*nuclei proprii pontis, npp*), from which begin the pons' own fibers (*fibrae proprii pontis*) consisting of two layers - the superficial (*stratum superficial pontis, sts*) and the deep (*stratum profundum pontis, stp*).

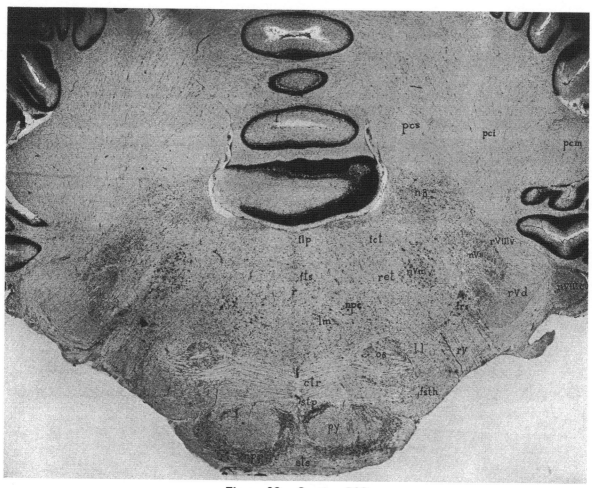

Figure 23 – Section 700

A Section through the pons Varolii, somewhat more Anterior (Section 760, Fig. 24)

The bottom of the *IV* ventricle (*vIV*) is covered by the ependyma, under which lies the central gray matter (*substantia grisea centralis, gc*). The lateral walls of the ventricle are formed by the fibers of the superior cerebellar peduncles (*pcs*). Below the floor of the ventricle passes the posterior longitudinal fasciculus (*flp*) and the tectospinal tract (*fts*).

In the tegmentum of the pons, among the cells of the reticular formation (*ret*) can be distinguished the well developed ventral nucleus of the tegmentum (*nucleus centralis tegmenti, nct*). The motor (*nVm*) and the sensory (*nVs*) nuclei of the trigeminal nerve have decreased somewhat in size. Below and lateral to the ventricle extend the fibers of the central tract of the tegmentum (*fct*).

The medial lemniscus (*lm*) is pushed slightly laterally; still more laterally lies the spinothalamic tract (*fsth*), and the lateral lemniscus (*ll*) with the powerfully developed nucleus of the lateral lemniscus (*nucleus lemnisci lateralis, nll*). In a more dorsal direction passes the rubrospinal tract (*frs*).

At the base of the pons can be seen the compact fascicule of the pyramids (*py*), surrounded by the pons' (*npp*) own extremely well developed nuclei, from which begin the pons' (*sts, stp*) own fibers extending into the medial cerebellar peduncles (pcm). Below the latter can be seen the large stem of the trigeminal nerve (*nervus trigeminus, V*).

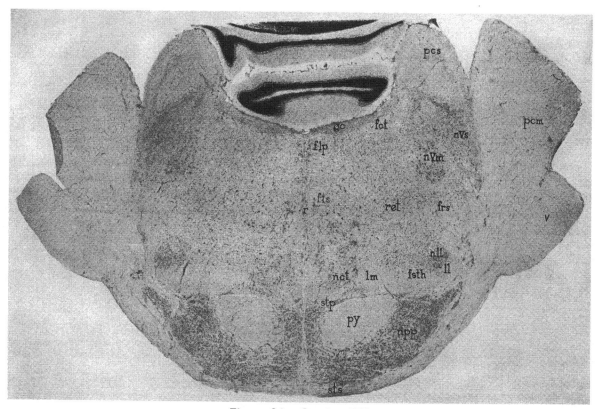

Figure 24 — Section 760

A Section at the Level of the Maximal Development of the Pons' Nuclei and Fibers (Section 820, Fig. 25)

The bottom of the *IV* ventricle (*vIV*) is covered by the ependyma, under which is the central gray matter (*gc*). The lateral walls of the IV ventricle are formed by the anterior cerebellar peduncles (*pcs*), toward the inside of which penetrates the locus coeruleus (*lc*).

Below the cavity of the *IV* ventricle lies the central tract of the tegmentum (*fct*), the posterior longitudinal fasciculus (*flp*), the tectospinal tract (*fts*), and the reticular formation (*ret*), in which there can be seen the enlarged central nucleus of the tegmentum (*nct*) and the oral nucleus of the pons (*nucleus pontis oralis, npo*).

Still further ventrally lie the medial lemniscus (*lm*), the spinothalamic tract (*fsth*), the lateral lemniscus (*ll*) with the well developed nucleus of the lateral lemniscus (*nll*). Medial to the nucleus of the lateral lemniscus passes the rubrospinal tract (*frs*).

The lower portion of the section is taken up by the pyramids (*py*), which divide into separate fasciculi. Clearly evident are the pons' own nuclei (*npp*) in which begin the pons' own fibers which are subdivided into layers: superficial (*stratum superficial pontis, sts*), complex (*stratum complexum, stc*), and deep (*stratum profundum pontis, stp*). These fibers form the medial cerebellar peduncles (*pcm*).

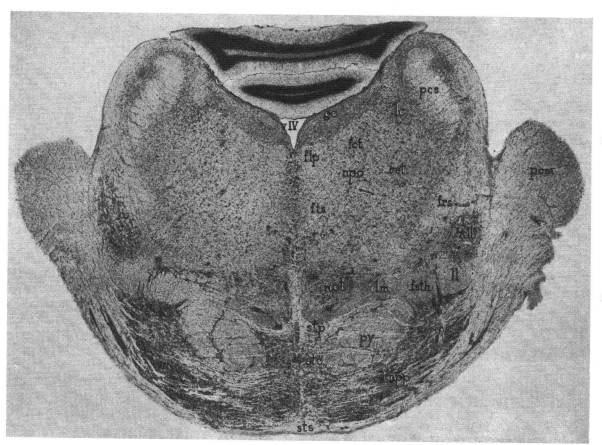

Figure 25 — Section 820

A Section at the Level of the Maximum Development of the Posterior Corpus Bigeminum (Which in the Dog Reaches Considerable Dimensions, Section 950, Fig. 26)

The *IV* ventricle has become narrower. It is penetrated by the cerebellar lobule. The floor of the ventricle is formed by a stratum of the central gray matter (*gc*).

Lateral to the *IV* ventricle lies the posterior corpus bigeminum (*corpus bigeminum posterius, cbp*), a nuclear formation. The posterior corpus bigeminum is surrounded by fibers, which form its capsule. Slightly more lateral to it lies the brachium of the posterior corpus bigeminum (*brachium corporis bigemini posterioris, bcbp*). The preparation well demonstrates how part of the fibers of the lateral lemniscus (*ll*) approach the posterior corpus bigeminum.

Below the floor of the *IV* ventricle lies the posterior longitudinal fasciculus (*flp*). Below the latter, one can see clearly the decussation of the fibers of the anterior cerebellar peduncle, or the decussation of Wernekinki (*decussatio pedunculorum cerebelli anteriorum s. decussatio Wernekinki, dW*) and the tectospinal tract (*fts*). In a more ventral direction lie the cells of the interpeduncular ganglion (*gangl. interpedunculare, gi*) and the fibers of the medial lemniscus (*lm*) and the spinothalamic tract (*fsth*).

In the reticular formation is the oral nucleus of the pons (*npo*), medial to which passes the central tract of the tegmentum (*fct*); below it is the *rubrospinal fasciculus* (*frs*).

The ventral portions of the section are taken up by the base of the cerebral peduncle (*pes pedunculi cerebri, pp*) which is emerging at this level. It is surrounded from below by the pons' own nuclei (*npp*) and the fibers, where one can see most clearly the superficial stratum (*sts*).

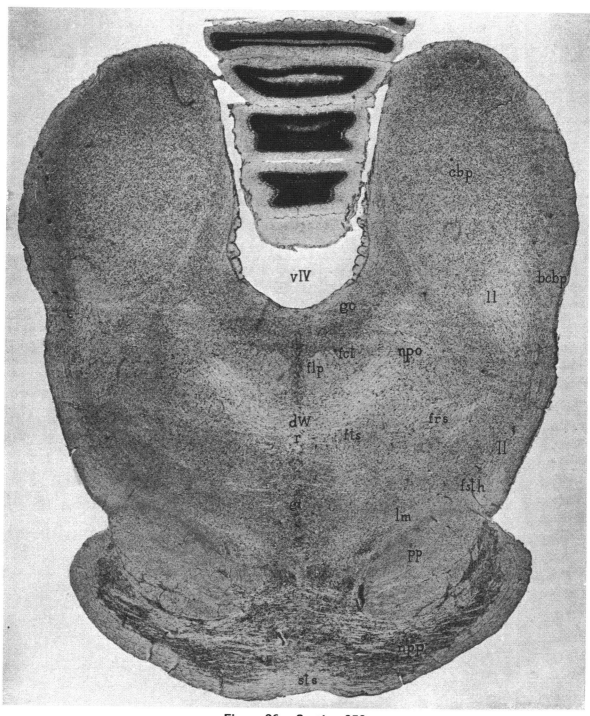

Figure 26 – Section 950

A Section through the Midbrain on the Level with the Corinissure of the Posterior Corpus Bigeminum (Section 990, Fig. 27)

The *IV* ventricle has now joined the sylvian aqueduct (*aquaeductus Sylvii, aS*) which is surrounded by the central gray matter (*gc*). Lateral to the central gray appears the nucleus of the mesencephalic root of the trigeminal nerve, formed by the vesicular, or round, cells (*nucleus radicis mesencephalicus s. ascendentis n. trigemini, nVa*), and its root. The superior parts of this section are taken up by the posterior corpus bigeminum (*cbp*); on its outer surface one can see the fibers of the brachium of the posterior corpus bigeminum (*bcbp*). The corpora bigemina are joined together by the commissure of the posterior corpus bigeminum (*commissura corporis bigemini posterioris, ccbp*) lying dorsal to the sylvian aqueduct.

The preparation shows how the small "bigeminal body" (*bb*) (Papez [59]) emerges from below the posterior corpus bigeminum; it sends its fibers to the nuclei of the pons. The "bigeminal body" can be considered the efferent system of the posterior corpus bigeminum. It is connected with the pons and the cerebellum and represents the subcortical tract for auditory motor reactions.

The fibers of the lateral lemniscus pass below the posterior corpus bigeminum.

The posterior longitudinal fasciculus (*flp*) lies below the sylvian aqueduct.

In the center of the section, the decussation of the fibers of the anterior cerebellar peduncle (decussation of Wernekinki, *dW*) is well marked. More ventrally can be seen the interpeduncular ganglion (*gi*), the medial lemniscus (*lm*), and the spinothalamic tract (*fsth*). Lateral to the decussation of Wernekinki is the tectospinal tract (*fts*), the reticular formation (*ret*) with the central tract of the tegmentum (*fct*), and the rubrospinal tract (*frs*).

The basal portion of the section is occupied by the fibers of the base of the cerebral peduncle (*pp*), by the pons' own nuclei (*npp*), and the pons' (*sts*) own fibers.

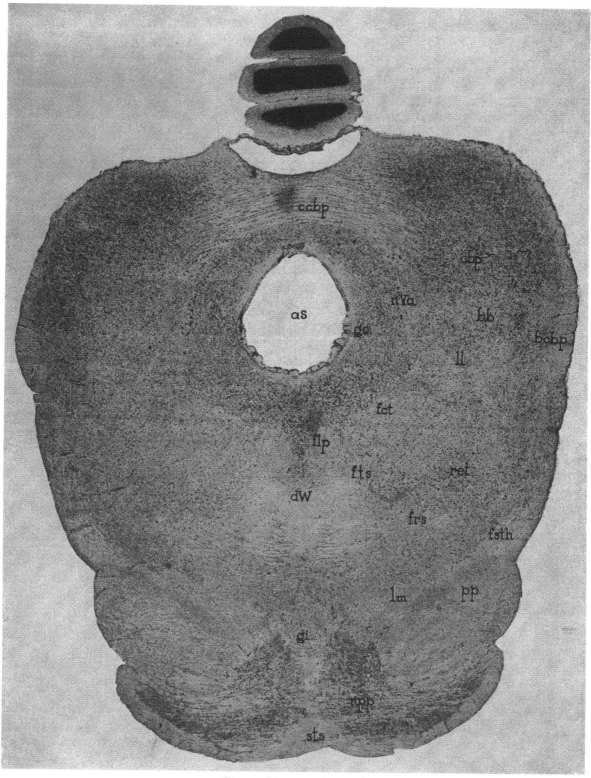

Figure 27 — Section 990

A Section through the Midbrain at the Level of the Nuclei of the Trochlear Nerve (Section 1020, Fig. 28)

The sylvian aqueduct (aS) is, as before, surrounded by a massive layer of the central gray matter (gc). Lateral to it Ides the nucleus of the mesencephalic root of the trigeminal nerve (nVa) and its root. Dorsal to the sylvian aqueduct lie the tubercles of the posterior corpus bigeminum (cbp), which are joined together by the commissure of the posterior corpus bigeminum (ccbp).

The fibers of the brachium of the posterior corpus bigeminum (bcbp) pass lateral to the posterior corpus bigeminum; the fibers of the lateral lemniscus (ll) pass below it.

Below the sylvian aqueduct lie the posterior longitudinal fasciculus (flp) and the nucleus of the trochlear nerve which emerges at this level (nucleus nervus trochlearis, nIV). More ventrally lie the tectospinal tract (fts), the decussation of the fibers of the anterior cerebellar peduncles (dW), and the well isolated interpeduncular ganglion (gi).

The ventral portions of the section are occupied by the pons' own nuclei (npp) and fibers (sts) and by the base of the cerebral peduncle. Above the later lies the substantia nigra of Soemmering (substantia nigra Soemmeringi, sn), the medial lemniscus (lm), the rubrospinal tract (frs), and the spinothalamic tract (fsth).

The lateral portions of the section are taken up by the well developed reticular formation (ret), through the medial area of which pass the fibers of the central tract of the tegmentum (fct).

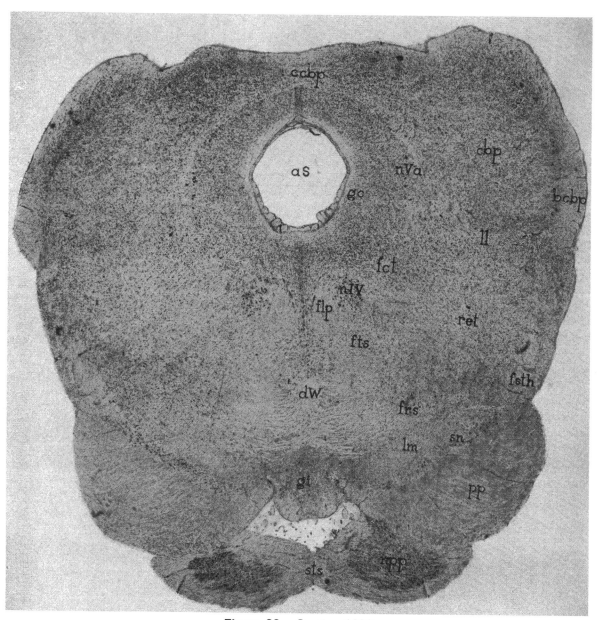

Figure 28 – Section 1020

A Section through the Midbrain at the Level of the Emergence of the Anterior Corpus Bigemini (Section 1040, Fig. 29)

The sylvian aqueduct (*aS*) is surrounded by a thick layer of the central gray matter (*gc*). Lateral to it is the ascending root of the *V* nerve and its nucleus (*nVa*), and also the fibers of the tectospinal tract (*fts*).

Above the sylvian aqueduct lie the anterior corpus bigeminum (*corpus bigeminum anterius, cba*) and the fibers of the anterior commissure of the anterior corpus bigeminum (*commissura corporis bigemini anterioris, ccba*).

Below the sylvian aqueduct is the now much smaller nucleus of the trochlear nerve (*nIV*), the nucleus of the oculomotor nerve (*nucleus n. oculomotorii, nIII*), which begins here, and the posterior longitudinal lemniscus (*flp*). Toward the outside of the latter passes the central tract of the tegmentum (*fct*).

As before, the reticular formation is well developed. In it stands out clearly the white nucleus (*nucleus album, na*) which represents the capsule of the red nucleus. Below the white nucleus lies the decussation of Wernekinki (*dW*) and the interpeduncular ganglion (*gi*). The ventral portions of the section are taken up by the base of the cerebral peduncle (*pp*). Above it lies the substantia nigra of Soemmering (*sn*). Above it is the medial lemniscus (*lm*) and the striopeduncular tract (*fasciculus striopeduncularis, fsp*). Further dorsally is the spinothalamic tract (*fsth*), the lateral lemniscus (*ll*) and the brachium of the posterior corpus bigeminum (*bcbp*).

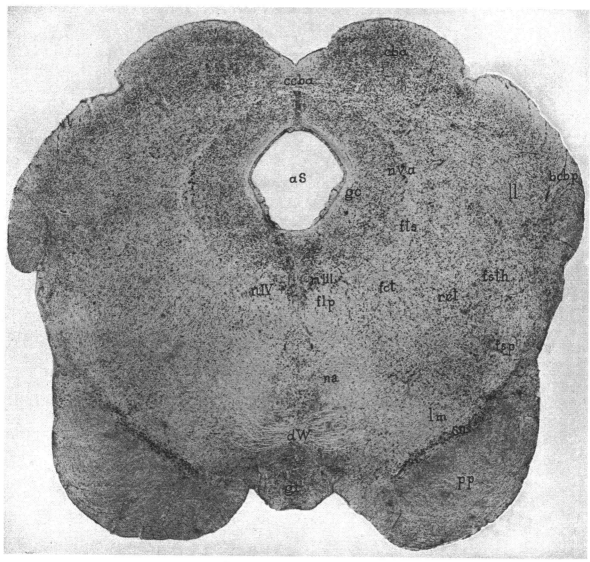

Figure 29 – Section 1040

A Section through the Midbrain at the Level of the Emergence of the Red Nuclei (Section 1090, Fig. 30)

The anterior corpus bigeminum (*cba*), located above the sylvian aqueduct, has a complicated structure consisting of a number of layers: *stratum zonale* (sz), *stratum griseum superficiale* (*sgs*), *stratum opticum* (*so*), through which pass the majority of the fibers of the optic tract to end in the gray layer (*stratum griseum medium, sgm*), *stratum album medium* (*sam*), *stratum griseum profundum* (*sgp*), and *stratum album profundum* (*sap*). Some of the fibers of the medial lemniscus (*lm*) and the lateral geniculate end in the deep layers of the corpus bigeminum. Out of these layers emerges the tectospinal tract (*fts*).

The corpora bigeminum are joined together by the commissure of the anterior corpus bigeminum (*ccba*).

The sylvian aqueduct (*aS*) is surrounded by a massive layer of central gray matter (*gc*); external to it lies the nucleus of the ascending or mesencephalic root of the trigeminal nerve (*nVa*).

Ventral to the central gray matter are the nuclei of the oculomotor nerve (*III*). The section clearly shows how the roots of the oculomotor nerve (*radicis nervi trigemini, rIII*) extend from the nuclei and partly decussate the red nuclei (*nr*). Lateral to the nuclei of the oculomotor nerve pass the fibers of the tectospinal tract (*fts*), which decussate later in the form of the fountain shaped decussation of Meynert (*decussatio Meynerti s. decussatio tectospinalis, dM*). Immediately below the latter can be seen the decussation of the fibers of the rubrospinal fasciculus, or the decussation of Forel (*decussatio Foreli, dF*). The fibers of the rubrospinal tract originate in the massive red nucleus (*nucleus ruber, nr*). This nucleus is the termination for some of the fibers of the superior cerebellar peduncle. Dorsolaterally from the tectospinal tract lies the central tract of the tegmentum (*fct*).

The base of the interpeduncular fossa is occupied by the interpeduncular ganglion (*gi*), lateral to which passes the habenulo-peduncular tract (*tractus habenulo-peduncularis, fhp*) and the massive fasciculi of the fibers of the base of the cerebral peduncle (*pp*). Above these fibers lies the substantia nigra of Soemmering, consisting of the ventral reticular zone (*substantia nigra zona reticularis, snr*) and the dorsal compact zone (*substantia nigra zona compacta, snc*). Dorsolateral to the compact zone of the substantia nigra can be seen the fibers of the medial lemniscus (*lm*), the striopeduncular tract (*fsp*), and the spinothalamic tract (*fsth*).

The lateral parts of the section are occupied by the well developed reticular substance of the tegmentum (*formatio reticularis tegmenti, ret*) and the brachium of the posterior corpus bigeminum (*bcbp*). The medial geniculate body appears in the outer portion of the section (*corpus geniculatum mediale, cgm*).

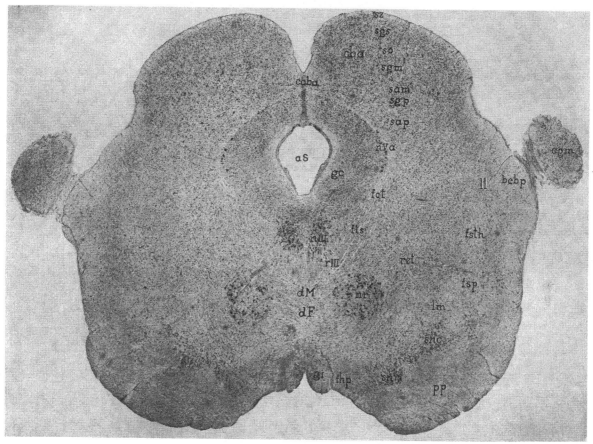

Figure 30 – Section 1090

A Section through the Mesencephalon at the Level of the Greatest Development of the Nuclei of the Oculomotor Nerve and the Red Nucleus (Section 1120, Fig. 31)

The cavity of the Sylvian aqueduct (*aS*) is surrounded by a wide layer of the central gray matter (*gc*), external to which lies the mesencephalic ascending root of the trigeminal nerve and its nucleus (*nVa*).

Dorsal to the sylvian aqueduct is the anterior corpus bigeminum (*cba*), consisting of various layers as described above. Between the corpora bigemini lies the commissure of the anterior corpus bigeminum (*ccba*).

Ventral to the sylvian aqueduct are located the well developed nuclei of the oculomotor nerve: the principal nucleus (*nucleus motorius n. oculomotorii, nIIIm*), the vegetative nucleus of Edinger-Westphal (*nucleus Edinger-Westphali, nIIIE*), and the unpaired nucleus of Perlia (*nucleus Perlia, nIIIP*). The root of the oculomotor nerve (*rIII*) goes in a ventral direction toward the interpeduncular fossa. Ventral to the nuclei of the oculomotor nerve lie the fountain shaped decussation of Meynert (the decussation of the fibers of the tectospinal tract, *dM*), and Forel's decussation (the decussation of the rubrospinal tract, *dF*). Further ventrally lie the mammillary peduncles (*pedunculi corporae mammillarae, pm*). Lateral to the decussations, on both sides, lies the massive red nucleus (*nr*), consisting essentially of large cells. There are very small cells in this section.

The ventral part of the preparation is taken up by the fibers of the base of the cerebral peduncle (*pp*). Above them lies the substantia nigra of Soemmering (*snr, snc*) and the fibers of the medial lemniscus (*lm*). Dorsolateral to the medial lemniscus passes the striopeduncular tract (*fsp*). More dorsally are located: the spinothalamic tract (*fsth*), the reticular substance of the tegmentum (*ret*), and the central tract of the tegmentum (*fct*). The outermost portion of the preparation is taken up by the medial geniculate body (*cgm*), which reaches considerable dimensions in the canine. Medial to the geniculate body is the brachium of the posterior corpus bigeminum (*bcbp*) which is now smaller in size, and the lateral lemniscus (*ll*). The medial geniculate body is surrounded by fibers which form a capsule (*capsula corporis geniculatum medialis, ccgm*).

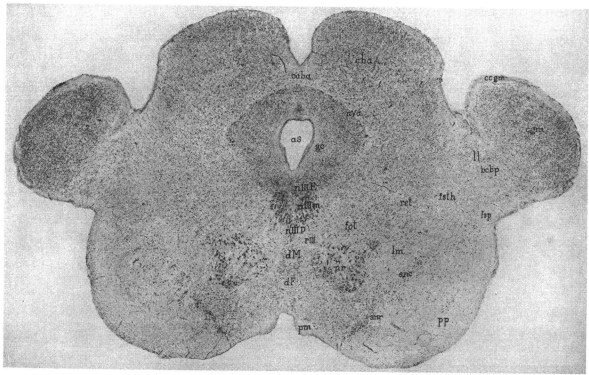

Figure 31 – Section 1120

A Section at the Level of the Maximal Development of the Medial and Lateral Geniculate Bodies (Section 1200, Fig. 32)

The cavity of the sylvian aqueduct (*aS*) is surrounded by the layer of the central gray matter which is now becoming smaller (*gc*).

Dorsal to the sylvian aqueduct lies the posterior commissure (*commissura posterior, cmp*) and its nucleus (*nucleus commissurae posterioris, ncp*). Above the posterior commissure lies the commissure of the anterior corpus bigeminum (*ccba*) and the anterior corpus bigeminum (*cba*) which has decreased considerably in size.

Ventral to the sylvian aqueduct are: the nucleus of Darkschevich (*nucleus Darkschewitschi, nDr*), the interstitial nucleus of Cajal (*nucleus interstitialis Cajali, nC*), and the now much smaller red nucleus (*nr*).

The ventral part of the preparation is occupied by the fibers of the base of the cerebral peduncle (*pp*), above which lie a small number of cells of the substantia nigra (*sn*) and the striopeduncular tract (*fsp*), which passes more laterally.

In the outer uppermost portion of the section lies the lateral geniculate body (*corpus geniculatum laterale, cgl*), which has a lamellar structure; the white matter alternates with the gray matter. The gray striae differ in structure; some are macrocellular, others are formed of smaller cells. The preparation clearly shows how the fibers of the optic tract (*tractus opticus, to*) approach the lateral geniculate body.

Underneath the lateral geniculate body lies the well developed medial geniculate body. Medial to the geniculate bodies is the optic thalamic (*thalamus opticus*). In this section can be seen: the suprageniculate nucleus (*nucleus suprageniculatus, scg*), a small portion of the pulvinar of the optic thalamus (*pulvinar, pul*), the posterior nucleus (*nucleus posterior thalami, post*), and the pretectal zone (*area praetectalis, prt*).

In the reticular substance (*ret*) passes the central tract of the tegmentum (*fct*) and lateral to it the spinothaiamic tract (*fsth*).

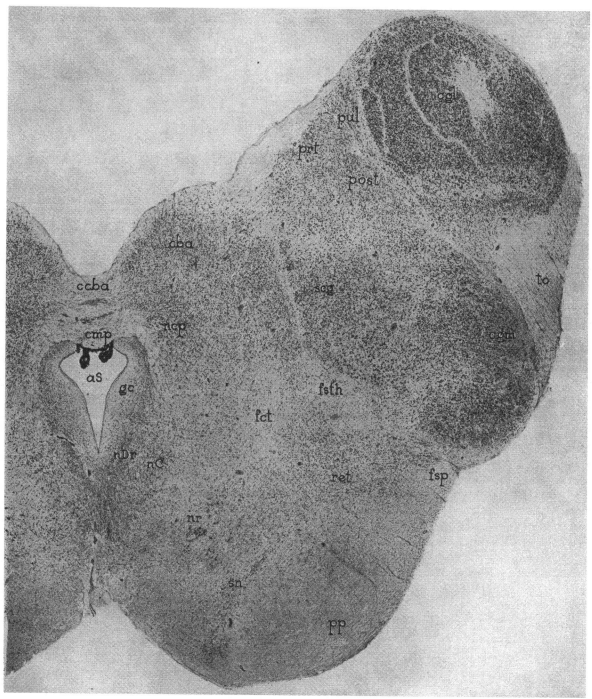

Figure 32 – Section 1200

A Section at the Level of the Opening of the Cavity of the Sylvian Aqueduct into the *III* Ventricle (Section 1260, Fig. 33)

The cavity of the *III* ventricle of the cerebrum (*ventriculus tertius cerebelli, vIII*) is surrounded by the periventricular system (*systema periventricularis, per*), consisting of fibers and small cells.

Dorsal to the cavity of the *III* ventricle lies the habenula, consisting of two nuclei: medial microcellular (*nucleus medialis habenulae, nhm*) and lateral macrocellular (*nucleus lateralis habenulae, nhl*). The habenula belongs to the epithalamus (*epithalamus*); from it extends the habenulopeduncular fasciculus (*tractus habenulopeduncularis s. fasciculus retroflexus Meynerti, frM*), connecting the epithalamus with the interpeduncular ganglion. This fasciculus is accompanied by the nucleus of the habenulopeduncular tract (*nucleus tractus habenulopeduncularis, hp*). Below this nucleus lies the interstitial nucleus of Cajal (*nC*).

The peduncles of the mammillary bodies (*pm*) lie ventral to the *III* ventricle. Lateral to these peduncles is the peripendicular nucleus (*nucleus peripeduncularis, npd*), the base of the cerebral peduncle (*pp*), and the striopeduncular tract (*fsp*).

The optic thalamus is represented in this section by the pulvinar (*pul*), the pretectal zone (*prt*), the posterior part of the lateral nucleus (*pars posterior nucleus lateralis, ltp*), the posterior nucleus (*post*), the suprageniculate nucleus (*scg*), the parafascicular nucleus (*nucleus parafascicularis, prf*), the lateral part of which forms the central nucleus of Luysi (*centrum medianum Luysi, cmd*), and the nucleus of the thalamic reticular zone (*nucleus reticularis thalami, nret*).

The subthalamic region is formed by the thalamic fasciculus or field H_1 of Forel (*fasciculus thalamicus, H_1*), the lenticular fasciculus or field H_2 of Forel (*fasciculus lenticularis, H_2*), by the cellular mass (*zona incerta, zin*) lying between them, and the subthalamic nucleus, or Luysils body (*nucleus subthalamicus s. corpus Luysi, cL*).

The outermost portion of the preparation is taken up by the optic tract (*to*), which divides the lateral geniculate body (*cgl*) into two separate nuclei. Below is the medial geniculate body (*cgm*), considerably decreased in size, and medial to it the spinothalamic tract (*fsth*).

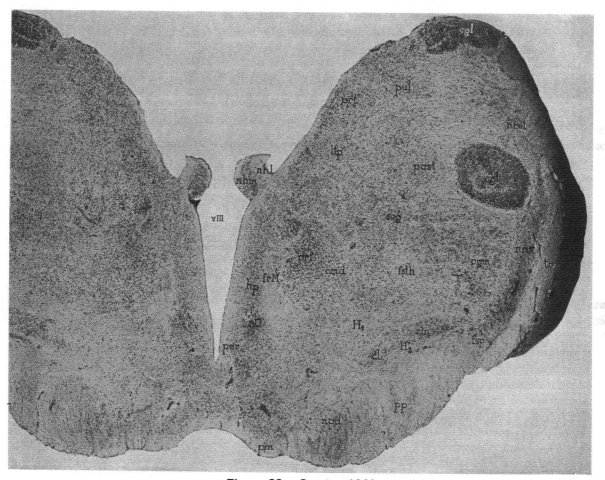

Figure 33 – Section 1260

A Section at the Level of the Maximal Development of the Mammillary Bodies (Section 1300, Fig. 34)

In the center of the preparation lies the cavity of the *III* ventricle (*vIII*) divided by the medial gray commissure (*commissura grisea media, cm*) into two parts. The cavity of the III ventricle is surrounded by the periventricular system (*per*).

The habenula, distinctly seen at the upper edge of the III ventricle, is clearly separated into two nuclei - the medial microcellular (*nhm*) and the lateral macrocellular (*nhl*). The white striae in the upper part of the habenula are the striae medullaris of the optic thalamus (*striae medullares thalami, smt*) or the olfactohabenular tract (*tractus olfactohabenularis*). In a ventral direction from the habenula extends the habenulopeduncular tract or the retroflex fasciculus of Meynert (*frM*) with its nucleus (*hp*).

The nuclei of the optic thalamus are well developed. In the dorsal part of the preparation lies the pulvinar (*pul*) and pretectal zone (*prt*); below this is the posterior part of the lateral nucleus (*ltp*). Near Meynert's fasciculus lies the medial dorsal nucleus (*nucleus medians dorsalis, md*). External to the latter is the central lateral nucleus (*nucleus centralis lateralis, cnl*), and below it is the *nucleus parafascicularis* (*prf*). In the ventral area of the optic thalamus is the suprageniculate nucleus (*scg*), which is much smaller here, and, appearing at this level are the arciform and lateral parts of the ventral nucleus (*pars arcuata, vnar, et pars externa, vne, nucleus ventralis*). The reticular nucleus (*nret*) of the optic thalamus is now larger; below it pass the fibers of the striopeduncular tract (*fsp*).

The subthalamic region is represented in the section by the field H_1 of Forel (H_1), the *zona incerta* (*zin*), field H_2 of Forel (H_2, and the subthalamic nucleus, or nucleus of Luysi (*cL*).

The ventral part of the section is made up of the nuclei of the hypothalamic region. In the paired mammillary body (*corpus mammillare*) can be distinguished two nuclei: the medial macrocellular (*nucleus medians corporis mamillaris, cmm*) and the lateral microcellular (*nucleus lateralis corporis mamillaris, cml*). Dorsally from the mammillary body, the fasciculus of Vicq d'Azyr (*fasciculus mamillothalamicus s. fasciculus Vicq d'Azyri, fmt*), connects the mammillary bodies with the anterior nucleus of the optic thalamus. Above the fasciculus of Vicq d'Azyr lies the supramammillary nucleus (*nucleus supramammillaris, scm*), the lateral hypothalamic field (*area hypothalamica lateralis, hpl*), the posterior hypothalamic nucleus (*nucleus hypothalamicus posterior, hpp*), and the interstitial nucleus of Cajal (*nC*).

Toward the ventral outer side are the fibers of the base of the cerebral peduncle (*pp*) with the peripendicular nucleus (*npd*) lying adjacent to it. The fibers of the cerebral peduncle gradually merge into the internal capsule.

The optic tract is pushed in a lateroventral direction, and the lateral geniculate body (*cgl*) is represented on the section by a small area in the dorsal part.

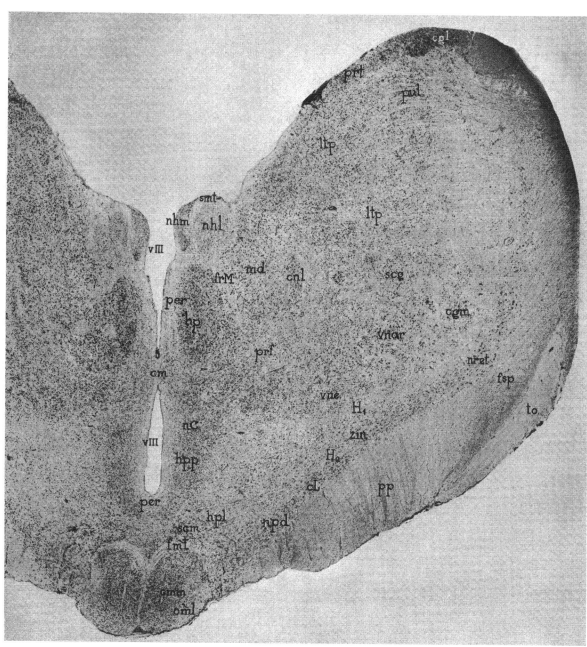

Figure 34 – Section 1300

A Section slightly Anterior to the Previous One, at the Level of the Maximal Development of Corpus Luysi (Section 1330, Fig. 35)

The cavity of the *III* ventricle (*vIII*) is divided by the now much larger medial commissure (*massa intermedia*). Among the cells of the latter can be distinguished the posterior paraventricular nucleus (*nucleus paraventricularis posterior, prp*) and the central medial nucleus (*nucleus centralis medialis, cnm*). Around the *III* ventricle lies the periventricular system (*per*). As before, the medial (*nhm*) and the lateral (*nhl*) nuclei are clearly discernible in the habenula. Below the habennla is the nucleus of the habenulopeduncular tract (*hp*).

The medial nuclei of the optic thalamus are represented by the medial dorsal nucleus (*md*), the parafascicular nucleus (*prf*), and the central lateral nucleus (*cnl*). The lateral nuclei form a considerably developed group among which stand out the pulvinar (*pul*), the intermedial part of the lateral nucleus which emerges at this level (*pars intermedia nucleus lateralis, lti*), the large posterior part of the lateral nucleus (*pars posterior nucleus lateralis, ltp*), and the reticular nucleus (*nret*). In the ventral group of thalamic nuclei can be distinguished the arciform (*vnar*), the lateral (*vne*) and the medial (*vnm*) parts.

As before, one can distinguish in the subthalamic region the field of Forel (H_1), the field of H_2 of Forel (H_2, the *zona incerta* (*zin*) and the rather large corpus Luysi (*cL*).

The hypothalamic region fills the ventral portions of the section and is represented by the lateral (*cml*) and medial (*cmm*) mammillary bodies, the lateral hypothalamic area (*hpl*), and the posterior hypothalamic nucleus (*hpp*). Above the mammillary bodies can be seen the fibers of the columns of the fornix (*fornix, f*).

In the lateral portion of the section, pass the fibers of the base of the cerebral peduncle (*pp*). Their merging into the internal capsule (*capsula interna, ci*) becomes more and more evident and laterally can be observed the external capsule and the cells of the claustraum (*claustrum, cls*) belonging to the telencephalon.

Below the base of the cerebral peduncle lie the optic tract and the posterior parts of the amygdaloid nucleus (*nucleus amygdalae, am*).

The medial wan of the inferior horn of the lateral ventricle (*ventriculus lateralis, vl*) is formed by the inferior part of Ammon's horn (*cornu Ammonis inferius, CAi*), belonging to the archeocortex and the dentate fascia (*fascia dentata inferior, FDi*). Below the amygdala, at the base of the cerebral hemisphere, lies the cortex of the entorhinal region (*regio entorhinalis, E*), which belongs to the interstitial cortex. The upper wall of the *III* ventricle (*vIII*) is formed by the dorsal parts of the dentate fascia (*fascia dentata superior, FDs*) and Ammon's horns (*cornu Ammonis superius CAs*), which closely adjoin the fornix (*fornix, f*) and the corpus callosum (*ccl*).

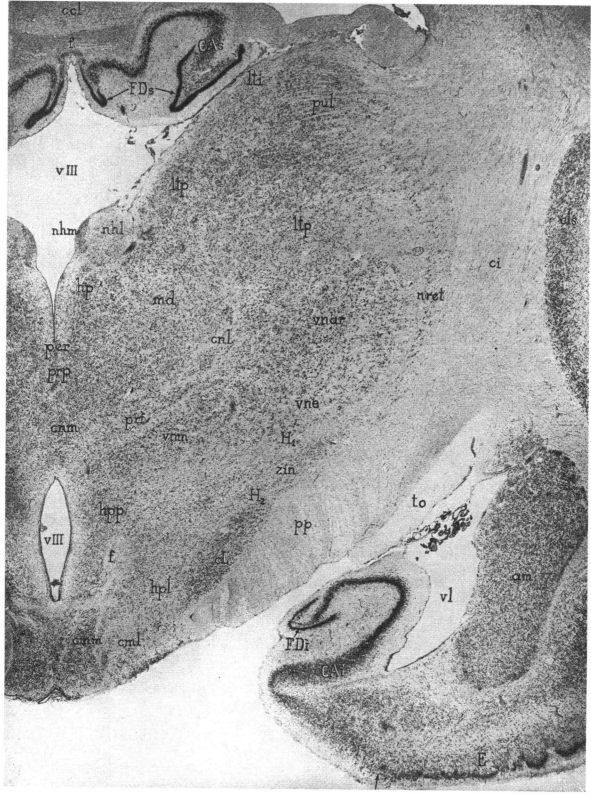

Figure 35 – Section 1330

A Section at the Level of the Infundibulum (Section 1380, Fig. 36)

The center of the preparation is occupied by the well developed medial commissure or massa intermedia in which are the midline nuclei, the anterior paraventricular nucleus (*nucleus paraventricularis anterior, pra*), the *nucleus intermediodorsalis* (*imd*), the rhomboid nucleus (*nucleus rhomboidalis, rhm*), and the central medial nucleus (*cnm*). The reuniens nucleus is clearly visible (*nucleus reunions thalami, reu*), and the medial nucleus of the optic thalamus (*md*) reaches its greatest development here.   Above lies the paratenial nucleus (*nucleus parataenialis, pt*), laterally the central lateral nucleus (*cnl*), and ventrally the Paracentral nucleus (*nucleus paracentralis, pcn*).   The lateral (*ltp, lti, lta*) and ventral (*vnar, vne, vnm*) groups of nuclei are well developed.   The nucleus of the reticular formation (*nret*), as before, is on the outer border of the lateral and ventral group of thalamic nuclei.

The subthalamic region is now somewhat smaller.   In the section can be seen the remains of the *zona incerta* (*zin*) of field H_1 and field H_2 of Forel (H_1 and H_2) and the subthalamic nucleus (*cL*), now smaller in size.

In the ventral portion of the preparation are clearly visible two isolated fasciculi of fibers: the superior or the fasciculus of Vicq d'Azyr (*fmt*), and the inferior or the fasciculus of the fornix (*f*).

The hypothalamic nuclei are represented on the section by the gray tuber (*tuber cinereum, tc*), the infundibulum (*in*), the posterior hypothalamic nucleus (*hpp*), and the lateral hypothalamic area (*hpl*).   The infundibulum forms the floor of the *III* ventricle (*vIII*).   The latter is surrounded by the periventricular system (*per*).

The outer portion of the section is taken up by the well developed fibers of the base of the cerebral peduncle (*pp*), which cross into the internal capsule (*ci*).

On this section there appears for the first time the lenticular nucleus (*nucleus lenticularis*), consisting of the globus pallidus and the putamen (*put*).

In the globus pallidus can be distinguished the external (*pallidum externum, pe*) and internal (*pallidum internum, pi*) members. Below the pallidum externum is the striopeduncular tract (*fsp*). The external capsule (*capsula externa, ce*) passes lateral to the putamen and separates the putamen from the cells of the claustrum (*cls*).   The latter is separated from the cortex of the islet by the extreme capsule (*capsula extrema, cex*). Below these formations lies the optic tract (*to*) and the amygdala (*am*).   The amygdala lies lateral to the inferior horn of the lateral ventricle (*vl*). The medial wall of the latter is formed by the inferior part of the horn of Ammon (*CAi*), medial to which can be seen the inferior part of the dentate fascia (*FDi*).   The base of the cerebral hemisphere is occupied by the periamygdalar region (*regio periamygdalaris, Pm*), belonging to the paleocortex, and the entorhinal area (*E*).

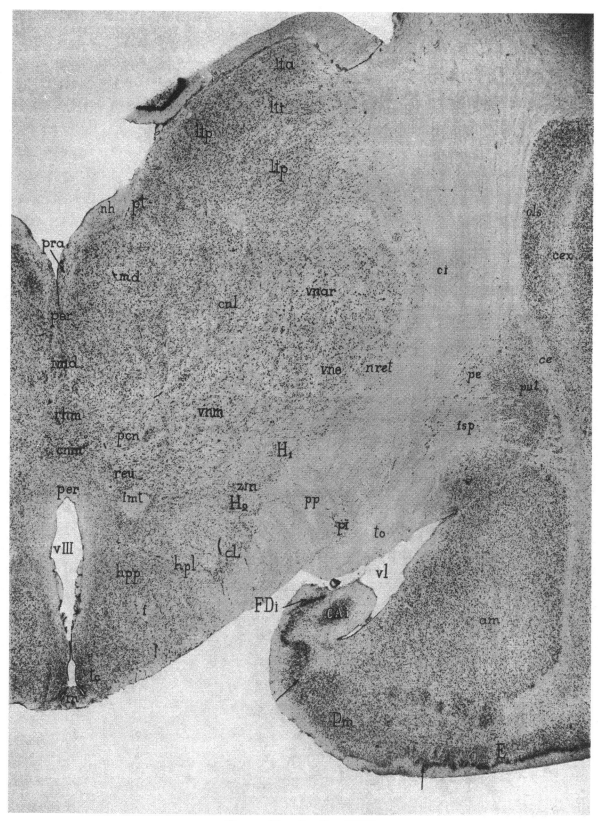

Figure 36 – Section 1380

A Section at the Level of the Maximal Development of the Central Lateral Nucleus of the Optic Thalamus (Section 1420, Fig. 37)

The fibers of the medullary stria of the optic thalamus (*smt*) pass over the lateral wall of the III ventricle (*vlll*), around which lies the periventricular system (*per*). Among the nuclei of the midline can be distinguished, as before, the anterior paraventricular (*pra*), *intermediodorsalis* (*imd*), *rhomboid* (*rhm*), central medial (*cnm*), and reunial (*reu*) nuclei. Outside these formations lie the medial group of thalamic nuclei (*pt, md, pcn*); at this level the greatest development is reached by the central lateral nucleus (*cnl*). Clearly discernible are the anterior (*lta*) and the intermediate (*lti*) parts of the lateral nucleus.

The ventral nucleus is represented by all four parts (*vna, vnar, vne, vnm*). The nucleus of the reticular formation (*nret*) passes external to the lateral and ventral group of nuclei. In the subthalamic region, which is now much smaller, can be distinguished field H_1 of Forel (H_1), the remains of *zona incerta* (*zin*), and the subthalamic nucleus (*cL*). In the hypothalamus can be clearly seen the medial nucleus with its two parts, dorsal (*nucleus hypothalamicus dorsomedialis, hpmd*) and ventral (*nucleus hypothalamicus ventromedialis, hpmv*), as well as the lateral hypothalamic field (*hpl*). Among the cellular formations of the hypothalamus are clearly discernible the fibers of the fornix (*f*) and the fasciculus of Vicq d'Azyr (*fmt*).

In the lateral parts of the preparation can be seen the fibers of the base of the cerebral peduncle (*pp*) and of the internal capsule (*ci*). External to the latter are the internal (*pi*) and external (*Pe*) members of the globuspallidus, the putamen (*put*), the external capsule (*ce*), the claustraum (*cls*), and the outermost external capsule (*cex*). The optic tract (*to*) is displaced in a ventral direction. The amygdala (*am*) is quite large. It is surrounded by the cortical lamina of the paleocortex, represented here by the periamygdalar region (*Pm*) and lateral to it the prepyriform region (*regio praepiriformis, Pp*).

In the upper part of the preparation can be seen a small portion of the corpus callosum (*ccl*) and the fornix (*f*).

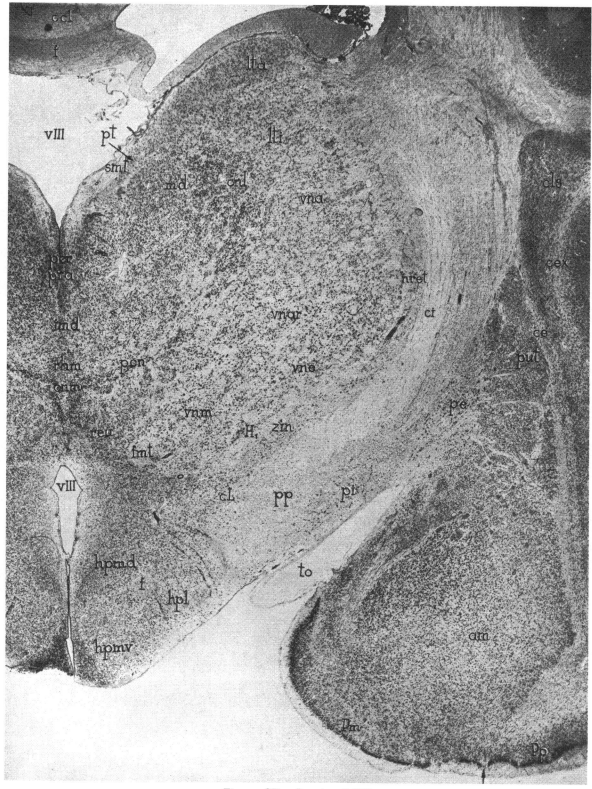

Figure 37 – Section 1420

A Section at the Level of the Emergence of the Caudate Nucleus (Section 1460, Fig. 38)

The fibers of the stria medullaris of the optic thalamus (*smt*) pass over the supralateral border of the optic thalamus. The massa intermedia decreases somewhat in size; one can distinguish in it the nuclei of the midline such as the anterior paraventricular nucleus (*pra*), the well developed rhomboid nucleus (*rhm*), and the central medial (*cnm*) and reunial (*reu*) nuclei.

In the medial group of thalamic nuclei, aside from the paratenial (*pt*), the medial dorsal (*md*), the central lateral (*cnl*), and the paracentral (*pcn*) nuclei, mentioned before, there appears the submedial nucleus (*nucleus submedium, smd*). Immediately below it can be seen the fibers of the mammillothalamic tract (*fmt*). The anterior lateral nucleus (*lta*) like a cap covers the anterior group of thalamic nuclei which appear in this section: the anterodorsal nucleus (*nucleus anterodorsalis, and*), the anteroventral nucleus (*nucleus anteroventralis, anv*), and the anteromedial nucleus (*nucleus anteromedialis, anm*).

The ventral thalamic nucleus is represented, as before, by all four groups (*vna, vnar, vne, vnm*). The reticular nucleus (*nret*) is slightly smaller in size.

In the subthalamic region can be seen the now much smaller field H_1 of Forel (H_1) and the remains of the *zona incerta* (*zin*).

The hypothalamic region lies ventrolateral to the cavity of the *III* ventricle (*vIII*). The latter is surrounded by the periventricular system (*per*). The hypothalamus is represented by the large medial nucleus, which shows the dorsal (*hpmd*) and ventral (*hpmv*) parts and the lateral hypothalamic field (*hpl*).

The outer part of the section is taken up by the fibers of the base of the cerebral peduncle (*pp*), which merge into the internal capsule (*ci*). The latter is increasing in size. The optic tract (*to*) passes the base of the cerebral peduncle. The putamen (*put*) reaches its greatest development here.

In this section can be seen the large cells of the globus pallidus, in which can be distinguished an internal (*pi*) and an external (*pe*) member. The amygdala (*am*) is formed by several groups of nuclei and is surrounded by the cortex of the periamygdalar (*Pm*) region; lateral to the cortex of the periamygdalar lies the prepyriform area (*Pp*).

The external capsule (*ce*) separates the claustrum (*cls*) from the putamen.

In the upper portion of the preparation appears the body of the caudate nucleus (*corpus nuclei caudati, ncd*).

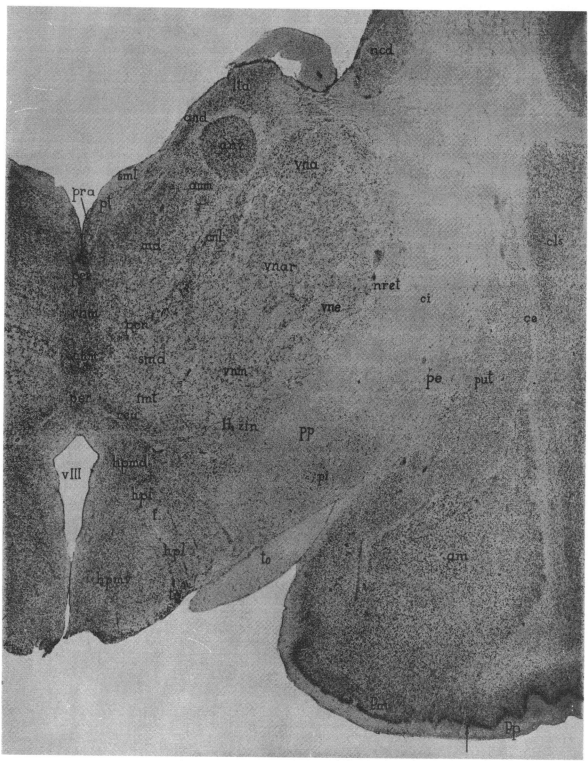

Figure 38 – Section 1460

A Section at the Level of the Optic Chiasm (Section 1490, Fig. 39)

One can clearly see the fibers of the stria medullaris of the optic thalamus (*smt*) on the lateral wall of the *III* ventricle. The roof of the ventricle is formed by the fibers of the fornix (*f*), which adjoin the corpus callosum (*ccl*). Outside the *III* ventricle can be seen the lateral ventricle (*vl*), on the side of which lies the body of the caudate nucleus (*corpus nuclei caudati, ncd*).

In the massa intermedia, which is now smaller, can be seen: the anterior periventricular nucleus (*pra*), the interanteromedial nucleus (*nucleus interantoromedians, iam*), and the central medial nucleus (*cnm*). The *nucleus reuniens* (*reu*) is clearly visible.

There are still remains of the paratenial (*pt*) and the medial dorsal (*md*) nuclei in the medial group of thalamic nuclei; laterally pass the fibers of the tract of the Vicq d'Azyr (*fmt*).

All three nuclei (*and, anv, anm*) of the anterior thalamic group stand out clearly. The ventral nucleus is represented by the anterior (*vna*), exterior (*vne*) and the middle (*vnm*) parts. In the outer portions of the thalamus can be seen its reticular nucleus (*nret*) now amaller in size.

In the hypothalamic region, immediately above the optic chiasm (*chiasma nervorum opticorum, ch*) lies the diffuse supraoptic nucleus (*nucleus supraopticus diffusus, nsp*), dorsal to it the anterior hypothalamic nucleus (*nucleus hypothalamicus anterior, hpa*) and the anterior filiform nucleus (*nucleus filiformis anterior, fa*). The exterior parts of the hypothalamus are represented, as before, by the lateral hypothalamic field (*hpl*) and the tangential nucleus (*tg*). The external portions of the preparation are occupied by the internal capsule (*ci*), the external (*pe*) and the internal (*pi*) members of the globus pallidus, the putamen (*put*), the external capsule (*ce*), and the claustrum (*cls*). The amygdala is much smaller, and its cells gradually change into the cortical lamina of the periamygdalar (*Pm*) and the prepyriform (*Pp*) regions.

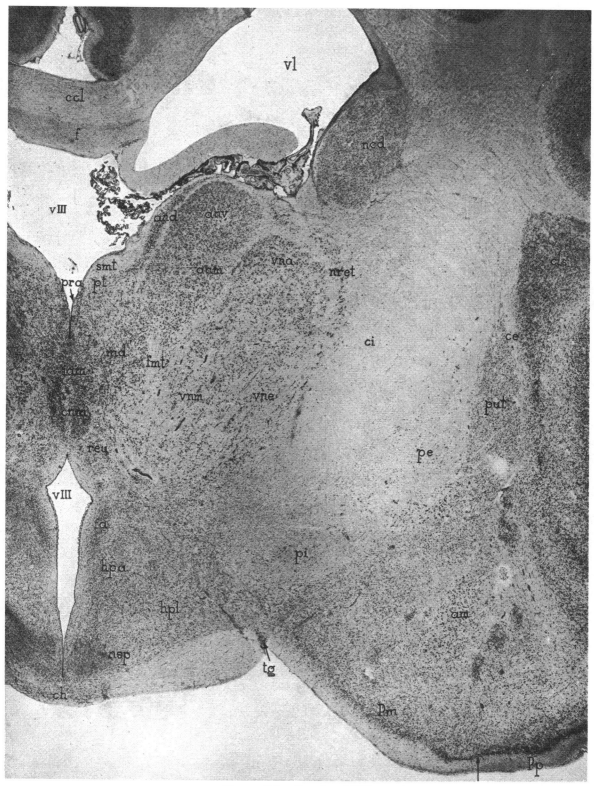

Figure 39 – Section 1490

A Section through the Optic Gniasm, slightly to the Front of the Previous Section (Section 1520, Fig. 40)

The optic thalamus is represented by the well developed anterior group of three nuclei (*and, anv, anm*). The fibers of the mammillothalamic tract (*fmt*) terminate in the anterior group of nuclei. The medullary striae of the thalamus (*smt*) pass medially from the anterodorsal nucleus. The nuclei of the midline include: the paratenial nucleus (*pt*), the paraventricular nucleus (*pra*), the interanteromedial nucleus (*iam*), and nucleus reuniens (*reu*). The ventral group of thalamic nuclei has decreased in size (*vna*). Outside it lies the reticular nucleus (*nret*).

The following stand out in the hypothalamic region: the anterior hypothalamic nucleus (*hpa*), the diffuse supraoptic nucleus (*nsp*), the anterior hypothalamic field (*hpl*), the anterior filiform nucleus (*fa*), the principal filiform nucleus (*nucleus filiformis principalis, fp*), and the tangential nucleus (*tg*).

At the bottom of the third ventricle (*III*) lies the optic chiasm (*ch*).

The outer parts of the section are taken up by the internal capsule (*ci*), now much larger in size, the external member of the globus pallidus (*pe*), the putamen (*put*), the external capsule (*ce*), the claustrum (*cls*), and the extreme capsule (*cex*). The base of the cerebral hemisphere is occupied by the cortical cells of the periamygdalar (*Pm*) and prepyriform (*Pp*) regions.

In the upper part of the section is the body of the caudate nucleus (*ncd*). The lateral ventricle (*vl*) is surrounded, from above and the outside, by the stratum subcallosum (*stratum subcallosum, ssc*), and from below by the fornix (*f*). The corpus callosum (*ccl*) lies above the fornix.

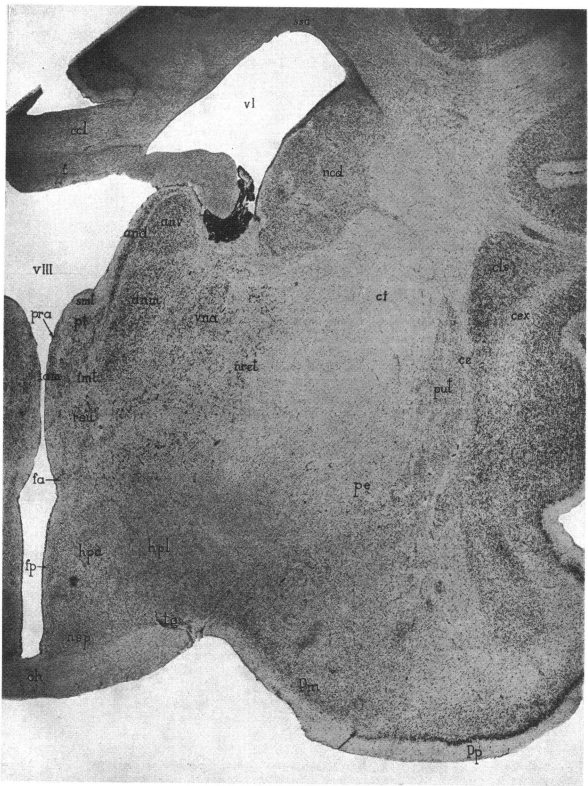

Figure 40 – Section 1520

A Section at the Level of the Anterior Commissure (Section 1580, Fig. 41)

The hemispheres are connected by the anterior conmissure (*commissura anterior, can*). Next to it lies the nucleus of the anterior commissure (*nucleus interstitialis commissurae anterioris, nca s.* "bed nucleus").

The terminal stria (*stria terminalis, st*) pass along the lateral wall of the *III* ventricle (*vIII*), below which lies the nucleus of the terminal stria (*nucleus interstitialis striae terminalis, nst*) and the now much amaller reticular nucleus of the thalamus (*nret*).

In the central portions of the section are located: the optic chiasm (*ch*), the medial preoptic area (*area praeoptica medians, hprm*), the lateral preoptic area (*area praeoptica lateralis, hprl*) and the tangential nucleus (*tg*). Lateral to them lies the innominate sdbstance of Reichert (*substantia innominata Reicherti, siR*), the cells of which blend into the cortical lamina of the diagonal region (*regio diagonalis, D*). Still further lateral lies the prepyriform region (*Pp*). The two last formations belong to the paleocortex.

The anterior genu of the internal capsule (*ci*) is of large dimensions. Lateral to it lies the external portion of the globus pallidus (*Pe*), the putamen (*put*) and the external capsule (*ce*), separating the putamen from the claustraum (*cls*). The claustrum is separated from islet cortex by the outermost capsule (*cex*).

Above the internal capsule lies the massive head of the caudate nucleus (*ncd*), which constitutes the external wall of the lateral ventricle (*vl*). The upper wall of the lateral ventricle is formed by the subcallosal stratum (*ssc*) and the corpus callosum (*ccl*) lying above it. The fornix (*f*) and the corpus callosum are firmly adherent in the midline.

Monroe's foramen (*foramen Monroi, fM*) which connects the *III* ventricle (*vIII*) with the lateral ventricle (*vl*) lies between the column of the fornix (*columna fornicis, cf*) and the head of the caudate nucleus.

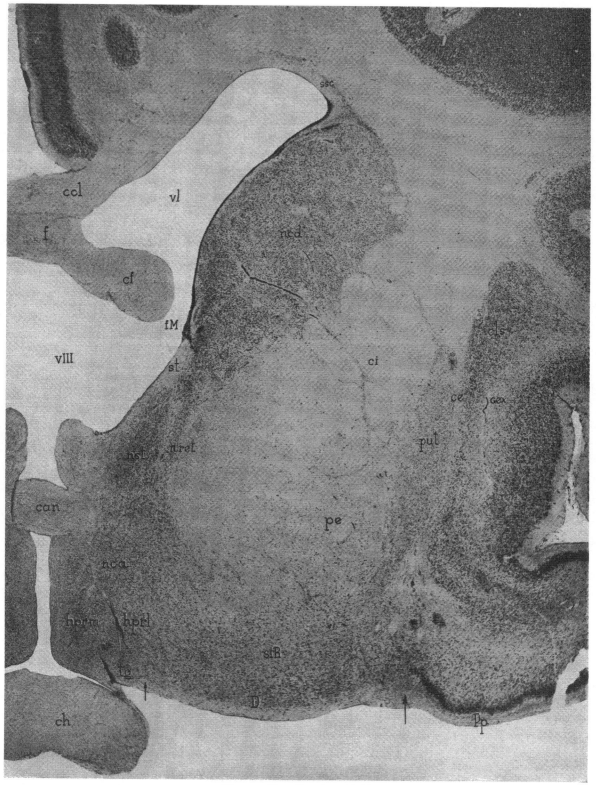

Figure 41 – Section 1580

A Section at the Level of the Emergence of the Mass of the Septum Pellucidum (Section 1620, Fig. 42)

The mass of the septum pellucidum (*massa septii pellucidi, spt*), together with the fornix (*f*), forms the internal wall of the lateral ventricle (*vl*). The roof of the latter is formed by the corpus callosum (*ccl*) and the subcallosal stratum (*ssc*). The massive head of the caudate nucleus (*ncd*) forms the external wall of the lateral ventricle. Below the caudate nucleus can be seen the anterior commissure (*can*). The internal capsule (*ci*) is slightly smaller and decussates in the shape of thin cellular shafts, which connect the caudate and the lenticular nuclei. Lateral to the internal capsule lie: the globus pallidus (*pe*), the putamen (*put*), the external capsule (*ce*), the claustrum (*cls*), and the outermost capsule (*cex*). In the lower portion of the section can be seen the optic nerve (*nervus opticus, II*), above which lie the cells of the preoptic area (*hpr*). Laterally from this area can be seen the cells of the innominate substance of Reichert (*siR*), which are adjoined by the cortex of the diagonal region (*D*) and which borders on the cortical lamina of the prepyriform region (*Pp*).

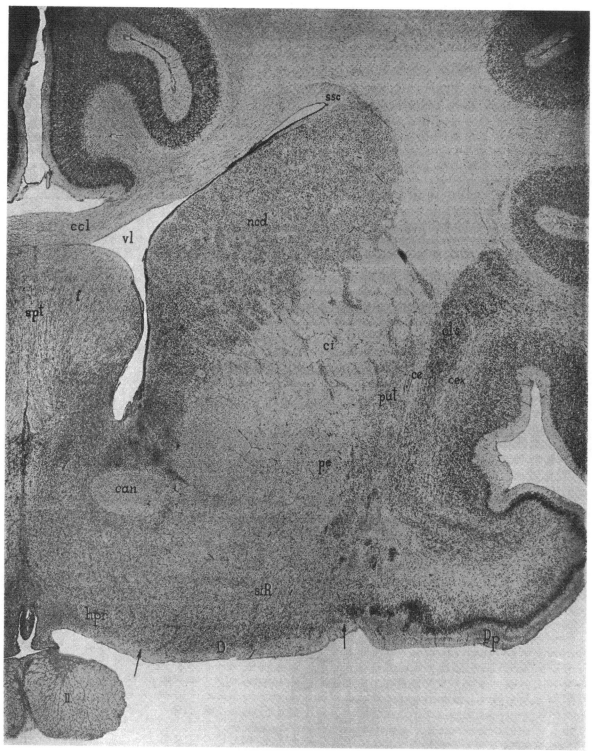

Figure 42 – Section 1620

A Section at the level of the Maximum Size of the Head of the Caudate Nucleus (Section 1820, Fig. 43)

The section shows that the lower regions of the head of the caudate nucleus (*ncd*) closely adjoin the cells of the putamen (*put*).   There is an increase in the number of cellular shafts which connect the two structures.   The external capsule (*ce*) separates the putamen from the claustrum (*cls*), and the outmost capsule (*cex*) separates the cells of the claustrum from the cortex of the islet.   The anterior commissure (*can*) is displaced into a more lateral and downward position, as compared with the preceding section.   The lateral ventricle (*vl*) is a closed cavity, the internal wall of which is formed by the fibers of the genu of the corpus callosum (*genu corporis callosi, gen*).   The upper wall of the lateral ventricle is formed by the stem of the *corpus callosum* (*ccl*) and the *subcallous stratum* (*ssc*); the outer wall is formed by the head of the *caudate nucleus* (*ncd*).   Below the genu of the corpus callosum can be seen the *taenia tecta* (*tt*), belonging to the archeocortex, and the cortex of the limbic region (*L2*).   Under the head of the caudate nucleus is the paleocortex: the olfactory tubercle (*tuberculum olfactorium, TO*) and lateral from it the prepyriform region (*Pp*).

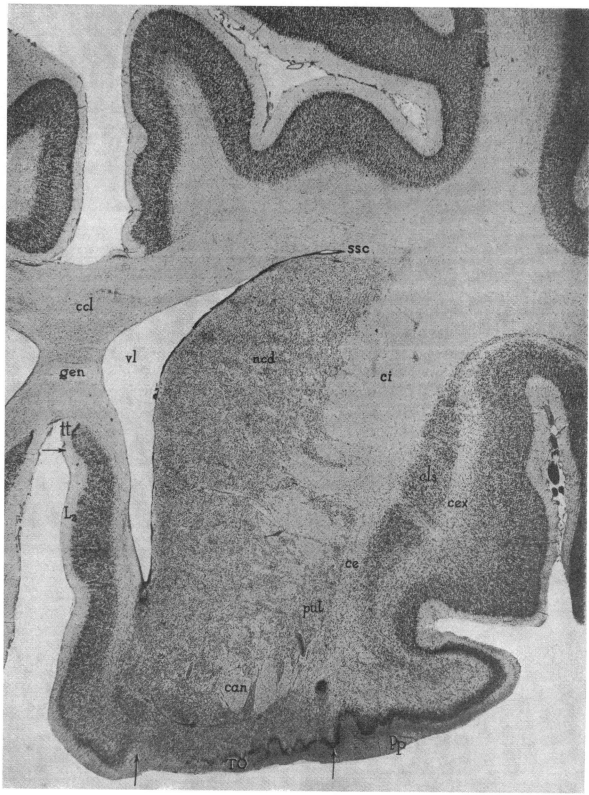

Figure 43 – Section 1820

THE STRUCTURE OF THE CANINE CEREBRAL CORTEX

The Sulci and Gyri of the Cerebrum

The absolute weight of the canine cerebrum ranges, on an average, from 54 to 150 grams. The ratio of the brain to the body, in terms of weight, is 1:37; in larger dogs, the ratio is 1:100 (according to Flatau and Jacobsohn [23]). The form, the size, and the weight of the canine cerebrum vary according to the breed, size, and weight of the animal.

The literature of the sulci and gyri of the cerebrum of the dog is copious (Kikin [36]; Leurat and Gratiolet, 1839; Miklukho-Maklai [752]; Betz [980]; Rudanovskiy [784]; Flautau [23]; Anthony [689]; Deshin [709]; Kappers [33]; Khachaturian [733]; and others) [*Editors' note: We could not find some of these references in the bibliography of the original Atlas. Consequently, we made substitutions to the best of our knowledge.*]. The designations of the sulci and gyri vary considerably; in this atlas, the terms used are in accordance with the designations of Filimonolr [713]. Filimonov's data on the variations of the sulci are also utilized.

The Sulci of the Lateral Surface of the Hemisphere (Fig. 44, 45)

The distribution of the sulci and gyri on the lateral surface of the hemisphere around the sylvian sulcus is characteristic for Carnivora including the canine. This distribution of the sulci determines the sequence of this presentation.

The sylvian sulcus (*sulcus Sylvii, sulcus pseudosylvius, s*) is a stationary and rather deep fissure, which begins in the place of transition of the anterior rhinal sulcus to the posterior of the so-called fossa of the sylvian sulcus (*fossa Sylvii*). The beginning of the sulcus varies in shape. In the majority of cases (61%), it has the form of a narrow slit or triangle drawn out and upwards, but it can also have the form of a polygon, or wide triangle. In most cases, the sylvian sulcus constitutes a direct continuation of the sylvian fossa in the shape of a narrow, straight fissure (Fig. 44, ill. 1). In case the sylvian fossa has an irregular configuration, the sylvian sulcus begins at one of the angles of the polygon, or consists of two branches (Fig. 44, ill. 2 or 3).

The ectosylvian suicus (*sulcus ectosylvius, es*), or the first arciform sulcus (*sulcus arcuatus primus*), bends around the sylvian sulcus and in most cases consists of three parts, frequently connected: the anterior (*sulcus ectosylvius anterior, esa*), the medial (*sulcua ectosylvius medium, esm*) and the posterior (*sulcus ectosylvius posterior, esp*). The anterior part is the longest one and the posterior is the shortest. The medial is usually curved, and in some cases rectilinear (Fig. 44, ill. 1). Radial processes (*processus acominis, a*) usually lie in places of transition of one part of the sulcus into the other.

Sometimes the medial and posterior parts of the sulcus are missing altogether (Fig. 44, ill. 4-6). In most cases (63%), the sulcus is not connected with the other sulci and is free in all its parts. In 16% of cases, there is a connection between the posterior section of this sulcus with the sylvian sulcus (Fig. 44, 6).

The suprasylvian sulcus (*sulcus suprasylvius, ss*), or the second arciform sulcus (*sulcus arcuatus secundus*), lies in an arch above the ectosylvian sulcus, and differs from it in that it is very constant. It is also made up of an anterior, a medial, and a posterior part extending parallel to the ectosylvian sulcus (*sulcus suprasylvius anterior, ssa, sulcus suprasylvius medium, ssm, sulcus suprasylvius posterior, ssp*, Fig. 44, ill. 1). According to Filimonov, the absence of any of its parts was not observed in any case. The variability of the suprasylvian sulcus is expressed in the configuration of the anterior section only (it is shortened, ends high, and has peculiar curves). Its connection is possible with the ectosylvian fissure, as well as with the system of *sulcus ansatus* (*an*) plus *sulcus coronalis* (*cor*) (17% of cases). These connections come about by means of the radial processes (*processus acominis, a*), lying mainly in the places of transition of one part of the sulcus into another (Fig. 45, ill. 1).

In the temporal region, there are two more inconstant sulci: *sulcus limitans posterior* (*lp*), located under the lower end of the suprasylvian sulcus which exists in 50% of the cases (Fig. 44, ill. 3), and the *sulcus posticus* (*p*), located between the posterior sections of the ectosylvian and the suprasylvian sulci, and extending parallel to them (Fig. 44, ill. 2, 3).

The lateral sulcus (*sulcus lateralis, l*) is a constant sulcus (Fig. 45, ill. 2). Most frequently (in 61% of the cases), the lateral sulcus is connected in front with the ansate sulcus (*sulcus ansatus, an*), and through the latter with the coronal sulcus (*sulcus coronalis, cor*), forming one uninterrupted fissure called the third arciform sulcus (*sulcus arcuatus tertius*). The lateral sulcus crosses, usually, into the ansate sulcus at a right angle. At the place

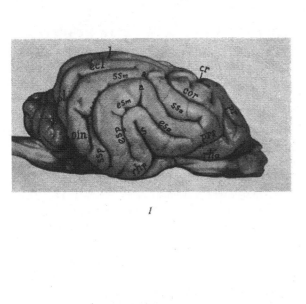

1

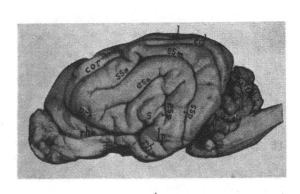

4

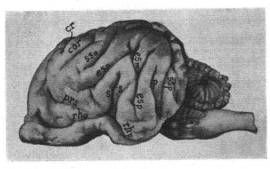

2

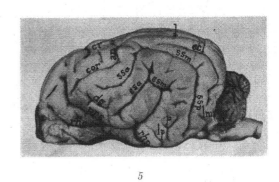

5

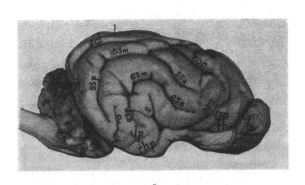

3

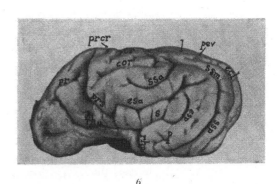

6

Figure 44 – The sulci of the lateral surfaces of the large hemispheres.

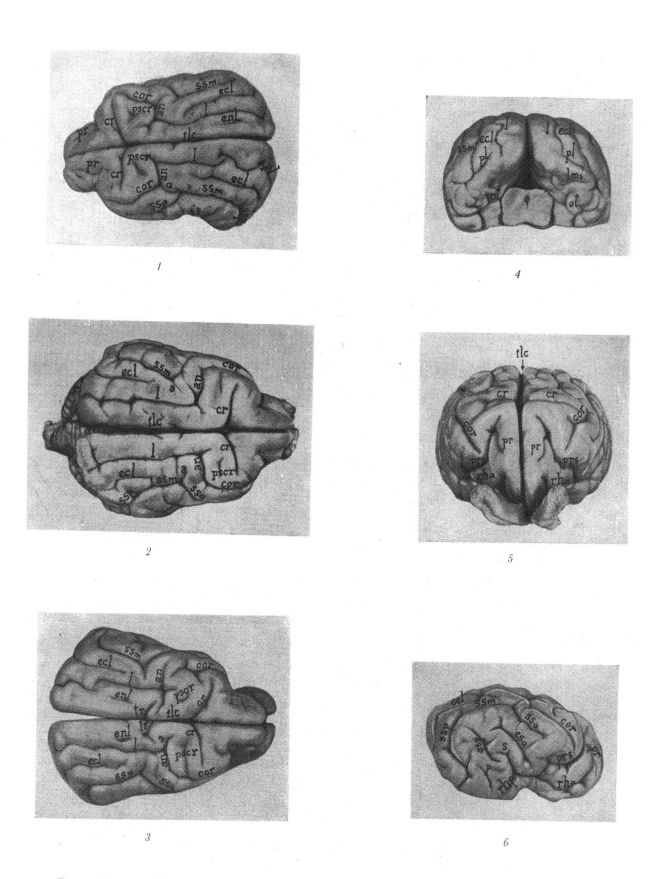

Figure 45 — The sulci of the dorsal, anterior and posterior surface of the large hemispheres.

of transition lies frequently the radial process (*processus acominis, a*) (Fig. 45, ill. 3). In 15% of the cases, the ansate aulcus is connected only with the lateral sulcus (Fig. 45, ill. 3). The posterior end of the lateral sulcus bends downward and forms the postlateral sulcus (*sulcus postlateralis, pl*), which is quite often (67% of the cases) connected with the lateral sulcus. Less frequently, the lateral sulcus is separated from the postlateral sulcus (Fig. 45, ill. 4).

The coronal sulcus (*sulcus coronalis, cor*) is very constant in its direction and form, but the structure of its posterior end varies considerably, i.e., the correlation with the ansate and the suprasylvian sulci. Filimonov detected ten basic types of connections, the most frequent type being the connection of *sulcus coronalis, sulcus ansatus,* and *sulcus lateralis* into one uninterrupted sulcus, as described above. The type of unification is, in itself, rather variable.

The entolateral sulcus (*sulcus entolateralis, enl; s. fissura confinis, Flatau*) is a short and inconstant sulcus (missing in almost 30% of cases). It lies between the lateral sulcus and the longitudinal fissure of the hemispheres (*fissura longitudinalis cerebri, flc;* Fig. 45, ill. 3).

The ectolateral sulcus (*sulcus ectolateralis, ecl*) is a constant sulcus, lying between the lateral and the postlateral sulcus on one side and between the medial and posterior part of the suprasylvian sulcus on the other side. It consists of two parts, the horizontal and the vertical, which merge in an arciform manner (Fig. 44, ill. 1). Sometimes one of the parts of the ectolateral sulcus is not sufficiently developed.

Filimonov describes four more small and inconstant sulci: *sulcus praeectolateralis verticalis (pev),* which lies in front of the ectolateral fissure (Fig. 44, ill. 6); *sulcus lateromedialis superior* and *inferior (lms* and *lmi),* which decussates with the posterior edge of the hemisphere, and lies on the external as well as on the internal surface (Fig. 45, ill. 4; Fig. 44, ill. 5); *sulcus occipitalis inferior (oin),* which extends in the direction of the lower end of the postlateral sulcus (Fig. 44, ill. 1).

The cruciate sulcus (*sulcus cruciatus, cr*) is a constant sulcus, cutting deeply through the upper edge of the hemisphere. It lies on the dorsal as well as on the medial surface of the hemisphere (Fig. 45, Fig. 46). On the medial surface, the sulcus bends acutely always backwards, where it merges (in 95% of cases) with the anterior end of the splenial sulcus. On the lateral surface, the sulcus extends down, vertically, or bends slightly forward. The sulcus never merges with the coronal sulcus.

Alongside of the cruciate sulcus lie two inconstant sulci: *sulcus praecruciatus (prcr)* and *sulcus postcruciatus (pscr)* (Fig. 44, ill. 6; Fig. 45, ill. 3).

Sulcus praecruciatus is especially inconstant and is completely absent in 35% of cases; often it is barely visible. The *sulcus postcruciatus* is more constant, being absent in only 4% of the cases.

The presylvian sulcus (*sulcus praesylvius, prs*) is the deepest constant sulcus of the anterior part of the external surface of the hemisphere (Fig. 44). It begins in the region of the anterior rhinal sulcus, merging with it in 95% of cases. Extending forward and upward, the sulcus lies toward the front of the anterior ectosylvian and cruciate sulci. Variants of the sulcus are negligible and have to do with its form, which is usually arciform with two protuberances. Sometimes, however, the curves may be missing or may appear as angles (Fig. 45, ill. 6), branching off and connecting with the anterior olfactory fissure (in 5% of cases the latter is not connected with the presylvian sulcus). At the rear of the presylvian sulcus lies the diagonal sulcus (*sulcus diagonalis, dg*) (Fig. 44, ill. 5). Anterior to the presylvian sulcus lie two inconstant sulci: *sulcus proreus (pr)* and *sulcus interprorealis (ipr).*

The proreal sulcus (*sulcus proreus, pr*) is inconstant, and in almost half the cases it is hardly visible or completely absent. This sulcus is mostly straight, extending parallel to the edge of the hemisphere; it may be connected with the presylvian sulcus (Fig. 45, ill. 5) or separated from it (Fig. 45, ill. 6).

The interproreal or the intraorbital sulcus (*sulcus interprorealis s. sulcus intraorbitalis, ipr*) extends parallel to the lower section of the presylvian sulcus. Its length ranges from 0.3 to 1 cm (Fig. 44, ill. 3). In most cases, however, this fissure is absent.

The Sulci of the Medial Surface of the Hemisphere (Fig. 46)

The sulcus of the corpus callosum (*sulcus corporis callosi, scc*) surrounds the corpus callosum from above. It is one of the least variable sulci and is almost always present.

The genual sulcus (*sulcus genualis, gn*) is constantly present, but varies considerably in form. The most frequent type is a long, arciform sulcus beginning in front, not far from the cruciate sulcus, and extending more or less parallel to the anterior edge of the hemisphere. Along either side of the genual sulcus are the ectogenual sulcus (*sulcus ectogenualis, egn*) and the entogenual sulcus (*sulcus entogenualis*). Below the genual sulcus lies the inconstant, often weakly developed rostral sulcus (*sulcus rostralis, ros,* Fig. 46, ill. 2).

The splenial sulcus (*sulcus splenialis, spl*) is a constant, well developed structure located above the sulcus of the corpus callosum. The anterior end of the uplenial sulcus usually merges with the cruciate sulcus (Fig. 46, ill. 1). Posterior to the point of transition of the anterior and medial parts of the splenial sulcus, the ascending ramus of the *sulcus splenialis (pas,* Fig. 46, ill. 2) frequently extends, running parallel to the cruciate sulcus.

Anterior to the ascending ramus can be found the less constant preascending ramus *sulcus splenialis (pas,* Fig. 46, ill. 2). Other small and inconstant sulci are located either immediately alongside the splenial sulcus or connected with it; the *sulcus transsecans (tr,* Fig. 45, ill. 3; Fig. 46, ill. 2), which is not connected to the uplenial sulcus and which transects the upper edge of the hemisphere; the ramus *horizontalis posterior sulcus splenialis* (*hps*, Fig. 46, ill. 2), which lies at the transition of the splenial sulcus into the retrosplenial sulcus, etc.

The retrosplenial sulcus (*sulcus retrosplenialis, rspl*), a constant feature, is the immediate continuation of the posterior end of the uplenial sulcus and is usually connected with it (Fig. 46, ill. 1, 2). In the majority of cases, it ends in the posterior rhinal sulcus. From both sulci extends the sulcus recurrens.

The suprasplenial sulcus (sulcus suprasplenialis, sspl) is a shallow, constant sulcus with a fairly regular form. It begins immediately behind the ascending ramus of sulcus splenialis, and taking a backward direction it bends gradually and extends more or less parallel to the splenial sulcus (Fig. 46, ill. 1). The suprasplenial sulcus sometimes merges, at its posterior end, with the retrosplenial sulcus. In front there is often found the inconstant sulcus praesuprasplenialis (psspl), located between the ascending and the preascending rami (Fig. 46, ill. 1).

The occipito-temporal sulcus (*sulcus occipito-temporalis, ot*) is very variable in form (Fig. 46, ill. 2). In a number of cases, it is connected with the suprasplenial sulcus.

The Sulci of the Lower Surface of the Hemisphere (Fig. 46)

The hippocampal fissure (*fissura hippocampi, hip, s. sulcus cornu Ammonis*) is a constant structure (Fig. 46, ill. 3). In its posterior part the fissure extends toward the rear of the splenium of the corpus callosum; its lower section separates the gyrus uncinatus from the gyrus hippocampus.

The rhinal sulcus (*sulcus rhinalis*) is exceptionally constant, although its beginning varies somewhat. One can distinguish an anterior rhinal sulcus (*sulcus rhinalis anterior, rha*) and a posterior rhinal sulcus (*sulcus rhinalis posterior, rhp*). The anterior sulcus begins at the olfactory sulcus and reaches the sylvian fissure; the posterior sulcus begins at the sylvian fossa, emerges on the medial surface of the hemisphere, where it either terminates separately (Fig. 46, ill. 2) or merges with the retrosplenial sulcus.

The Cerebral Gyri (Fig. 47-48)

Characteristic of the majority of the gyri, as well as sulci of the lateral surface of the hemisphere, is their concentric position.

The sylvian gyrus (*gyrus Sylvius, s. gyrus arcuatus primus*) lies around the sylvian fissure. Toward the front of the latter lies the anterior part (*pars anterior, Sa*) and toward the back the posterior part (*pars posterior, Sp*). The lower border of this gyrus is formed by the olfactory fissure and the upper border by the ectosylvian sulcus.

The ectosylvian gyrus (*gyrus ectosylvius, s. gyrus arcuatus secundus*) is located between the ectosylvian and suprasylvian sulci and consists of three parts: anterior (*gyrus ectosylvius anterior, Esa*), medial (*gyrus ectosylvius mediusm, Esm*), and posterior (*gyrus ectosylvius posterior, Esp*). Anteriorly the ectosylvian gyrus merges into the orbital gyrus (*gyrus orbitalis, Or*); in front it is bordered by the presylvian sulcus, above by the coronal sulcus, and below by the rhinal sulcus.

The suprasylvian gyrus (*gyrus suprasylvius s. gyrus arcuatus tertius*) is located between the suprasylvian sulcus on one side and on the other the coronal sulcus, the anterior part of the lateral sulcus, and the ectolateral sulcus. Like the preceding gyrus, it divides into three parts: *gyrus suprasylvius anterior (Ssa), gyrus suprasylvius medius (Ssm), gyrus suprasylvius posterior (Ssp)*. The anterior portion of the suprasylvian gyrus is usually called the coronal gyrus (*gyrus coronalis, Cor*).

A number of authors use the term *gyrus compositus posterior* for the lower portion of the posterior part of the ectosylvian and suprasylvian gyri.

The ectolateral gyrus (*gyrus ectolateralis, Ecl*) lies between the ectolateral sulcus on one side, and the lateral and postlateral sulcus on the other.

The marginal gyrus (gyrus marginalis s. gyrus arcuatus quartus) lies between the coronal, lateral, and postlateral sulci on one side, and the splenial sulcus, located on the medial surface of the hemisphere, on the other side. The the marginal gyrus lies on the medial as well as the external surface of the hemisphere. The marginal gyrus is divided into the following gyri:

1. The sigmoid gyrus (gyrus sigmoideus), which lies around the cruciate sulcus and consists of two parts: the anterior part (pars anterior gyri sigmoidei, s. gyrus cruciatus anterior, Sga), located toward the front of the cruciate sulcus, and the posterior part (pars posterior gyri sigmoidei, s. gyrus cruciatus posterior, Sgp), lying toward the back of the cruciate sulcus. The coronal sulcus constitutes the outer lower borderline of the sigmoid gyrus.

2. The presplenial gyrus (gyrus praesplenialis, Prslp), which lies between the cruciate sulcus and the processus of the splenial sulcus.

3. The entolateral gyrus (gyrus entolateralis, En1) which lies between the lateral and the entolateral sulcus.

4. The suprasplenial gyrus (gyrus suprasplenialis, Pspl), located between the entolateral and the suprasplenial sulcus.

5. The postsplenial gyrus (gyrus postsplenialis, Pspl), located between the postlateral and the retrosplenial sulci.

6. The splenial gyrus (gyrus splenialis, Spl), lying between the splenial and the suprasplenial sulcus.

The frontal pole of the hemispheres is taken up by the proreal gyrus (gyrus proreus, Pr, s. prorea), lying on the external as well as the internal surface of the hemispheres. The proreal gyrus on the external surface is bordered by the presylvian sulcus and on the internal surface by the genual sulcus.

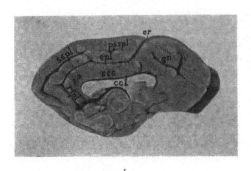

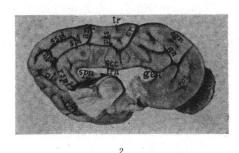

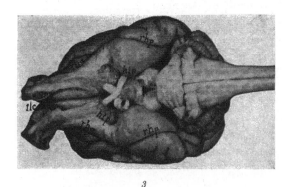

Figure 46 - Sulci of the medial and inferior surfaces of the large hemispheres.

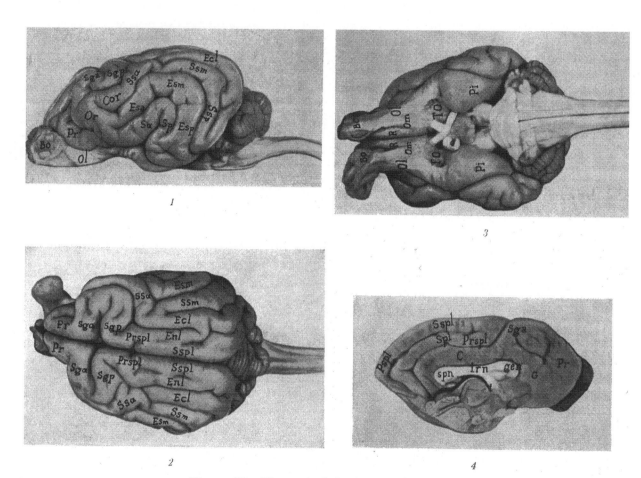

Figure 47 - The gyri of the large hemispheres.

The arcuate gyrus (gyrus fornicatus) is located above the corpus callosum, between the sulcus of the corpus callosum on the one side and the genual, splenial and partly the posterior rhinal sulci on the other side.

In the arcuate gyrus can be distinguished the following parts: the genual gyrus (gyrus genualis, G), located between the genu of the corpus callosum and the genual sulcus, and the lumbar gyrus (gyrus cinguli, C), located between the body of the corpus callosum and the splenial sulcus. The continuation of the arcuate gyrus at the base of the cerebrum constitutes the hippocampal gyrus (gyrus hip- pocampus s. gyrus piriformis, Pi), which borders laterally on the posterior rhinal sulcus. Toward the front, the hippocampal gyrus merges into the unciform gyrus (gyrus uncinatus). The anterior part of the medial surface of the hemisphere is occupied by the olfactory bulb (bulbus olfactorius, BO), the straight gyrus (gyrus rectus, R), and the internal and external olfactory gyri (gyri olfactorii medialis, Om, et lateralis, ol) (Fig. 47, ill. 3).

The projection of the gyri upon the skull of the dog is indicated in Fig. 48.

The Cellular Structure of the Cerebral Cortex (Fig. 49-51)

In accordance with the classification of Filimonov [715], the cerebral cortex of the dog, as other mammals, can be divided into five basic zones: (1) the neocortex, (2) the archicortex, (3) the paleocortex and intermediate cortex consisting of (4) periarchicortex, as well as (5) peripalaeocortex.

The area of the canine neocortex equals 84.2% of the area of the entire hemisphere, while the size of the complex of the palaeocortex, the archicortex, and the cortex intermedius equals 15.8%. These data are an indication that in such well developed subprimates as the dog the area of the neocortex reaches considerable dimensions. It is interesting that in man, according to the Brain Institute, the neocortex occupies 95.6% and the complex of the paleocortex, archicortex, and the cortex intermedius is only 4.4% of the area of the entire cerebral cortex.

The description of the areas of the paleocortex, the archicortex, and the cortex intermedius is given here according to the data of Filimonov.

In examining the neocortex and dividing it into areas and fields, and also in plotting the map of cytoarchitectural fields, we decided not to use numerals, believing it more expedient to use letters for the designation of the cytoarchitectural fields of the canine cortex. The designations in letters exclude the possibility of erroneous homologies of diverse architectural formations among mammals. The nomenclature in numerals can lead, involuntarily, to the admission of a total homology of the cytoarchitectural fields in the representatives of various orders. It is hardly possible to homologize in all mammals, as did Brodmann [700], such "inconstant" formations as, for instance, the frontal and temporal fields.

More successful are the attempts to homologize the areas of the neocortex, which correspond to the basic cortical territories of the analysers. However, the possibility of homologizing diverse structures is limited here as well; thus, if there is a possibility for some kind of homology in respect to the territory of the optic, auditory, cutaneous, and motor analysors, it is quite impossible to homologize, to the same extent, the frontal or the insular region of the cerebrum in the canine or in primates.

The designation in letters permits emphasis on the fact that a given field belongs to this or that analyser. Some of the regions investigated by us (the insular, limbic, and frontal) cannot be definitely referred to some analyser in view of the fact that there are not enough data - our own or those in the literature - on the connections and functions of these areas. Therefore, it is impossible at the moment to give the designations of all the fields of the cortex according to the analyser principle, although such a principle of designation would no doubt be more rational. On the strength of these circumstances, we adhered to the designations based on the Latin names of the regions. A capital letter refers to the area which has to do with this or that field. The field itself is marked by a capital letter together with a small number. For instance, O_1 stands for area occipitalis prima or the first occipital field. In naming the fields the numbers increase as they progress from the occipital pole to the frontal and there, wherever this is possible, upward from below.

The letter O designates the occipital region (regio occipitalis), T - the temporal region (regio temporalis), P - the parietal region (regio parietalis), Pc - the postcoronary region (regio postcoronalis), Pro - the precoronary region (regio praecoronalis), F - the frontal region (regio frontalis), L - the limbic region (regio limbica), I - the insular region (regio insularis).

The nuclear zones of the optic, auditory, cutaneomechanical (somatic sensory), motor analysors are characterized by some structural generalities. The nuclei of the diverse analysors are not homogeneous as to their cellular structure, and they consist of a number of fields. In the nucleus of each analysor there is a portion containing the very large cells of pyramidal form, especially in layer V, which no doubt suggests the existence in every analysor of its own efferent systems for the realization of different efferent outputs. There is a great deal of similarity in the character of the cellular elements in the correlation of the layers in the fields of the various analysors. The six-layer level structure of the cortex, with division of its diameter into an upper level (layers I, II, III and IV) and lower level (layers V and VI), is characteristic for the majority of fields.

The view that there is great similarity in the structure of the cortical ends of the diverse analysors is supported by Pavlov [144], who considers the cortex an undivided united system.

For the dog, as well as for primates, an established characteristic is the fine structural differentiation of the

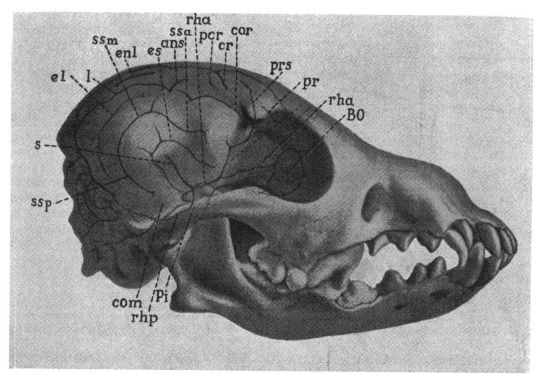

Figure 48 - The projection of the sulci and gyri upon the skull of the dog (according to Flatau). hemispheres.

cerebral cortex into regions and fields, and the fields in some instances into smaller structural units or subfields. Typically, for instance, the fields of the optic analysor have a comparatively narrow cortex, rich in small cells and with a clearly developed layer *IV*, whereas the fields of the auditory analysor have a broad cortex and a clear radial striation of the entire diameter of the cortex.

The borders between the regions and the fields are most in the depths of the suici where sulci exist. In this case, the borderline is more or less clear. It is more difficult to establish the borderline between the fields on the open surface; here there is a gradual transition of one structure into another, and certain sectors often have characteristics of the two adjacent fields. This, for example, is characteristic for the borderline between fields O_1 and O_2 of the optic analysor between the gigantopyramidal field Prc_1 and field Prc_2 of the motor analysor, between field Prc_1 and field Pc_1 of the cutaneous (somatic sensory) analysor, between field T_1 of the auditory analysor and the temporal-entorhinal field TE_2, as well as between a number of other structures.

As to their morphology, some fields can be regarded as transitional structures from one cytoarchitectural formation to another (i.e., the occipito-parietal field *OP*, the temporal-postcoronary field *TPc*, etc.). Filimonov has formulated the principle of the intermediate formations, pointing out that between the cortical territories of dissimilar origin (i.e., between the neocortex and the archeocortex, the neocortex and the paleocortex) lie entire regions which he calls intermediate cortex (cortex inter-

medius).

The existence of a zone of gradual transition from one cellular structure into another possibly can be explained from the point of view of the teachings of Pavlov [144] on the stratification of the cortical ends of the analysors among themselves. There is no doubt about the stratification in respect to the cortical ends of the cutaneous and motor analysors, which has been demonstrated by a nuMber of investigators (Asratian [975]; Anokhin [973]; Rosenthal [680]; Robiner [589]; Adrianov [969] and others).

However, it is rather doubtful that this type of stratification of the fields of the neocortex in the dog is the result of one developing around the other in the final stage of differentiation. It is well known that in lower organized animals there are considerably more such intermediate territories. For instance, in the rabbit and the cat, according to the data of Gurevich, Khachaturian, and Khachaturov [726] as well as Kukuyev [1012], the motor field 4 has a clearly developed internal granular layer (layer *IV*). In the dog, there is a more distinct isolation of the nuclear zones, and a more complicated differentiation of structure within the nuclei of the analysors. However, even at this level of development there remain, as we have seen, transitional structures. In the canine, as seen in the experiments of Luciani and Pavlov, the regions are not precisely demarcated as to their functions.

The neocortex of the canine cerebrum characteristically has few structural pecularities. For many areas, there is characteristically an imprecise division of the depths of the cortex into layers. In some areas layer *II* is barely separated from layer *III*, which can be explained by the similarity of the form of the cellular elements of these layers. An isolated layer *IV* may be absent; as a result, it is difficult to decide on the presence of typical granulations of many neocortical areas.

The majority of nervous elements of the cortex are of pyramidal or irregular (flattened or polygonal) shape. Many cells are anomalously oriented in respect to the surface of the cortex. This results in an insufficient radial striation. With rare exceptions, it is characteristic for areas of the neocortex that the cortex changes abruptly into the white matter located below.

The structure of an area on the wall of a sulcus usually differs, more or less, from the structure of that very same area on the open surface. The width of the cortex decreases especially at the expense of the lower layers; the cells of the width of the cortex lie closer together, and layer *IV* is clearly isolated. These characteristics stand out especially in the structure of the floor of sulci. The structure of the area on the wan and the floor of the sulcus remains more constant than that on the free surface.

Most of the cortex of the posterior half of the hemispheres (toward the back of the sylvian fissure and its imaginary continuation perpendicular to the median sulcus of the hemisphere) is formed by cells smaller than those of the cortex of the anterior half of the hemispheres. In the cortex of the anterior portion of the hemispheres, there are a considerable number of large cells in layer *III*, and especially in layer *IV*. They are characteristic not only of the gigantopyramidal area Prc_1 but also most of the areas of the postcoronal region - the territory of the cortex of the cutaneous analysor (for areas Pc_1, Pc_2, Pc_3, which adjoin the area Prc, and the transitional area TPc).

In plotting the map of the cytoarchitectural areas of the canine cerebral cortex with the purpose of clarifying the topography of the nuclei of some analysors, we referred to the literature as well as our own data from physiological and morphological experiments.

In part, the study of the cytoarchitecture of the nuclear zones of the motor and auditory analysors was accompanied by the investigation of the connections and functions of the above-mentioned analysors by the methods of conditioned reflexes and clinical observation, together with extirpation of either the entire nuclear zone or its separate sections, and subsequent morphological control (Adrianov [968, 969]; Mering [914, 915]).

Let us compare our own data on the location of diverse areas with data from the cytoarchitectural maps of Campbell [704], Klempin [737], Gurevich and Bykhovskaya [725], and from the works of Kukuyev [645], Svetukhina [1079], and others (Fig. 49, 50 and 51).

According to our data, the area of the optic analysor actually includes optic areas O_1 and O_2, which basically coincide, as to territory, with areas 17 and 18 on the map of Klempin, as well as of Gurevich and Bykhovskaya.

Area *OP* (area 19 on the maps of these authors) we consider a transitional structure from the occipital to the parietal cortex.

Areas T_1, T_2, T_3, and T_4 belong to the auditory analysor. Area T_1, located in the posterior part of the suprasylvian gyrus, corresponds to the anterior section of area 21 on the map of Gurevich and of Bykhovskaya, and to sub-areas *21Ba*, *21Bb*, and *21c* on the map of Klempin, but it does not extend beyond the borders of the ectosylvian sulcus. Area T_2 corresponds to area 22, and area T_3 to the medial part of area 50. A part of area 50, located in the anterior portion of the ectosylvian gyrus, is defined by us as a transitional field from the cortex of the temporal region to the area of the postcoronal formation (area *TPc*). This has many more characteristics common to the areas of the postcoronal region than to the areas of the temporal region. Area T_4, lying in the middle part of the suprasylvian gyrus, corresponds to the lower section of area 7 (subarea 7c).

Areas TE_1 and TE_2 (corresponding approximately to areas 20 and 36a on the maps of Klempin and Gurevich and Bykhovskaya) cannot be referred to the territory of the auditory analysor, and we consider them areas in transition toward formations of the intermediate entorhinal subarea. Obviously, they cannot be referred to the territory of the auditory analysor and area 52.

The insular region (*regio insularis*) actually consists of two insular areas, I_1 and I_2, and two parainsular areas, PI_1 and PI_2. Area I_1 corresponds to area 13a on the map of Klempin and partly to area 13 on the map of Gurevich and Bykhovskaya, although in contrast to the latter we do not expand area I_1 over the posterior section of the sylvian gyri. Our conclusion finds support in the investigations of Filimonov [714], who assumes that in man a part of the islet enclosed between the *sulcus circularis insulae superior* and *sulcus circularis insulae posterior* can be homologous only to the anterior parts of the sylvian and the ectosylvian gyri of the canine hemispheres. Area I_2 corresponds to area 14 on the map of Gurevich and Bykhovskaya. According to Klempin's and Gurevich's data, the cortex of the islet is surrounded by area 52, which they refer to the temporal region; on the basis of our investigations, we are unable to agree. The structure located on the sylvian gyrus, around the islet, we regard as parainsular areas PI_1 and PI_2 (52a and 52b according to Klempin's designations).

A part of the parietal region (*regio parietalis*) is the single area *P*. Area *P* corresponds to subarea 7a and 7b on the map of Klempin, and to considerable parts of area 7 on the map of Gurevich and Bykhovskaya (except for the lower part of the area 7, which according to our data is occupied by temporal area T_4).

We referred area 5 to the formation of the postcoronal region, and on the basis of the similarity in cellular structure it was designated area Pc_1. Data in the literature on the connections of the temporal region (Lisitsa [1122]; Babayan [1096]) support these assumptions. At

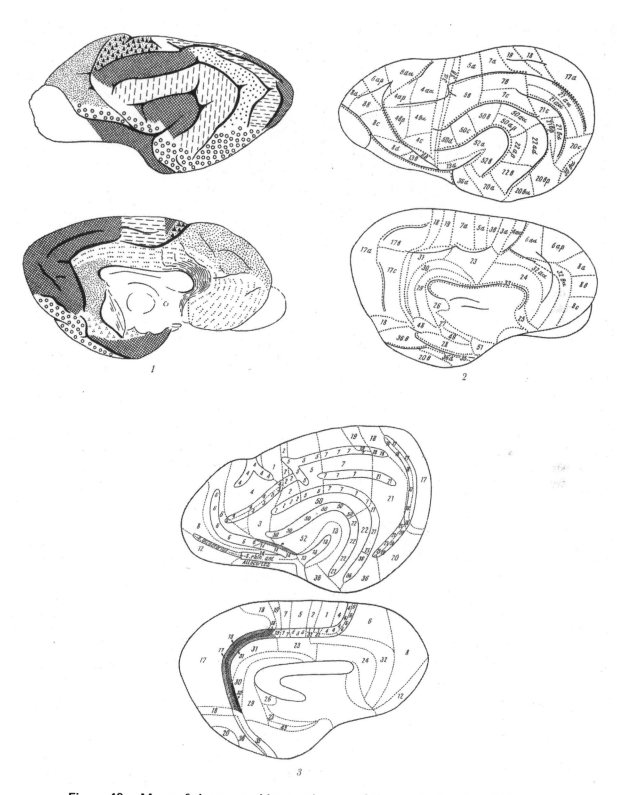

Figure 49 – Maps of the cytoarchitectural areas of the cerebral cortex of the dog.

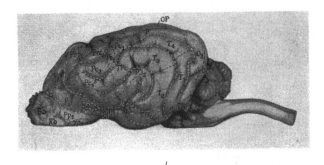

1

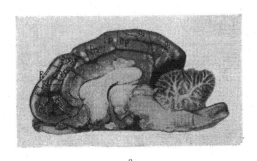

2

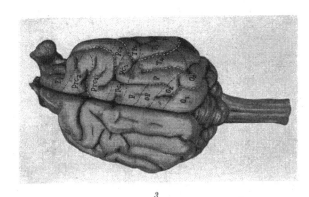

3

Figure 50 — A map of the cytoarchitectural areas of the cerebral cortex of the dog (after Adrianov and Mering). Illustration 1 : The lateral surface of the hemisphere. Illustration 2 : The medial surface of the hemisphere. Illustration 3 : The dorsal surface of the hemisphere.

Figure 51 – A map of the cytoarchitectural areas of the cerebral cortex of the dog (after Adrianov and Mering).

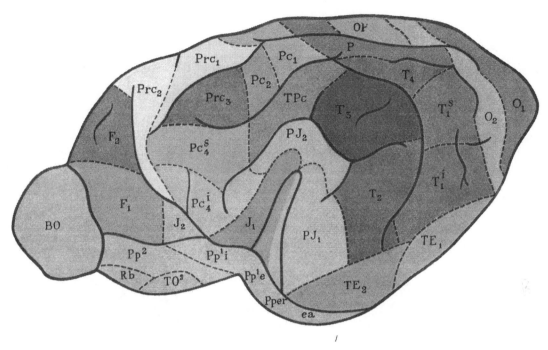

Illustration 1: The lateral surface of the hemisphere.

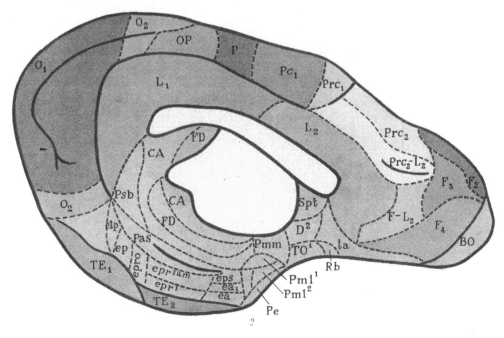

llustration 2: The medial surface of the hemisphere.

Figure 51 (cont.)– A map of the cytoarchitectural areas of the cerebral cortex of the dog (after Adrianov and Mering).

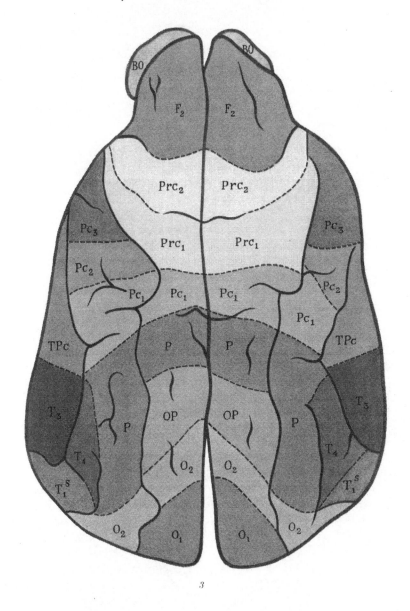

Illustration 3 : The dorsal surface of the hemisphere.

area 5, fibers begin which project toward globus pallidus and substantia nigra, and also fibers which enter into the pyramidal tract. When area 7 is destroyed, such connections cannot be traced. At the same time, it is a well known phenomenon that fibers extending toward the above mentioned areas begin in the areas of the precoronal and postcoronal regions.

The postcoronal region consists of four areas of its own: Pc_1, Pc_2, Pc_3, Pc_4, and the transitional area TPc. As to the composition and topography of this region, our findings differ sharply from those of Klempin, as well as of Gurevich and Bykhovskaya, who also disagree among themselves, as mentioned before.

In topography, area Pc_1 is closest to area 5. Area Pc_2 coincides with the lower part of area 2 on the map of Gurevich and Bykhovskaya, and with the middle part of area 3 on the map of Klempin. Area Pc_3 corresponds partly to the upper section of area 4 (sub-area 4b) on the map of Klempin. Area Pc_4 corresponds to areas 3 and 43 on the map of Gurevich and Bykhovskaya and to subarea 4c on the map of Klempin.

The precoronal region (regio praecoronalis) represents, according to morphological and physiological investigations, the territory of the motor analysor. It consists of two areas - Prc_1 and Prc_2. The borders of the precoronal region, isolated as a whole, correspond more than anything else to the borders of the motor cortex (motor cortex) isolated by Campbell [704].

Area Prc_1 corresponds to subarea $4a\alpha$ and $4a\beta$ on the map of Klempin and area 1, and also to part of area 4 on the map of Gurevich and Bykhovskaya.

Contrary to the data of Klempin, area 4 does not spread below the coronal sulcus. Area 4 does not extend over the anterior section of the sigmoid gyrus, as was pointed out by Gurevich and Bykhovskaya. Area Prc_2 corresponds to sub-area 6a on the map of Klempin, and to the anterior section of area 4 and partly to area 6 on the map of Gurevich and Bykhovskaya.

The borders of area Prc_1, according to our investigations, correspond most closely to the borders of area 4 traced in the canine by Kukuyev and Svetukhina, and the borders of area Prc_2 to the borders of area praegigantopyramidalis according to Svetukhina.

The frontal region consists of four of its own areas (F_1, F_2, F_3, and F_4) and one transitional area $F-L_2$. Areas F_1, F_2, F_3, and F_4 correspond roughly to area 8 on the map of Klempin and areas 8 and 12 on the map of Gurevich and Bykhovskaya. Area $F-L_2$ corresponds to subareas 32b and partly 32a on the map of Klempin, and the anterior section of area 32 on the map of Gurevich and Bykhovskaya.

The new division of the frontal region suggested by Svetukhina [1079] seems more correct. Our definitions of the borders of the areas of the frontal region on the external surface of the hemisphere (areas F_1 and F_2) coincide, essentially, with those of Svetukhina.

Our data on the composition and topography of the areas of the limbic region differ from the data of Klempin, Gurevich and Bykhovskaya, all of whom include in this region a number of areas: 23, 24, 29, 30, 31, and 32.

In accordance with our data, it is possible to isolate the posterior limbic area L and the anterior limbic area L_2. Between these areas, there is no doubt a transitional zone, which we cannot, however, consider a separate area. The subdivision of the limbic region diametrically into several areas seems to us rather debatable.

The division of the canine limbic region into areas, longitudinally, as well as diametrically across the limbic gyrus, presents a difficult and disputable project. Our data support the opinion of Blinkov [1101], who notes that in the supraterrestrial Garnivora the limbic area is much less differentiated than in primates; in it can be isolated the anterior agranular section and the posterior region, characterized by the presence of an analogue of layer IV.

The Occipital Region (Regio Occipitalis) (Fig. 52-56)

There are many studies in the literature devoted to the connections and functions of the visual analysor in the dog. The connections of the optic region were described in great detail in the works of Tseleritskiy [877], Troshin [803], Bekhterev [2], Kononova [843], Brouwer [5], Rioch [588], and others. These reports describe the termination of the central optic tract in the cortex of the occipital region in the canine hemispheres.

Munk [758], Bekhterev [823], Agadzhaniants [819], and Minkowski [852] determined that the removal of the occipital region on the medial surface of the hemisphere is accompanied by the loss of objective sight, while the extirpation of the external surface of the hemisphere leads to a temporary lowering of visual functions, to partial blindness (the so called amblyopia), named by Munk "psychic blindness." Pavlov has shown that the basis for "psychic blindness" is a disorder in the analytico-synthetic function of the optic analysor.

The nature of the optic function of the dog has been thoroughly investigated by Orbeli [761], Frolov [833], and Shenger-Krestovnikova [866], among others. By applying the method of conditioned reflexes it was shown that the dog differentiates sharply between diverse degrees of intensity of light, surpassing man in this respect. The dog also possesses an acute sense of differentiation in the shapes of objects; however, this sense is far less perfect than man's. Whether a dog sees colors is questionable (Samoilov and Feofilaktova [864]; Nagel [854]; Orbeli [856]; Leontovich [848]).

Pavlov and his pupils (Toropov [874]; Kudrin [874]; and others) consider the occipital part of the hemispheres as the central zone of the optic analysor. When this area is completely or almost completely removed, the dog loses its objective vision, which requires a higher analysis and a synthesis of visual stimuli. Such animals retain simpler functions, such as the differentiation of light intensity and the ability to form a conditioned reflex in respect to the general lighting of the room. A minimum disruption in the activity of the optic analysor is expressed in a limitation of the optic field.

The research of Marquis and Hilgard [850], Smith [868], and Kriazhev and Tsind [844] was devoted to the investigation of conditioned visual reflexes after the removal of the cortex of the occipital area in the dog. Marquis and Hilgard, as well as Smith, drew the conclusion that there is relatively far reaching compensation of visual functions after extirpation of the occipital region. Kriazhev and Tsind, on the other hand, noted that if a minimum portion of the visual cortex remains, the dogs have only an elementary ability to react to visual stimuli; ability to discern objects as well as differentiate intensity of light disappears completely.

The zone of the optic analysor consists of two, strictly speaking, visual areas (O_1 and O_2) and of one transitional area (OP), located on the medial and lateral surface of the hemisphere.

The areas of the occipital region are characterized by their comparatively narrow cortex, rich in small cells (area OP is somewhat of an exception), and by the indistinct separation of layer II from layer III, a clearly discernible layer IV, and clear stria in layer V.

The Parietal Region (*Regio Parietalis*) (Fig. 57, 58)

The efferent tracts of the parietal region in the canine were investigated in great detail by Lisitsa [1122]. He demonstrated that the efferent projection systems of the parietal region are differentiated in carnivora. Fibers project out of the anterior parietal region (area 5 on the map of Gurevich and Bykhovskaya) toward globus pallidus, the optic thalamus, into the lateral portion of the base of the cerebral peduncle, toward the anterior corpus bigeminum, into stinstantia nigra, the Pons varolii and the pyramidal tract. After removal of the posterior occipital region (area 7 on the map of Gurevich and Bykhovskaya) it is possible to trace degenerated fibers extending into the internal capsule and a small number of fibers extending into the base of the cerebellar peduncle and the Pons varolii.

Babayan [1096] also noted differences in the efferent tracts of areas 5 and 7. Thus, area 5 is connected with substantia nigra, the globus pallidus, the lateral pyramidal tract, the middle part of the lateral nucleus and the ventral nucleus of the optic thalamus. Area 7 is connected with the posterior portion of the labeled nucleus and the anterior corpus bigeminum.

The existence of connections between the cortex of the parietal region and globus pallidus was proved by Bekhterev [2], Grunstein [26], and a number of other scientists. The presence of connections of the parietal region with the caudate nucleus is doubted by many scientists.

The functional importance of the parietal region of the cortex of the large hemispheres of the canine has not been completely investigated. Luciani [1123] regarded this region as a site of higher psychic functions, where all sensory zones of the cortex overlap. Demoor [708], proceeding from Flechsig's conception of projective and associational zones, regarded the parietal region as a posterior associational center. The collaborators of Pavlov proved objectively the uselessness of defining regions of lower and higher functions in the cerebral cortex. Orbeli [855] showed in a dog in which the upper portions of the hemispheres had been removed that conditioned reflexes to sound and light were formed quickly, whereas it was impossible to obtain conditioned reflexes to cutaneous and cold stimuli.

Bekhterev [2] concluded that the occipital and parietal regions overlap throughout a considerable expanse. Many investigators refer to the relation of the posterior sections of the parietal region to vision (Tseleritskiy [877]; Agadzhaniants [819]; Minkowski [852]; Sarkissow [790]).

In the parietal region we discern only area P (corresponding approximately to area 7 on the map of Gurevich and Bykhovskaya).

The Temporal Region (*Regio Temporalis*) (Fig. 59-66)

Insufficient data exist in the literature on the connections of the auditory analysor of carnivora (Bekhterev [2]; Larionov [910], Poljak [336]; Rioch [588]; Mettler [917]; Woolard and Harpman [937]; Ades [483]; Mering [915] and others). Data on the localization of the auditory region in the cortex of the hemispheres of carnivora are quite contradictory. Some investigators (Munk, 1881 [*Editor's note: The Munk reference could not be found in the bibliography.*] and others) thought that the auditory area in the dog is located in the posterior portions of the ectosylvian, suprasylvian, and postlateral gyri. Other investigators, using the method of electroencephalography, showed that the cortical auditory zone lies in the upper portion of the sylvian gyrus and in the middle and partly anterior portion of the ectosylvian gyrus (Bremer and Dow [891]; Tunturi [931]). Woolsey and Walzl [938], Ades [881], Rose and Woolsey [925], Bremer, Bonnet and Terzuolo [890] also have shown the existence of the so called secondary auditory areas.

Mering [915] showed that the central auditory tract consists of two fasciculi, the superficial and the deep. The superficial fasciculus can be traced as a compact, very thin layer from the lateral and upper surface of the medial geniculate body to the free surface of the cortex of the posterior and middle sections of the suprasylvian gyrus.

The deep fibers of the auditory radiation extend from the medial geniculate body as a compact fasciculus; they pass into the sublenticular part of the medial capsule and approadh, usually in the form of thin laminae, the cortex of the middle sections of the ectosylvian and suprasylvian gyri.

Further morphophysiological comparisons have revealed that the medial and posterior sections of the ectosylvian and suprasylvian gyri constitute the zone of the auditory analysor. This is divided into four temporal areas.

The activity of the canine auditory analysor was thoroughly studied by Pavlov and his pupils. Dogs differentiate keenly the sounds of various frequencies, catching the difference in sound up to $1/8$ of a tone (Zelenyi [939] and Andreyev, 1928, 1934 [885, 886]). Here too the dog far surpasses man in its ability to distinguish sounds of various intensities. The upper limit of the auditory perception in the dog amounts to 37,000-38,000 cycles per second, which is more than twice the upper limit of auditory perception in man.

In respect to synthetic activity, the ability of the canine auditory analysor is much less developed than in man. Thus, for instance, the differentiation of a four-period, successive sound complex is very slowly analyzed, which shows that this is a problem sometimes far beyond the capacity of a dog (Ivanov-Smolenskiy [903]; Zimkina and Zimkin [940]; Skipin [928]; Mering [916]); for man such a problem poses no difficulty whatsoever.

Makovskiy [913], Elyason (1908), Krzhyzhanovskiy (1909), Burmakin [893], Babkin [889], Kudrin [845], Voskresenskiy [936] disclosed that the removal of the center of the auditory analysor (the auditory sphere of Munk) is accompanied by various degrees of disruption of the analytico-synthetic activity of the auditory analysor. This may vary from its complete disappearance to the disruption of only the fine differentiations of sounds. Pavlov concluded, on the basis of his investigations, that in the center of the auditory analyser occurs the analysis and synthesis of simultaneous as well as successive complex conditioned stimuli.

The center of the auditory analyser consists of four cytoarchitectural areas – T_1, T_2, T_3, and T_4. It lies on the external surface of the hemisphere.

These areas dharacteristically have a thick cortex, rich in cells (an exception is area T_4, distinct radial striations over the entire diameter of the cortex, a wide upper level, a multi- and microcellular layer II and a columnar arrangement of cells in layer VI.

The Insular Region (*Regio Insularis*) (Fig. 67-72)

Very little information has been published on the functional value of the insular region of the canine hmmisphere. Bekhterev [2] and his pupils (Trapeznikov [1042]; Larionov [910]; Gorshkov [1110]; and Belitskiy [1100]) demonstrated that destruction of the antero-inferior section of the third and fourth primary gyri (*gyrus sylvius*

anterior, *gyrus ectosylvius anterior*, and *gyrus compositus anterior*) results in a more or less acute weakening of the taste sense and a disorder in chewing. According to these authors, the above-mentioned regions have direct efferent connections with the nuclei of the glossopharyngeal nerve in the medulla oblongata. Adler [1090], Gerebtzoff [1109], and Woolsey have subsequently assumed that the insular region surrounding the sylvian sulcus must be regarded as a cortical gustatory zone.

The insular region occupies the sylvian gyrus and the posterior inferior section of gyrus proreus, on which lie actually two insular areas (I_1 and I_2) and two parainsular areas (PI_1 and PI_2).

The area of the insular region is characterized by its wide cortex (especially at the expense of the inferior layers), good radial striations, distinct separation of layer II, the absence of layer IV as an independent layer, and the gradual transition into white matter.

It is characteristic of these areas that the boundary cells are located close together.

The Postcoronal Region (*Regio Postcoronalis*) (Fig. 73-80)

In conformity with the research of Pavlov and his pupils, one has to regard the postcoronal area of the hemispheres (the coronal gyrus, the anterior and partly the middle sector of the ectosylvian gyrus), as the zone of the cutaneous analysor. In this area occurs the analysis and synthesis of so-called cutaneo-mechanical stimuli (caused by touching the skin, etc.) The relation of this region in the dog to the analysis of temperature and pain stimuli seems debatable.

The connections of the cortical end of the cutaneous analysor have not been sufficiently investigated. It is well known that the postcoronal region receives the fibers from the lateral as well as the ventral group of nuclei of the optic thalamus, where the spinothalamic tract and the medial lemniscus end.

The function of the cutaneo-mechanical analysor was investigated in detail in the laboratories of Pavlou, Krasnogorskiy [1011], Arkhangelskiy [974], Voskresenskiy [963], and Kupalov [952]. It is not very difficult to obtain in the dog spacial differentiation of cutaneo-mechanical stimuli at the place of contact. Differentiation of cutaneous irritation through frequency of contact is usually very difficult for the dog.

In case of removal of the zone of the cutaneomechanical analysor, one can observe the disappearance for a more or less prolonged time of cutaneo-mechanical conditional reflexes. Gradual restoration of function, which is usually not complete, can possibly be explained by the activity of scattered elements of the analysor. In the removal of the zone of this analysor, the greatest damage is done to differentiation of successive cutaneomechanical complex stimuli (Voskresenskiy [963]).

Krasnogorskiy determined that in the dog the centers of cutaneo-mechanical and motor analysors are topographically delimited. At the same time, since both analysors play a basic role in the realization of motor reactions, and since in the case of removal of one of them the activity of the other is often interrupted (Rosenthal [1031]; Asratian [975]; Anokhin and Chernevskiy [973]; Zhuravlev [966]), one has to admit the possibility of an especially wide and close overlapping of the central zones of the cutaneo-mechanical and motor analysors in the cortex of the hemispheres of the canine and other carnivora. Another indication of this is the closeness of the structures of the areas of the postcoronal region and the areas of the precoronal region (the center of the motor analysor) and finally the electrophysiological investigations of somatic sensation in the dog and cat (Dusser de Barenne and McGulloch [947]; Marshall, Woolsey and Bard [954]; Woolsey [965]; Robiner [589]; Hamuy, Bromiley and Woolsey [948]; Zubek [967]; Scherrer and Oeconomos [961]; and others).

According to our investigations, the postcoronal region occupies the coronal gyrus, the anterior sections of the lateral suprasylvian and ectosylvian gyri. This region has four areas of its own: Pc_1, Pc_2, Pc_3, Pc_4, and area TPc, a transitional area toward the temporal region.

All the areas of the postcoronal region have a cortex rich in cells. The cortex is of medium width with a clear stria of translucence in layer V. There can be observed, against the general background of small cells, a considerable number of large cells of pyramidal form in layer III, and especially large cells, closer in size to the pyramidal cells of Betz, in layer V. A great number of large pyramidal cells are in areas Pc_1 and Pc_2, and also in the transitional area TPc. All areas are characterized by a sharply defined boundary with white matter.

Area Pc_4 (Area Postcoronalis Quarta) (Fig. 76, 77)

Area Pc_4 lies in the anterior sections of the ectosylvian and sylvian gyri (Fig. 50 and 51). The anterior boundary (with area Prc_2) extends partly along the presylvian sulcus and partly along the free surface of the ectosylvian gyrus parallel to the presylvian sulcus. The superior boundary (with area Pc_2) coincides with the anterior portion of the suprasylvian sulcus; the posterior (with area TPc) and inferior (with area I_1) boundaries extend over the free surface of the ectosylvian and sylvian gyri.

Area Pc_4 can be divided into two subareas: Pc^s_4 (subarea postcoronalis quarto superior) and pci4 (subarea postcoronalis quarts. inferior).

Precoronal Region (Regio Praecoronalis) (Fig. 81-83)

The precoronal region occupies the sigmoid gyrus of the hemispheres. On the basis of the research of Pavlov's school, this region must be regarded as the central zone of the motor analysor, inside of which occurs the analysis and synthesis of stimuli coming from skeletal musculature.

The precoronal region receives fibers from the lateral and ventral groups of nuclei of the optic thalamus, which is the terminus of the basic mass of fibers of the medial lemniscus. The latter conducts kinesthetic stimuli. An essential characteristic of this region is that the basic mass of fibers of the pyramidal or the corticospinal tract begin in this cortical area. The fibers projecting to the motor nuclei of the craniocerebral nerves (the corticobulbar tract) also begin in the precoronal region. These fibers are represented by axons of neurons of layer V of the precoronal region, which pass through the corona radiata and the genu of the internal capsule into the middle portion of the base of the cerebellar peduncle (where they lie medial to the fibers of the pyramidal tract) and end at cranial motor nuclei III, IV, V, VI, VII, IX, X, XI, XII of the opposite as well as partly on the same side.

Cells of the precoronal region give rise to fibers which end at neurons of the ventrolateral group of nuclei of the optic thalamus, globus pallidus, and substantia nigra. These connections belong to the extrapyramidal portion of the nervous system.

Numerous investigations of the functions of the motor region of the cortex by the method of electrostimulation (Tyshetskiy [167]; Fritsch and Hitzig [995]; Ferrier [22]; Pasternatzkiy [1026]; Tarkhanov [1039]; Bekhterev [2]; Vorotynskiy [172]; Bari [976]; et al.) revealed that motor centers of the body and extremities are located in the sigmoid gyrus.

Reports on the boundaries and topography of these areas as derived by electrostimulation are rather contradictory. However, the majority of investigators produced motor movement by electrical stimulation of the posterior section of the sigmoid gyrus. Before the research of Pavlov's school, the problem of the functional nature of the motor region remained unsolved. Some investigators regarded the motor region of the cortex only as a motor efferent zone, while others regarded it as a sensory, afferent zone. A pupil of Pavlov, Krasnogorskiy [1011] using the method of conditional motor reflexes, proved objectively the sensory nature of the analyser of the motor region.

The research of Protopopov [1029], Asratian [975], Rosenthal [1031], Anokhin [973, 687], Shumilina [1034, 1033] and Adrianov [968, 969, 970] was devoted to the functional significance of the motor analysor. These investigators combined the method of conditioned motor reflexes with removal of the motor region of the hemispheres on the dog. The majority of investigators arrived at the conclusion that removal of the center of the motor analysor is accompanied, at first, by an abrupt interruption of motor reactions, especially in conditioned motor reflexes requiring complicated analysis and synthesis of kinesthetic stimuli (for instance sitting up, extending of the paw, etc.). They also pointed to the relation of the motor region of the canine hemispheres to the regulation of tonic reactions which are brought about at various levels of the brainstem, for example, the increase of extensor tonus, the disorder of plastic tonus, etc. (Woolsey [1044]; Lisitsa and Pentsik [1015]; Tower [1040]; Adrianov [969, 970]). There exist data on the functional differentiation of the center of the motor analysor in the canine as measured by the degrees of participation of its diverse areas in the complex of the above mentioned reactions and in bringing about visual functions (Adrianov, 1953).

The research of Trapeznikov [1042], Ivanov [1005], Bekhterev [2] and Gerver [718] pointed to the participation of the motor region of the hemispheres in the activity of the internal organs. According to the data of Fulton [24], the motor region, and above all its anterior section, the so called premotor zone, sbyuld be regarded as a place of overlapping of somatic and vegetative projections in the cortex of the hemispheres. Recently there appeared new data (Airapetiants [682]) on the role of the motor region of the canine brain, in the activity of the analysor of the internal milieu.

The center of the motor analysor occupies the territory of the sigmoid gyrus, in which are located areas Prc_1 and Prc_2.

The areas of the precoronal region are characterized by a rather narrow cortex, the absence of the internal layer of granules (of layer IV), and a wide layer III.

The Frontal Region (*Regio Frontalis*) (Fig. 84-89)

The function of the frontal region is still unknown. Numerous investigators who have concerned themselves with the study of the functional aspect of the frontal region have failed to rank it with any of the well known analysors even though this region receives a great number of afferent fibers from the optic thalamus.

Some investigators foresaw the frontal region as a special "center of intellectual life" Zhukovskiy [1087]; Franz [1061]; Bianchi [1052]), whereas Luciani and Seppilli [747] and Munk [758] did not recognize a specific relation of the frontal lobes to higher psychic functions. They assumed that the frontal region regulates movements of various muscles, mostly of the trunk and the occiput. Later on, numerous investigators of the highest nervous activity of lobectomized and lobotomized animals (Tikhomirov [1081]; Babkin [1050]; Afanasyev [1049]; Usiyevich, Kudriashov, and Sovietov [1083]) ruled out the existence of a section with special higher functions behind the frontal region of the canine cerebrum. However, there is no doubt about the participation of this region in the processes of highest nervous activity, and also, according to Shustin [1035, 1073] in bringing about trace reactions and regulating the vocal conditioned reactions and reflexes that depend on the relation of various stimuli.

Soon after an operation on the frontal regions, there was noted in most cases a weakening and disruption of the processes of internal inhibition in various analysors, which leads to disinhibition of differentiation (Konorski [1010] [*Editors' note: The Konorski reference could not be found in the bibliography. Consequently, we made a substitution.*]), disorders of deferred reactions (Lawicka [1066]), the appearance of so-called pendulum-like movements (Shumilina [1034]), and an increased inertia of nervous processes. However, according to the majority of authors, the quality of the activity of the cortex after the removal of the frontal regions remains, essentially unchanged. Some authors assume that the frontal region has a definite relation to reactions of an extrapyramidal type (Langworthy in 12x28). Shumilina [1034] regards the frontal region as an extrapyramidal cortical area. Using the method of electrostimulation of the posterior section of the frontal region Gerver [718] has succeeded in obtaining a concomitant turning of the eyes and the head to the side opposite from the stimulation (the so called anterior adversive area). The large number of efferent connections of the frontal region (with nuclei of the Pons, the red nucleus, and substantia nigra) can also be regarded as proof that this region possesses extrapyramidal functions, and thus plays a definite part in the activity of the motor analysor.

There are indications that connections exist between the frontal region and the hypothalamus (through the dorsomedial nucleus of the optic thalamus - Clark and Meyer [509]). This supports the existing assumption of the participation of this region in vegetative reactions.

The areas of the frontal region lie on the external, medial, and inferior surface of the hemisphere, and occupy the gyrus proreus (prorea) and the foremost section of the fornicate gyrus. On the external surface of the hemisphere, the frontal region is bounded by the anterior rhinal and presylvian sulci, and on the surface by the genual sulcus.

Within the frontal region, one can discern four areas and one transitional frontolimbic area. The areas are characterized by a weak differentiation of layers, wide layers I and III, the absence of a distinct layer IV, and a clearly defined boundary with white matter.

In areas F_1 and F_3, the cortex is of medium width and rich in large cells. Areas F_2 and F_4 are characterized by a narrow cortex and the absence of large cellular elements.

Limbic Area (*Regio Limbica*) (Fig. 90-93)

The connections and functions of the limbic region have not been thoroughly studied. A number of authors point to the direct connections of the limbic gyrus with the olfactory tubercle, the septum translucidum, the mammillary bodies (Smith [1141]), the stria olfactoria medialis (Kappers [33]; Savich [1137]), the reticular formation (Ward [1146]), and the subiculum (Adey [1089]).

In reporting his study of the function of the limbic region, Kasyanov [1117] suggested that the posterior limbic region has an intimate relation to the localization of nutritional, gustatory, and olfactory centers. In addition, he pointed out the connections of the posterior limbic subregion with the areas of the anterior limbic subregions, with area 4, and with the retrosplenial areas.

The work of Smith [1141] and Kremer [1120], carried out by means of electrostimulation, and that of Babkin and Kite [1097], who removed the posterior limbic region in the dog, suggest the participation of the limbic region in various vegetative reactions of the organism including the activity of the cardiovascular, respiratory, secretory, and digestive systems. Zambrzhitskiy [1148] assumes that the limbic region is responsible for the analysis and synthesis of chemical signals from the external and possibly the internal environment, on the basis of his study of the structure of the limbic region and a comparative anatomical analysis of the literature.

The differences in structure of the anterior and posterior portions of the limbic region point to their different functions.

The limbic region, which lies on the internal surface of the hemisphere, consists of two limbic areas L_1 and L_2 occupying the free surface of the limbic gyrus. In the posterior half of the limbic gyrus, they join the peritectal areas Pt_1 and Pt_2, and in the anterior half they join area Pt_3. All of these are located on the superior portion of the sulcus of the corpus callosum. Along the entire spread of the inferior portion of the splenial sulcus, there stands out clearly the formation L_1, which has signs of a limbic area as well as of areas which are located above the splenial sulcus. The structure of the free surface of the limbic gyrus on the same level has a number of insignificant modifications, but we do not see any purpose in regarding them as separate areas and subareas (Fig. 92).

Area O_1 (*Area Occipitalis Prima*) (Fig. 52)

Area O_1 occupies the posterior part of the marginal gyrus, and is surrounded on all sides by area O_2 (Fig. 50 and 51). On the outer surface of the hemisphere, the borderline of area O_1 crosses the free surface of the postsplenial gyrus and passes medial to the postlateral sulcus. On the internal surface of the hemisphere, the borderline extends over the free surface of the suprasplenial and the uplenial gyrus, dips into the depth of the retrosplenial sulcus, and emerges on the free surface in the posterior part of the postsplenial gyrus.

The upper level of the cortex is wider and has more cells than the lower level. The majority of cells are of a small, rounded, triangular, or irregular shape. The most typical characteristic of area O_1 is the exceptional width of layer *IV* and the palisade-like appearance (a gathering of the cells into small columns) of layer *VI*. The border of the white matter is clearly defined. The diameter of the cortex of area O_1 on an average equals 1.7 mm.

Layer *I* is narrow and has few cells; the cells present are small, rounded, and elongated. The boundary with layer *II* is uneven.

Layer *II* is poorly separated from layer *III*. The complex of layer *II + III* is narrow, consisting of small cells mostly of triangular shape.

Layer *IV* is wide and within it, there is a predominance of granular cells, divided into three sublayers: Sublayer IV^1 is narrow and full of cells; sublayer IV^2 has fewer cells, with single large cells of a rounded and irregular form; sublayer IV^3 is rich in cells.

Layer *V* is narrow and has few cells; it contains both small cells and the single layer cells of Meynert.

Layer *VI* is composed of triangular, spindle-shaped cells arranged in columns.

The most typical structure of area O_1 is on the internal (medial) surface of the hemisphere.

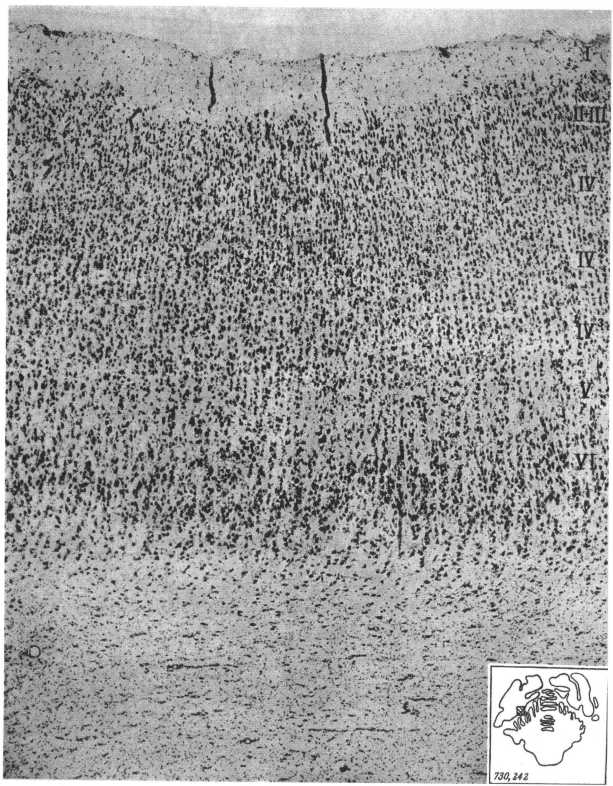

Figure 52 – Area *O₁*.

Area O_2 (*Area Occipitalis Secunda*) (Fig. 53, 54)

Area O_2 surrounds area O_1 on both surfaces (Fig. 50 and 51). On the external surface, it occupies the ectolateral and a part of the lateral gyrus. On the medial surface, it occupies the anterior parts of the suprasplenial and splenial gyri. It then enters the splenial sulcus (where it borders on area L) and emerges in the posterior parts of the postsplenial and splenial gyri. The anterior boundary of area O_2 passes in its upper paxt across the free surface of the lateral gyrus, where it joins area OP. In its middle portion, it extends deep inside the ectolateral sulcus; in the lower portion, along the free edge of the ectolateral gyrus, area O_2 is separated from T_1. On the medial surface of the hemisphere the border of area O_2 extends across the free surface of the suprasplenial, splenial (with the area OP), and postsplenial gyri, and partly in the depth of the splenial and retrosplenial sulci (with area L_1 and the areas of the entorhinal region).

The upper level of the cortex is considerably wider than the lower one, and has many more cells. In general, one may observe medium and large pyramidal cells among the microcellular elements in layer III; the radial striations are well defined. The boundary with white matter is clear. The average width of the cortex is 1.8 mm.

Layer I is narrow, consisting of small cells of a rounded or oval form diffusely arranged.

Layer II is also narrow and is poorly separated from layer III; it consists of small cells similar in shape to pyramidal cells.

Layer III is wide and is subdivided into two layers: The narrower sublayer III^{1+2} consists predominantly of small cells of a triangular and pyramidal shape; the wider sublayer III^3 consists of larger pyramidal cellular elements which occasionally reach considerable dimensions.

Layer IV is relatively narrow, and is not clearly separated from layer III and V; it consists of small cells mostly of a round form.

Layer V is light and narrow; here and there stand out separate large cells of a round or irregular shape and less frequently of a pyramidal form.

Layer VI is wide; the cells are arranged in siman columns.

Area O_2, in contrast to area O_1, characteristically has a much wider layer III and a narrower layer IV, a smaller number of cells in layer VI and clearer radial striations. Owing to these distinguishing features as enumerated above, the boundary between areas O_1 and O_2 is relatively clear.

In some places near the boundary of area O_2 with area O_1 there appear pyramidal cells of very large dimensions (Fig. 54) in layer III and V.

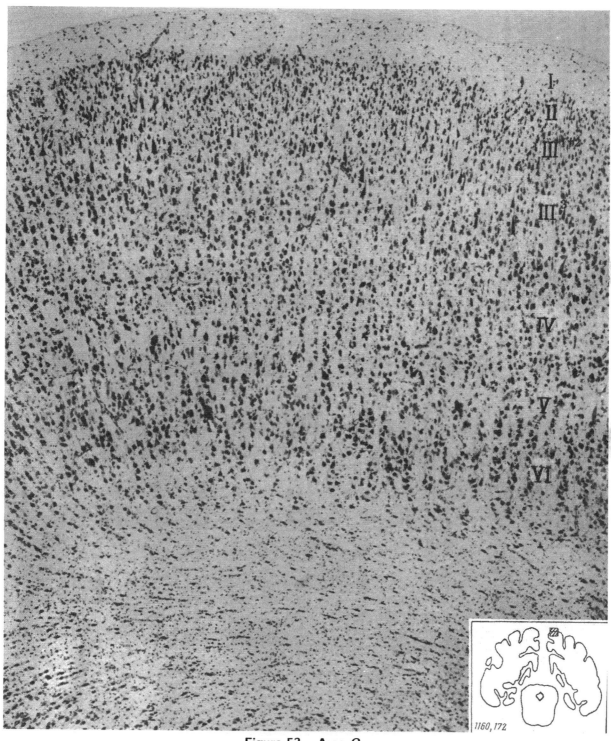

Figure 53 – Area O_2.

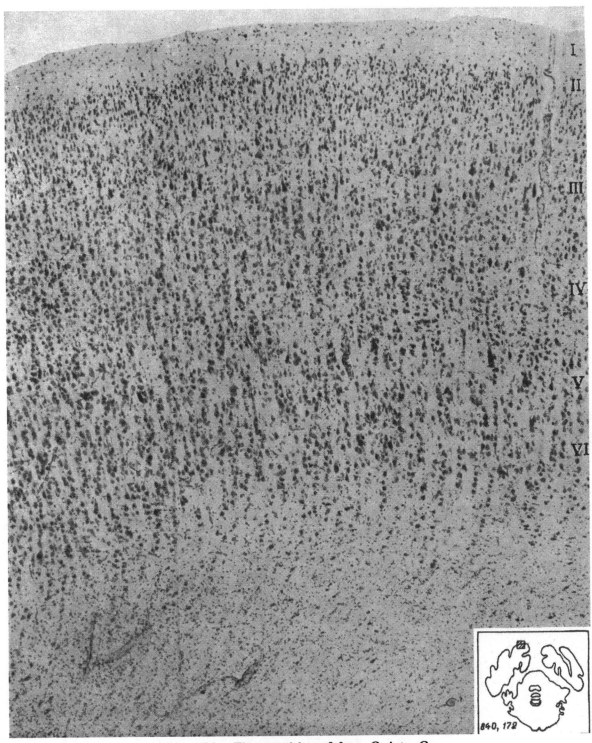

Figure 54 – The transition of Area O_1 into O_2.

Area *OP* (*Area Occipto Parietalis*) (Fig. 55, 56)

Area *OP* lies in the middle portion of the marginal gyrus, occupying the external and the medial surfaces of the hemisphere. It is bounded by the lateral and the splenial sulcus (Fig. 50 and 51). The anterior boundary (with area *P*) and the posterior boundary (with area O_2) extend across the free surface of the marginal gyrus. Area *OP* is a transitional structure having characteristics of the occipital as well as the parietal areas (area *P*).

The cells of the upper level of the cortex are smaller than the cells of the lower level. The majority of cells of the upper portion have a triangular or a pyramidal shape (except for layer *IV*). There is a predominance of rounded and spindle-shaped cellular elements in the lower level, which is less rich in cells. The cells are arranged in regular rows over the entire width of the cortex, which results in a clearly defined radial striation. The border with white matter is quite distinct. The average width of the cortex is 1.8 mm.

Layer *I* is of medium width. It is relatively rich in cells of a rounded and irregular shape and diffusely arranged.

Layer *II* is narrow and multicellular. It consists of small pyramidal and triangular cells. The boundary with layer *III* is rather distinct.

Layer *III* is wide and consists of cellular elements of mostly pyramidal and triangular shape. It is subdivided into two sublayers of approximately the same width: Sublayer III^{1+2} consists of small cells; the cells are larger in sublayer III^3. Medium sized pyramidal cells are found in these sublayers.

Layer *IV* is narrow; it consists of small rounded cells, poorly separated from the adjacent layers.

Layer *V* is clear. It is of medium width and consists of rather large cells of an irregular form.

Layer *VI* is narrow and consists of sparsely distributed polymorphous cells of small size extending in vertical rows.

Area *OP* differs from area O_2 in that it has larger cells in layer *II*; it has a narrower layer *III* containing a smaller number of large cells, and has a rather multicellular upper portion.

Layer *VI* consists of much smaller cells than those in the comparable layer of area O_2 (Fig. 56).

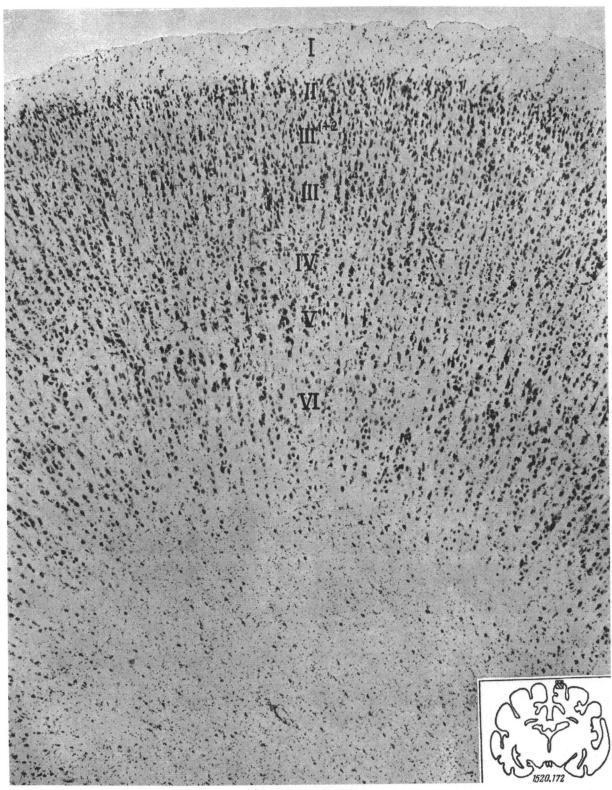

Figure 55 – Area *OP*.

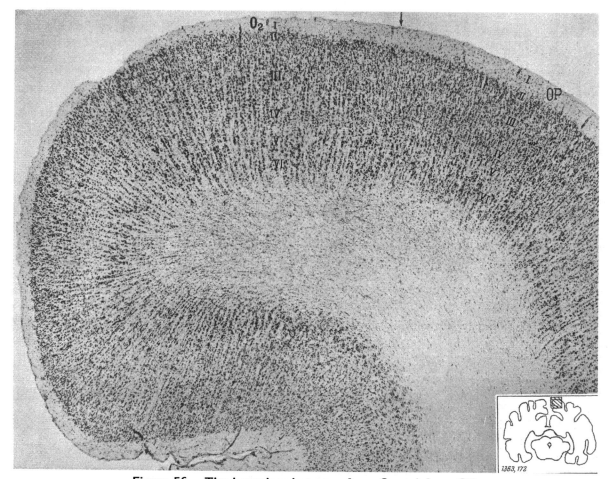

Figure 56 – The boundary between Area *O₂* and Area *OP*.

Area P (Area Parietalis) (Fig. 57, 58)

Area *P* lies on the external and medial surface of the hemisphere occupying the middle section of the marginal and suprasylvian gyri, and also the anterior section of the ectolateral gyrus (Fig. 50 and 51). On the external surface of the hemisphere the anterior boundary of area *P* (with area Pc_1) passes across the free surface of the suprasylvian and lateral gyri. The lower border of area *P* (with area T_4) is in the depth of the ectolateral sulcus; the upper border (with area *OP* and O_2) is partly in the depth of the lateral sulcus. On the medial surface of the hemisphere, the anterior and posterior boundaries of area *P* extend over the free surface of the marginal gyrus (with areas Pc_1 and *OP*); the lower medial border is in the depth of the splenial sulcus (with area L_1).

The cells of the rather narrow upper level of the cortex are smaller than the mass of fewer cells of the lower level. The upper level is richer in cells than the lower. One can see clearly striae of translucence in layers *III* and on the general background of the cortex, which is very rich in cells. Layer *IV* is clearly discernible. The radial striations extend across the entire thickness of the cortex; however, these striations are much coarser in the lower layers. The boundary with white matter is quite distinct. The diameter of the cortex on an average is 1.9 mm.

Layer *I* is of medium width and consists of small cells of a granular or oval form arranged diffusely.

Layer *II* is clear and multicellular, composed predominantly of small cells of a pyramidal form; the boundary with layer *III* is, in places, not sufficiently distinct.

Layer *III* is of an average width and consists of small and medium cells mostly of a pyramidal form. The size of the cells gradually increases within the layer. The middle section of layer *III* is lighter, which permits us to divide it into three sublayers: Sublayer III^1 is rich in cells, mostly of small size; sublayer III^2 is rarefied; sublayer III^3 consists of rather large cells.

Layer *IV* is narrow and rich in cells of a rounded and pyramidal form. The boundaries with layers *III* and *V* are quite distinct.

Layer *V* can be divided into two sublayers: Sublayer V^1 consists of pyramidal cells of a medium size but larger than in layer *III*; sublayer V^2 is relatively sparsely composed of cells of an irregular form.

Layer *VI* is relatively thick, and rich in rather large polymorphous cells; its boundary with layer *V* is distinct.

Area *P* is closer in structure to the areas of the optic analysor than to the areas of the analysor of general sensation (the postcoronal area). In contrast to area *OP*, differentiation of layers in area *P* is clearly evident; especially discernible are layers *III* and *IV*. Layer *VI* is richer in cells; the radial striations of the lower level are weakly developed (Fig. 58).

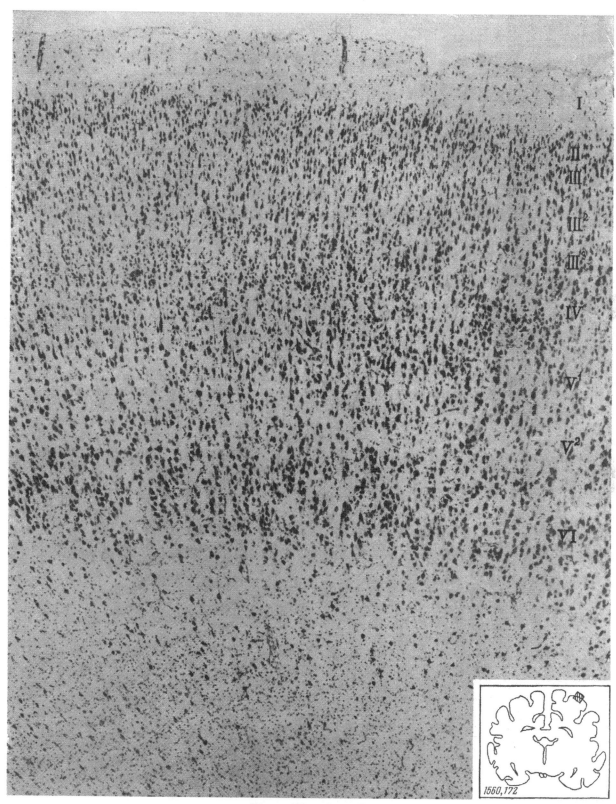

Figure 57 – Area *P*.

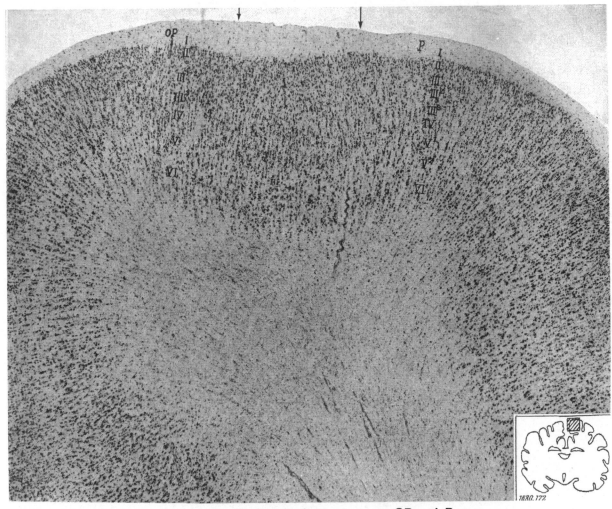

Figure 58 – The border between areas *OP* and *P*.

Area T_1 (*Area Temporalis Prima*) (Fig. 59)

Area T_1 is located in the posterior portion of the suprasylvian gyrus (Fig. 50 and 51).   Its posterior boundary, for the greater part, extends along the base of the ectolateral gyrus where area T_1 borders on area O_2; the lower boundary goes along the free surface of the ectolateral convolution, not quite reaching the posterior edge of the hemisphere separating area T_1 from area TE_1; the anterior boundary extends in the depth of the posterior section of the suprasylvian sulcus, separating area T_1 from areas T_2 and T_3.   The superior boundary extends across the free surface of the suprasylvian gyrus, approximately in the location of the transition of its middle and posterior sections, where area T_1 borders on area T_4.

Of all the temporal areas, the cortex of area T_1 is richest in cells; this is especially characteristic for layer V where, in contrast to other temporal areas, translucent striations do not appear.

The width of the cortex is 2.2 mm.   The upper level is richer in cells.   Its cells are smaller than in the lower portion and are closer in form to the pyramidal cells; the lower level of cortex consists of cellular elements, mostly spindle-shaped or irregular in form.   The differentiation of layers is poor.   Radial striations are more clearly defined in the upper portion.

Layer I is of medium width and consists of small cells of rounded shape; its boundaries with layer II are uneven and undulant.

Layer II consists of a large number of small cells.   Their form is closer to pyramids; layer II is poorly separated from layer III.

Layer III is wide.   Its cells increase in size in the depth of the layer.   In this connection, there can be observed a division into three sublayers: Sublayer III^1 consists of small cells; sublayer III^2 is less dense; sublayer III^3 consists of larger cells.

Layer IV does not stand out as an independent layer; its cells mingle with the cells of layers III and V.

Layer V is of medium width and usually consists of small cells, less frequently of large cells, mostly of an irregular shape.   In places, it is rarefied.

Layer VI is richer in cells than layer V and consists of small and medium-sized polymorphous cells; it is well separated from layer V by a light stria.

Area T_1 can be divided into two subareas: the superior subarea T^s_1 and the inferior subarea T^i_1.   In the latter, the superior portion cannot be divided into substrata.   Laterally, area T_1 changes into area O_2, differing from the latter in that it has a wider cortex, a somewhat more microcellular layer III, less distinct isolation of layer IV, and less evidence of translucence in layer V.

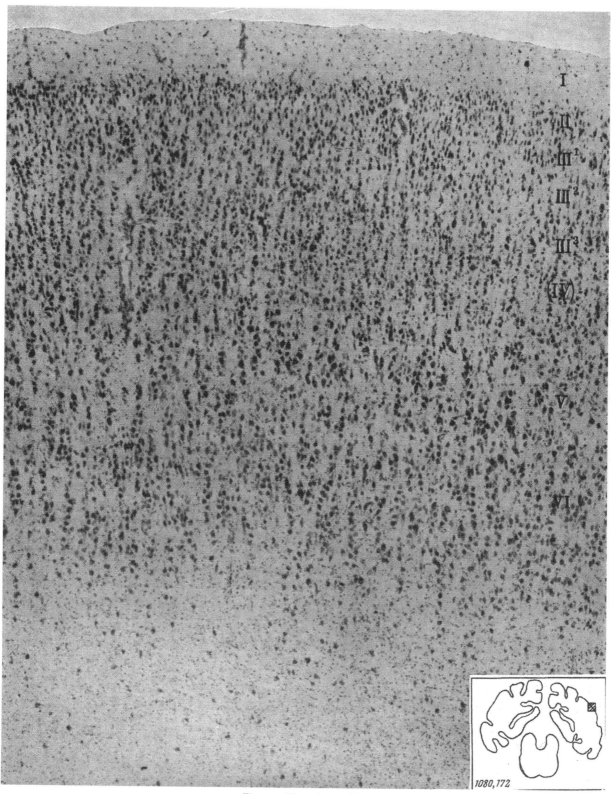

Figure 59 – Area T_1.

Area T_2 (*Area Temporalis Secunda*) (Fig. 60)

Area T_2 is located in the posterior portion of the ectosylvian gyrus (Fig. 50 and 51). The posterior boundary (with area T_1) extends over the floor of the posterior sector of the suprasylvian sulcus. The lower boundary (with the area TE_2) extends along the free surface of the posterior portion of the ectosylvian gyrus; the anterior boundary (with area Pl_1) is in the depth of the posterior sector of the ectosylvian sulcus; the auperior boundary with area T_3 extends partly across the free surface of the ectosylvian gyrus (approximately in the place of transition of the posterior and middle portions), and partly along the apical portion of the ectosylvian sulcus. The cortex of area T_2 is rich in cells; the cells of the upper level are similar in size to the cells of the lower portion. The horizontal striation is indistinct. The boundary with white matter is clearly defined. The diameter of the cortex averages about 2.2 mm.

Layer *I* is wide and is composed of small and medium cells of an irregular form. The boundary with layer *II* is uneven but less undulating than in area T_1.

Layer *II* is rich in cells; there is in it a predominance of medium-sized cells of spindle and triangular form. The boundary with layer *III* is indistinct.

Layer *III* is of medium width but narrower than in area T_1; it consists of medium sized cells which increase in size as they penetrate into the depth of this layer.

Layer *IV* is not clearly isolated; its cells penetrate into layers *III* and *V*.

Layer *V* is wide, consisting of medium sized cells of irregular form, and of single large cells. It contains two sublayers: Sublayer Vi is richer in cells and its cells are larger than the ones in the sublayer V^2. The latter contains well defined striae of translucence.

Layer *VI* is wide, and rich in large cells of irregular form arranged in vertical rows.

Area T_1 differs from area T_2 in that it has less well defined radial striations, is somewhat less multicellular, and contains more large cells. In the upper portion, the striae of translucence in layer V^2 are more distinct.

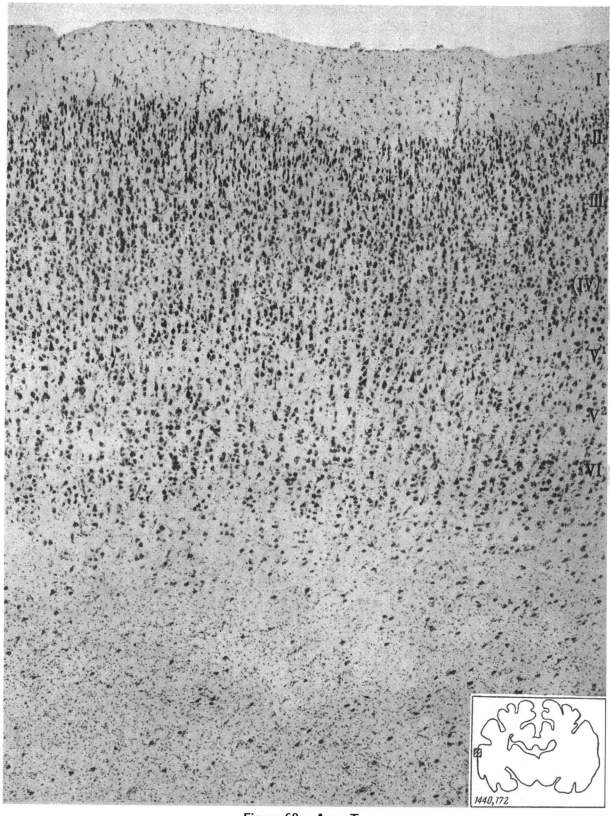

Figure 60 – Area *T₂*.

Area T_3 (*Area Temporalis Tertia*) (Fig. 61)

Area T_3 lies in the middle section of the ectosylvian gyrus (Fig. 50 and 51). Its posterior and anterior boundaries (with area T_2 and area TPc) extend partly along the free surface of the ectosylvian gyrus and partly along the apical process of the ectosylvian sulcus. Its inferior boundary (with area Pl_2) extends along the lower portion of the middle part of the ectosylvian sulcus, and the superior boundary (with areas T_4 and T_1) is along the base of the middle portion of the suprasylvian sulcus.

The cortex of area T_3 is rich in cells. Basically, the majority of cells are small and of a triangular or irregular form. The lower level of the cortex is of considerable width. The radial striations are distinct; the differentiation of layers is not clear and the boundary with white matter is abrupt. The width of the cortex is on an average 2.4 mm.

Layer I is of medium width and relatively rich in small cells.

Layer II is rich in small cells, similar in form to pyramidal cells. This layer is poorly separated from layer III.

Layer III is wide; it consists of small cells of irregular shape and has almost no large cells.

Layer IV is absent as an isolated layer. The cells of the layers III and V penetrate into it diffusely.

Layer V is very wide and is divided into two sublayers: Sublayer V^1 is rich in small and medium cells; there are single large cells. Sublayer V^2 contains striae of translucence.

Layer VI is wide and contains many cells of pyramidal form, which are strangely oriented to the cortical surface. It is richer in cells here than in area T_2.

In the posterior section, area T_3 consists of smaller cells than in the anterior section, where there appear single large cells of a pyramidal form in layers III and V; these cells are smaller than similar cells in area T_4. The cortex of area T_3 is wider than the cortex of area T_2; in contrast to the latter, there is a more distinct radial striation in area T_3. It is richer in cells. The cells are smaller than the cells of area T_2. In structure, T_3 resembles area T_1 but has more cells and somewhat inferior radial striations.

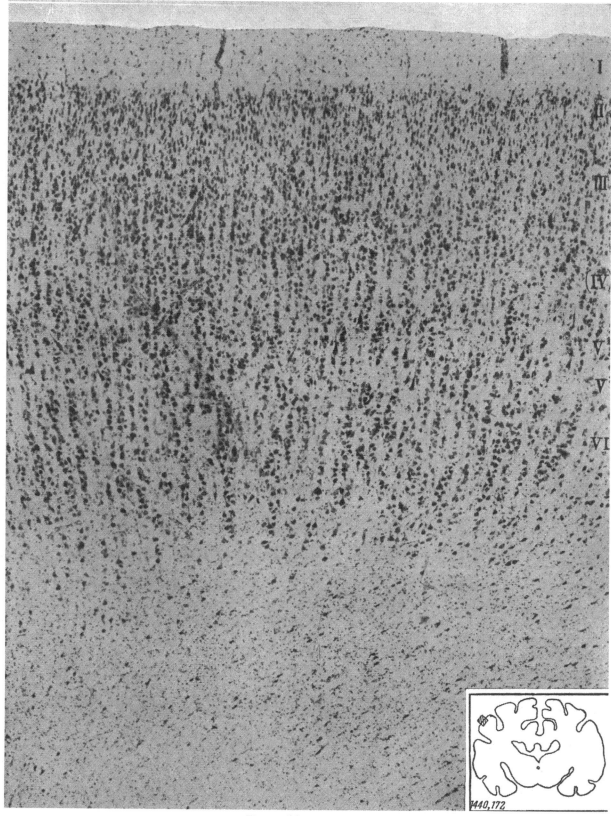

Figure 61 – Area T_3.

Area T_4 (*Area Temporalis Quarta*) (Fig. 62, 63)

Area T_4 is located in the middle section of the suprasylvian gyrus and surrounds area T_3 like a horseshoe (Fig. 50 and 51). The superior and anterior boundary with area P passes, partly, along the floor of the anterior sector of the ectolateral sulcus and partly along the free surface of the suprasylvian gyrus. The inferior boundary (with area T_3) extends inside the middle sector of the suprasylvian sulcus, and the posterior boundary (with area T_1) along the free surface of the suprasylvian gyrus.

The cortex of this area is rich in cells. Differentiation of the layers is well defined. This is related to the fact that most of the cells in layers *III* and *V* are large and of a pyramidal form, while the basic mass of cells in layers *II* and *IV* are small and of an irregular, triangular, and rounded form. There is possibly a stria of translucence in layer *V*. The radial striations extend over the entire thickness of the cortex. The boundary with white matter is clearly defined. In comparison with the other temporal areas, area T_4 contains the greatest number of large cells. The width of the cortex is on an average 1.8 mm.

Layer *I* is narrow and relatively rich in small cells.

Layer *II* is also narrow and very rich in small cells mostly of triangular shape; this layer is well separated from layer *III*.

Layer *III* can be divided into two sublayers: Sublayer III^{1+2} is rarefied and consists of small and medium-sized cells, mostly of pyramidal form and becoming larger on the inner aspect of the sublayer; sublayer III^3 consists of a large number of large cells of pyramidal form.

Layer *IV* is more clearly defined than in other temporal areas; the majority of cells are of a rounded and irregular form.

Layer *V* is of medium width; it is divided into sublayer V^1 consisting of large cells of pyramidal form, and sublayer V^2 which is less rich in cells.

Layer *VI* contains many spindle-shaped and triangular cells.

Compared with area T_3 the horizontal striations in area T_4 are well defined; there are considerably more large cells in layer *III* and *V*; layer *II* is better separated from layer *III*; layer *IV* is more clearly isolated.

Area T_4, in comparison with the adjacent area P, contains considerably more large cells (especially in layers *III* and *IV*); layer *IV* is less distinct in this area and layer *VI* has fewer cells (Fig. 63).

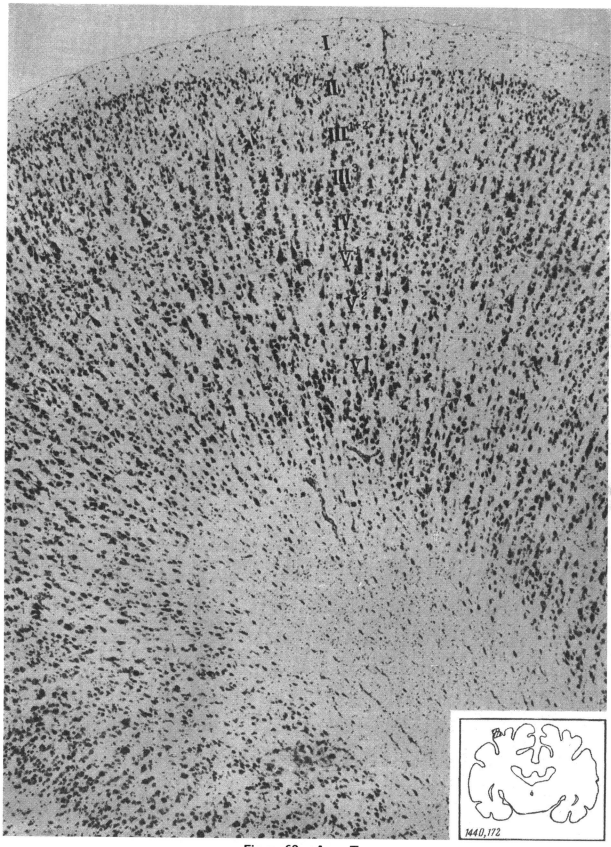

Figure 62 – Area T_2.

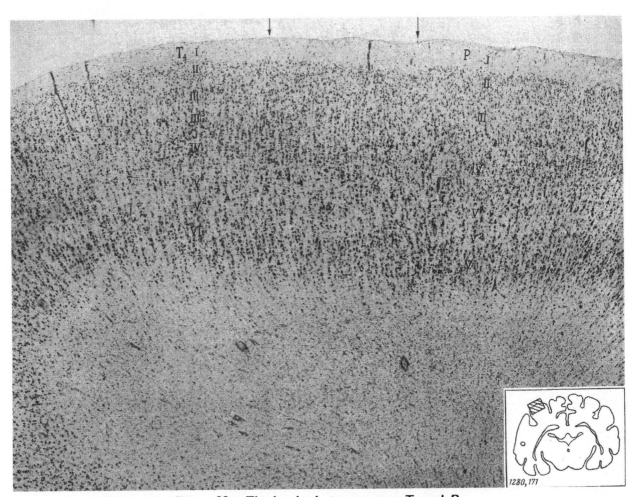

Figure 63 – The border between areas T_4 and P.

Transition of Cortical Areas from Temporal into the Entorhinal Region (TE_1 and TE_2) (Fig. 64-66)

Areas TE_1 and TE_2 are characterized primarily by the fact that layer II is of a mammillary form which is typical for the cortex of the entorhinal region bordering on these areas. The radial striations are very indistinct.

The cortex of areas TE_1 and TE_2, in contrast to the adjacent areas T_1 and T_2, contains a small number of cells. The majority of neurons are of an irregular form; layer II has a mammillary appearance and layer III does not divide into sublayers (Fig. 64).

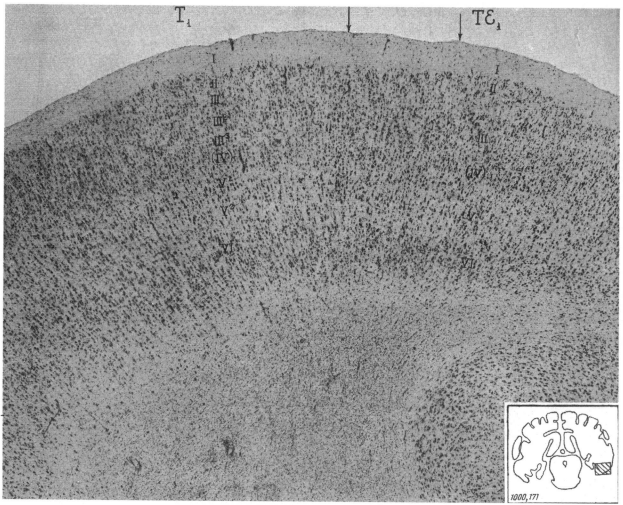

Figure 64 – The border between areas T_1 and TE_1.

Area *TE₁* (*Area Temporoentorhinalis Prima*) (Fig. 65)

Area TE_1 lies in the very lowest section of the suprasylvian gyrus, on the external as well as on the medial surface of the hemisphere (Fig. 50 and 51). The anterior boundary with area T_2, the superior boundary with area T_1, and the posterior boundary with area O_2 extend along the free surface of the suprasylvian gyrus. The boundary with the entorhinal subregion passes deep inside of the posterior rhinal sulcus.

The cortex of this area is not rich in cells. The lower portion is more rarefied and contains a great number of large cells of an irregular and rounded form (especially in layer V), as compared with areas T_1, T_2, T_3, and T_4. The horizontal and vertical radial striations are indistinct. The boundary with white matter is clearly defined. The diameter of the cortex is on an average 1.9 mm.

Layer I is very wide and contains small, rounded cells.

Layer II is composed of cells of diverse form, gathered into separate groups; it is well separated by a light stria from layer III, as if elevated above it.

Layer III is rather wide and consists of cells of various sizes and irregular form.

It is difficult to isolate layer IV as an independent layer. It is penetrated by cells of layers III and V.

Layer V is of medium width and rarefied. It contains separate large cells of an irregular form.

Layer VI has a distinct boundary with layer V, inasmuch as it is composed of smaller cells. It contains many cells which are oriented in a different direction toward the surface of the cortex.

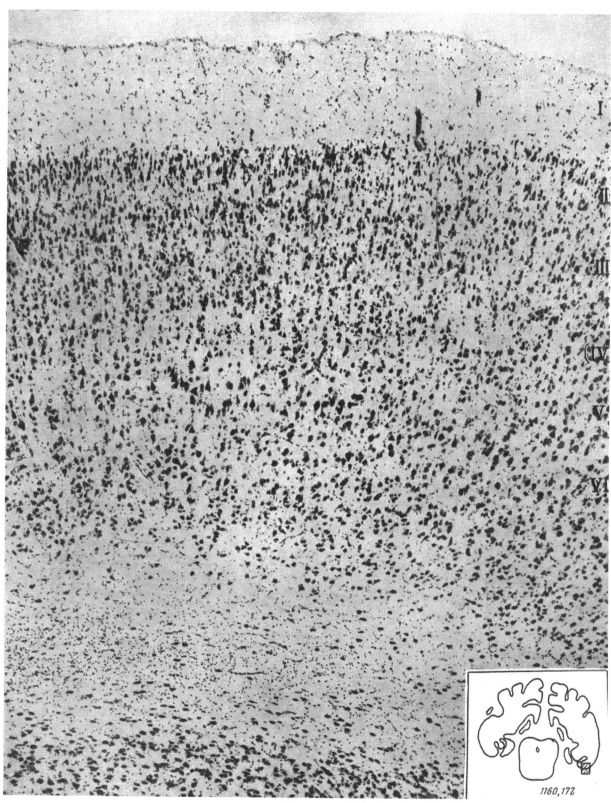

Figure 65 – Area *TE₁*.

Area *TE₂* (*Area Temporoentorhinalis Secunda*) (Fig. 66)

Area TE_2 lies on gyrus compositus posterior. The superior boundary (with areas Pl_1 and T_2) and the posterior boundary (with area T_2) extend along the free surface of the gyrus. The inferior boundary (with areas of the entorhinal region) extends in the depth of the posterior rhinal sulcus (Fig. 50 and 51).

Area TE_2 has a wide cortex (the width is approximately 2.2 mm). The cortex has few cells (except for layer II). The majority of cells are of irregular shape and medium size. Differentiation into layers is indistinct. The transition into the white matter is gradual.

Layer I is of medium width; it contains small, rounded cells sparsely distributed.

Layer II is rich in cells, mostly of triangular form, gathered into separate groups projecting into layer I, in the shape of "papillae."

Layer III is wide, rarefied, and consists of cells of an irregular and triangular form. The size of the cells increases gradually toward the inner portion of the layer.

Layer IV is missing.

Layer V is of medium width and has few cells, especially in its lower region. It is poorly separated from layer III. Its cells are somewhat larger than the cells of layer III.

Layer VI is wide, owing to the considerable number of elongated small cells; the boundary with layer V is quite clear. The transition of layer VI into the white matter is very gradual.

Area TE_2 differs from area TE_1 in that it has a wider cortex, more gradual transition into white matter, and a greater accumulation of large cells.

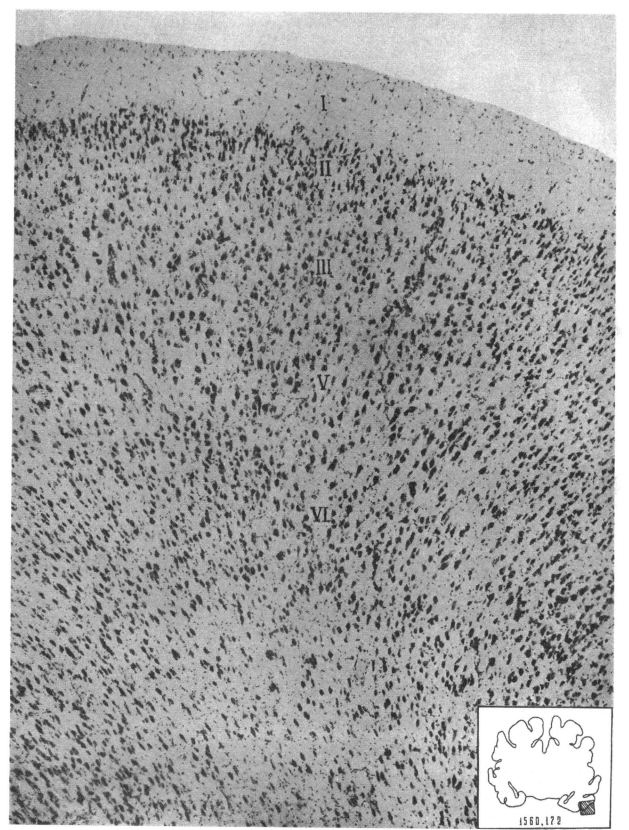

Figure 66 – Area *TE₂*.

Area I_1 (*Area Insularis Prima*) (Fig. 67)

Area I_1 lies in the anterior section of the sylvian gyrus and on the anterior wall of the sylvian sulcus (Fig. 50 and 51). The inferior boundary of area with the formations of the prepyriform region extends along the rhinal sulcus. Posteriorly area I_1 is bounded by the sylvian sulcus. The anterior and superior boundaries of the area extend along the surface of the anterior section of the sylvian gyrus, parallel to the anterior portion of the ectosylvian sulcus.

Area I_1 has a wide cortex (width 2.5 mm) with few cells. The lower level is considerably wider than the upper. The cells of the upper level are basically small and of a triangular form, while the majority of the cells of the lower level have an irregular form and reach large dimensions.

Layer *I* is of medium width, formed of small cells.

Layer *II* is narrow. It is rich in cells mostly of triangular form. It is well separated from sublayer III^{1+2} which contains few cells. The boundary with layer *I* is uneven.

Layer *III* is wide and is divided into two sublayers: Sublayer III^{1+2} contains a small number of small cells of triangular form; sublayer III^3 is richer in cells, which also are larger, and this sublayer blends gradually into layer *V*.

Layer *IV* is missing.

Layer *V* is wide and contains two sublayers: Sublayer V^1 is rich in rather large cells, larger than those of layer *III*; sublayer V^2 has a few cells and shows a stria of translucence.

Layer *VI* also is wide. It is composed of cells of various sizes. It is subdivided into a rather multicellular upper layer and a less multicellular lower layer. The transition into white matter is gradual.

A considerable part of area I_1 occupies the wall and the floor of the sylvian sulcus, and here its structure is somewhat different from that on the free surface. The cortex is narrower and there are no radial striations; the majority of the cellular elements show rounded or irregular forms, and rather large cells in layer *V*. The cells of layer *VI* blend immediately into the cells of the claustrum (Fig. 72).

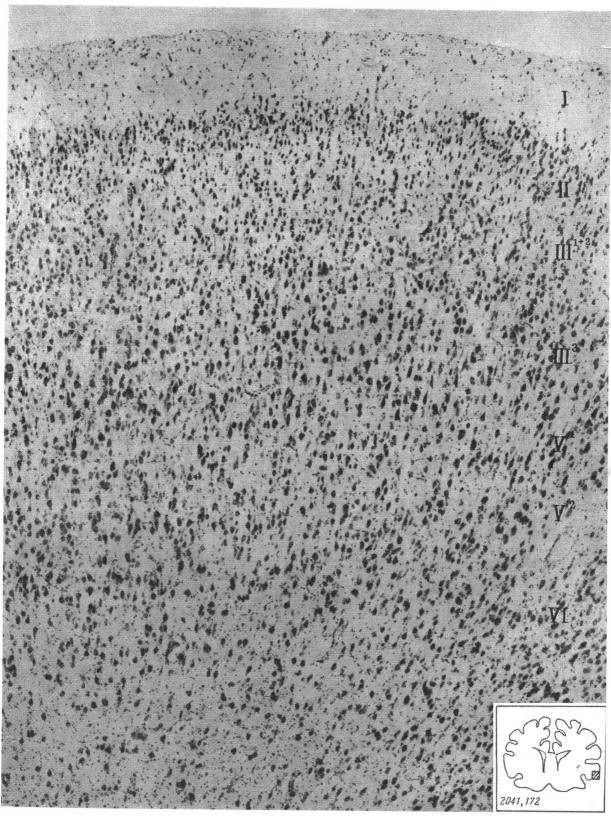

Figure 67 – Area *I₁*.

Area I_2 (*Area Insularis Secunda*) (Fig. 68)

Area I_2 lies on the external surface of the hemisphere in the posteroinferior part of gyrus proreus (Fig. 50 and 51). The area has a triangular form, bounded by the sector of the anterior rhinal sulcus and the presylvian sulcus. The anterior boundary (with area F_1) extends along the free surface of gyrus proreus.

Area I_2 has a wide cortex (the width is approximately 2.6 mm). The upper portion is rich in small cells, mostly of triangular form. The lower portion is wide and has few cells, mostly rounded and irregular in form. The radial striations are far more distinct in the lower level.

Layer *I* is wide and relatively rich in cells of predominantly small size.

Layer *II* is rich in cells of small and medium size gathered into separate groups. As a result of this the boundary with layer *I* has an undulating appearance.

Layer *III* is wide and rich in cells of relatively small size. Layer *IV* is missing.

Layer *V* is wide, consists of a small number of medium sized cells, and is rarefied in its entire thickness.

Layer *VI* is wide and richer in cells than layer *V*. It consists of medium sized cells varying in form and adjoining the cells of the claustrum.

Area I_2 differs from area I_1 in that it is richer in cells in the upper layers and the cells vary greatly in size and form.

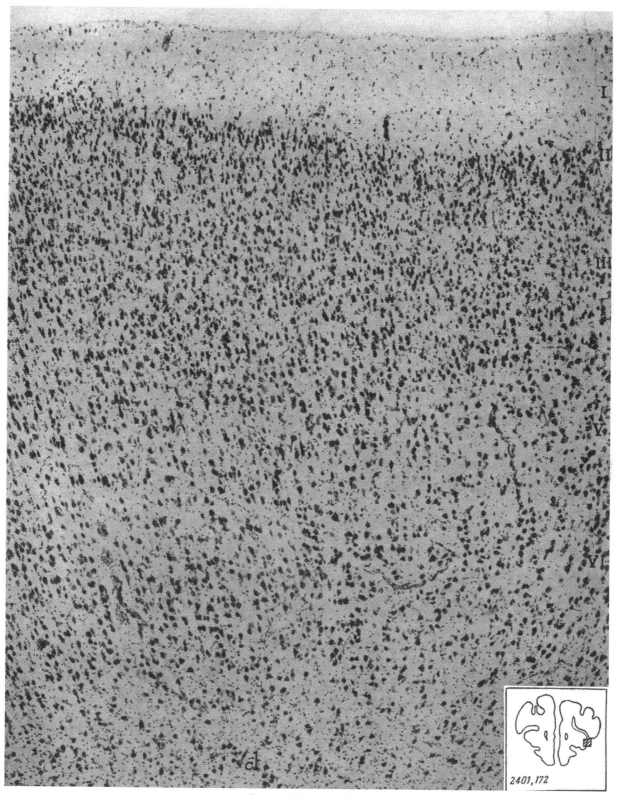

Figure 68 – Area I_2.

Area PI₁ (Area Parainsularis Prima) (Fig. 69)

Area PI_1 lies on the external surface of the hemisphere in the posterior portion of the sylvian gyrus (Fig. 50 and 51). The anterior boundary of area PI_2 (with area I_2) extends within the depth of the sylvian sulcus. The superior boundary (with area PI_2) is along the surface of the sylvian gyrus. The posterior boundary (with area T_2) extends partly across the free surface of the inferior section of the ectosylvian gyrus and partly deep inside of the posterior ectosylvian sulcus.

Area PI_1 has a wide cortex (the width is 2.6 mm). The cortex is rich in cells especially in the upper portions. The cells of the upper level are predominantly triangular; the cells of the lower level are predominantly rounded. The area is characterized by radial striations extending across the entire thickness of the cortex, a very wide layer III, and translucence in layer V. The boundary with the white matter is gradual.

Area PI_1 has a wide cortex (the especially in the upper portions. triangular; the cells of the lower characterized by radial striations cortex, a very wide layer III, and the white matter is gradual.

Layer I is of medium width and consists of small rounded cells.

Layer II is composed mostly of smaller cells. Its boundary with layer I is undulating. Layer II appears as if it were elevated above layer III.

Area III is very wide and is divided into three sublayers: Sublayer III^1 is rich in smaller cells; sublayer III^2 consists of small and medium sized cells and is translucent in its middle section; sublayer III^3 has fewer cells, which are larger than those in sublayers III^1 and III^2.

Layer IV as an independent layer is missing. It is represented by small granular cells located between the cells of layer III.

Layer V is wide, has fewer cells, and divides into two sublayers: Sublayer V^1 is composed of scattered cells, both medium sized and large; sublayer V^2 has stria of translucence in which there are separate large cells.

Layer VI is rich in cells of various sizes. It is clearly separated from layer V. As it blends into white matter the number of cells gradually decreases.

In comparison with area I_1 area PI_1 is characterized by its greater number of cells, a greater width of layer III, and a more distinct division of layers. It differs from area T_2 in that it has a wider cortex, clearer separation of layer II from III, a much wider layer III, and a gradual transition into white matter.

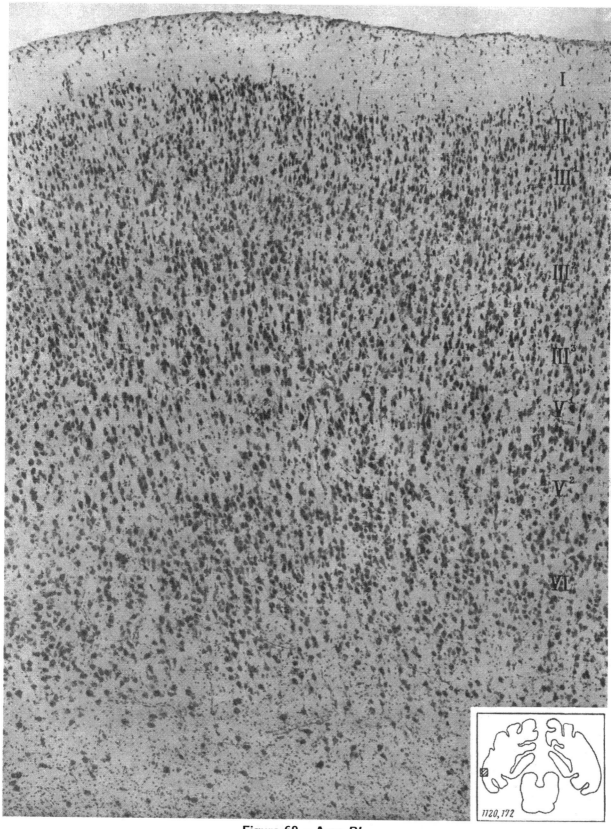

Figure 69 – Area *PI₁*.

Area PI₂ (Area Parainsularis Secunda) (Fig. 70)

Area PI_2 is located on the external surface of the hemisphere in the superior part of the sylvian gyrus, in the shape of a horseshoe, above area I_1 and PI_1 (Fig. 50 and 51). The anterior, superior, and posterior boundaries extend deep within the ectosylvian sulcus, separating area PI_2 from areas TPC, T_3, and T_2. The inferior boundary extends across the surface of the sylvian gyrus, parallel to the ectosylvian sulcus.

Area PI_2 has a wide cortex (about 2.5 mm) with clearly visible radial striations. The upper layers are richer in cells than the lower layers; the lower layers are wider than the upper layers. The majority of the cells of the upper layers are of triangular and pyramidal form. In the lower layers, there is a predominance of cells of a rounded and irregular form. The cortex shows striae of cellular accumulations in layer II, III, and V. The transition into white matter is gradual.

Layer I is of medium width.

Layer II consists of a large number of cells of small size. It is clearly isolated from layer III by the translucent stria.

Layer III is wide, rich in cells, and distinctly divided into three sublayers: Sublayers III^1 and III^3 contain somewhat fewer cells than the clearly defined sublayer III^2; sublayer III^2 is composed of larger cells than sublayer III^3.

Layer IV is missing.

Layer V is wide and is divided into two sublayers: Sublayer V^1 is rich in cells of medium size mostly irregular but occasionally triangular, with a few single larger cells; sublayer V^2 is formed by a stria of translucence.

Layer VI is wide and contains a great number of cells of various forms. It is not distinctly separated from layer V, and the number of cells gradually decreases toward the white matter.

Area PI_2 differs from area PI_1 in the structure of layer III. Sublayers III^1 and III^3 in area PI are less rich in cells than sublayer III^2; area PI_1 sublayer III^2 is rather translucent.

In area PI_2, as compared with area PI_1, layer IV is missing. Also area PI_2 is characterized by a finer radial striation. In comparison with area I_1 the layers in area PI_2 are better differentiated: there is a translucence on the boundary of layers III and III and in sublayer III^3, and a fine radial striation (Fig. 72).

Area PI_2 differs from area T_3 in that it shows clearer separation of the layers, it has larger cells in layer III and V, and the transition into white matter is gradual rather than abrupt.

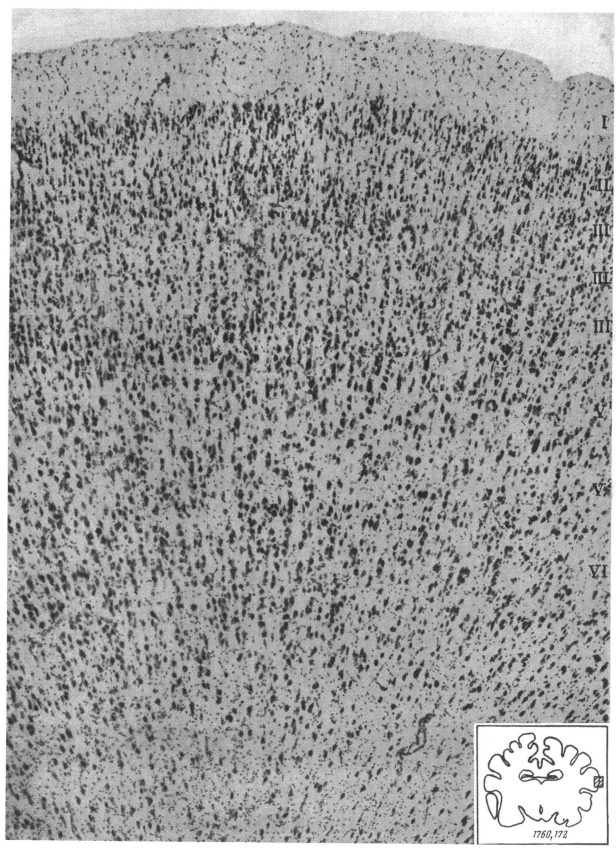

Figure 70 – Area *Pl₂*.

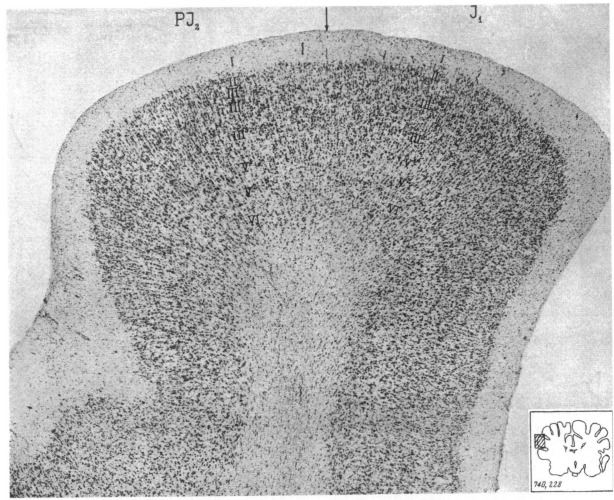

Figure 71 – The border of areaas I_1 and PI_2.

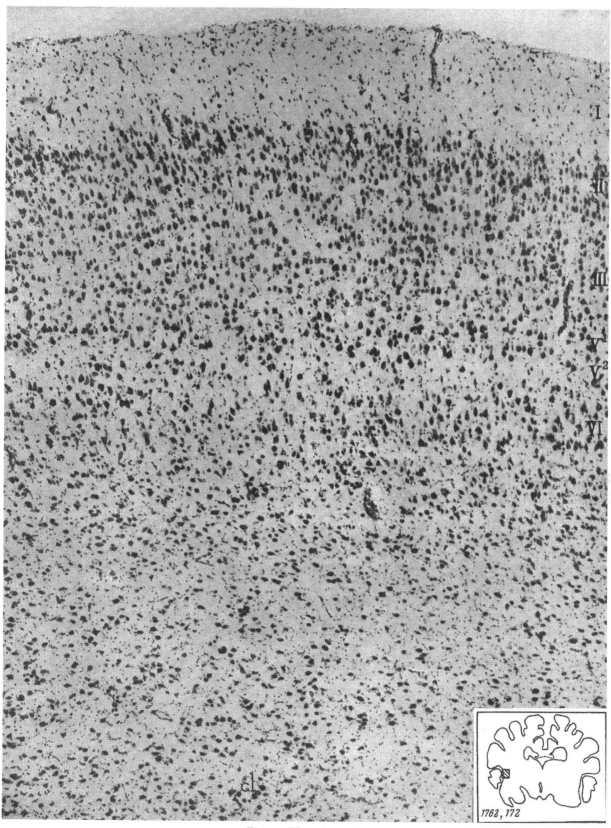

Figure 72 – Area *I₁*.

Area Pc₁ (Area Postcoronalis Prima) (Fig. 73)

Area Pc_1 is located on the external and medial surface of the hemisphere, occupying the posterior part of the coronal gyrus and the anterior section of the marginal gyrus (Fig. 50 and 51). On the external surface of the hemisphere, the lower boundary passes across the anterior sector of the suprasylvian sulcus, separating area Pc_1 from area TPc; the anterior boundary (with area Prc_1 and Pc_2) and the posterior boundary (with area P) extend over the free surface of the above mentioned gyri. On the medial surface of the hemisphere, the inferior boundary extends in the depth of the anterior portion of the uplenial sulcus (separating area Pc_1 from the limbic areas).

The cortex of this area is rich in cells, especially in the upper portion. The basic mass of cells are of an irregular and polyangular form. A subdivision of the cortex into layers is clearly visible. There are a great number of large cells in layers III and V, similar in size to the pyramidal cells of Betz in layer V. In the lower layers, there is a clearly defined radial striation. The boundary with white matter is abrupt. The diameter of the cortex averages 1.7 mm.

Layer I is narrow and relatively rich in cells.

Layer II is narrow, rich in cells, mostly of small size and rounded and irregular form. It is rather clearly separated from layer III.

Layer III is wide; the size of its cells increases as one penetrates deeper into the layer. This makes it possible to divide this layer into three sublayers: Sublayer III^1 contains small cells of a pyramidal and polyangular form; sublayer III^2 is formed of larger cells than sublayer III^1, in sublayer III^3, there are sometimes large cells of a triangular and an irregular form.

Layer IV contains small cells of irregular form. It is penetrated by the cells of layers III and V.

Layer V is not wide, and is divided into two sublayers: Sublayer V^1 contains numerous very large cells occurring in groups or singly, and similar in size and form to the gigantic pyramidal cells of Betz; sublayer V^2 has few cells.

Layer VI is of medium width and contains a great number of medium-sized, triangular and spindle-shaped cells, arranged in radial rows.

Of all postcoronal areas, area Pc_1 has the most cells and contains the greatest number of large cells. Area Pc_1 differs greatly in structure from the adjoining area P. Area Pc_1 contains a great number of cells, especially in layers II and III. Its cells are much larger than the cells in area P. Layer V contains very large cells similar in size to the gigantic pyramidal cells of Betz.

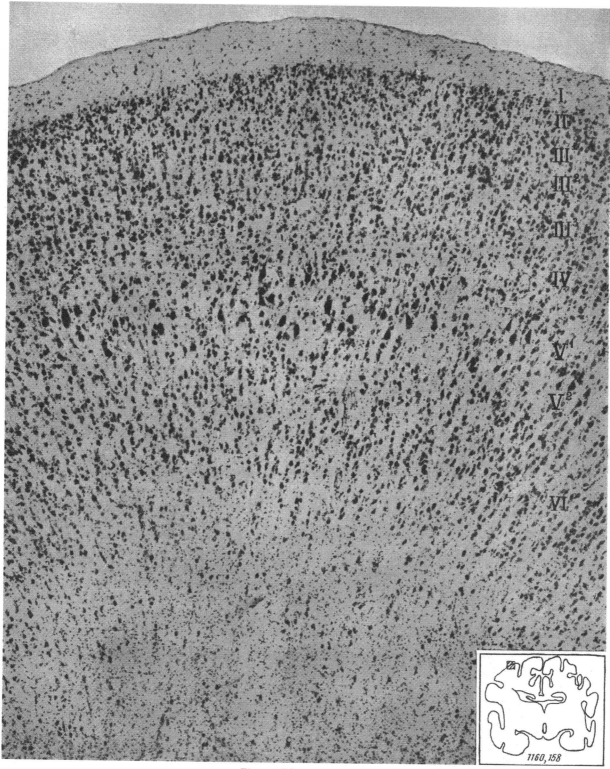

Figure 73 – Area Pc_1.

Area Pc_2 (*Area Postcoronalis Secunda*) (Fig. 74)

Area Pc_2 is located in the middle portion of the coronal gyrus (Fig. 50 and 51). The lower boundary, separating area Pc_2 from area TPc, extends along the anterior section of the suprasylvian aulcus. The superior boundary is in the depth of the coronal sulcus; the anterior (with area Pc_3) and the posterior (with area Pc_3) boundaries extend over the free surface of the coronal gyrus.

Of all postcoronal areas, area Pc_2 has the smallest nuMber of cells. The cortex of this area is of medium width (1.8 mm). The upper part is relatively rich in cells and the lower part is rarefied and somewhat wider. By far the greatest number of cells of layers *II*, *III*, and *V* are of a triangular and pyramidal form. Layers *IV* and *VI* are composed of rounded and spindle-shaped cells. Layer *V* contains single, very large cells of a pyramidal form. Radial striations are more distinct in the lower level.

Layer *I* is narrow and relatively rich in cells.

Layer *II* is narrow and is composed of small triangular and irregular cells. It is well separated from layer *III* by a stria of translucence.

Layer *III* is of medium width and is divided into two sublayers: Sublayer *II* III^{1+2} has fewer small and medium sized cells; sublayer III^3 contains a great number of large cells of a pyramidal form.

Layer *IV* is poorly developed. It is penetrated by large cells of layers *III* and *V*.

Layer *V* is wide and has few cells. One finds in it single very large cells of a pyramidal form.

Layer *VI* is of medium width and is relatively rich in cells of avail and medium size, arranged in columns, It is well separated from the less dense layer *V*.

Area Pc_2 differs from area Pc_1 in that it has fewer cells, less pronounced differentiation of the layers, larger cells in layer *III* and fewer very large cells in layer *V* (Fig. 79).

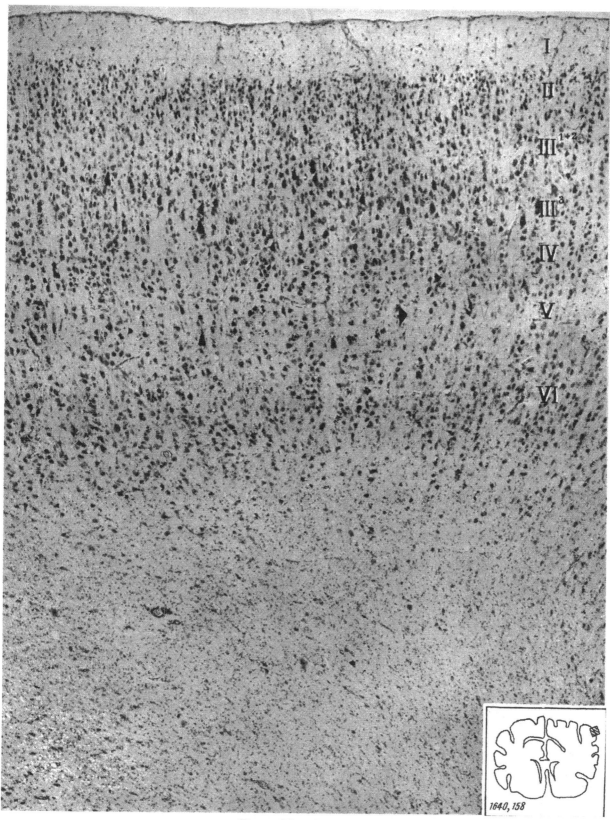

Figure 74 – Area *Pc₂*.

Area Pc₃ (Area Postcoronalis Tertia) (Fig. 75)

Area Pc_3 lies in the anterior portion of the coronal gyrus (Fig. 50 and 51). The superior boundary (with area Prc_1) extends along the coronal sulcus; the posterior boundary (with area Pc_2) is along the free surface of the coronal gyrus; the inferior boundary (with area Pc_4) is partly along the anterior sector of the suprasylvian sulcus and partly along the free surface of the coronal gyrus.

The width of the cortex of area Pc_3 is 1.6 mm. The upper portion (especially layers *II* and *III*) is rich in cellular elements of various forms; the lower portion is less rich in cells. One finds rather large cells in layer *III* and *V*, closer in form to the pyramidal cells, but there are fewer of them than in areas Pc_1 and Pc_2. The cortex is characteristic for its radial striation, which extends over all layers, for an abrupt boundary with white matter, and for a clearly expressed stria of translucence in layer *V*.

Layer *I* is narrow and rich in cells of a rounded form.

Layer *II* consists of a great number of small cells, mostly of irregular form and is poorly separated from layer *III*.

Layer *III* is rich in cells. Their size increases as one penetrates deeper into this layer. As a result, one can distinguish sublayer III^{1+2}, consisting of cells of small and medium size, and sublayer III^3 consisting basically of large cells.

Layer *IV* is narrow and is composed of cells of predominantly rounded and irregular form. It is penetrated diffusely by cells of layers *III* and *V*.

Layer *V* is rarefied and composed of medium sized cells. One also finds in it single large and even gigantic cells of a pyramidal form.

Layer *VI* is rich in cells of various forms; it is distinctly separated from layer *V*.

Area Pc_3 differs from area Pc_2 in that it has fewer large cells in layers *III* and *V*, more cells in the upper portions, and a clearer isolation of layer *IV*.

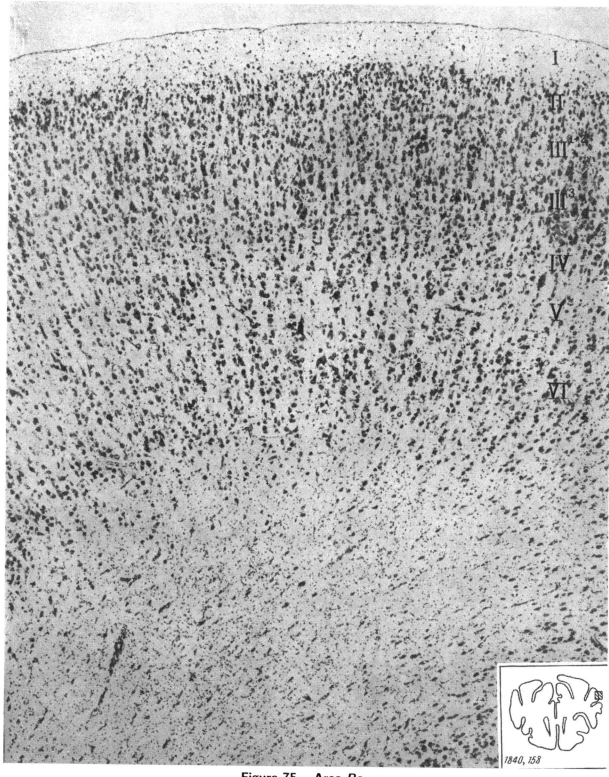

Figure 75 – Area Pc_3.

Subarea Pc^s_4 (*Subarea Postcoronalis Quarta Superior*) (Fig. 76)

Subarea Pc^s_4 is characterized by a cortex of medium width (1.8 mm), rich in cells. The upper portion is much wider than the lower and contains a great number of cells, mostly of triangular and less frequently of an irregular form. In layers *III* and *V* there are large cells of a pyramidal form but there are fewer of them and they are smaller than in the corresponding layers of areas Pc_1, Pc_2, and Pc_3. The radial striations extend across the entire diameter of the cortex. The boundary with white matter is clearly defined.

Layer *I* is of medium width and contains fewer cells than areas Pc_1, Pc_2, and Pc_3.

Layer *II* is composed of small, densely grouped cells, and as a result, it is well separated from layer *III* which is less rich in cells.

Layer *III* is wide and consists of two sublayers: Sublayer III^{1+2} contains fewer and smaller cells than sublayer III^3; sublayer III^3 is rich in cells of medium size. One finds in them single large cells of a pyramidal form.

Layer *IV* is composed of a considerable number of smaller cells of a rounded form. The separation from layers *III* and *V* is less abrupt.

Layer *V* is of medium width and is divided into two sublayers: Sublayer V^1 is rich in cells and contains single large cells of a pyramidal form; sublayer V^2 has fewer cells.

Layer *VI* is rich in cells of medium size and of a rounded and irregular form. It is well separated from layer *V*, which has fewer cells.

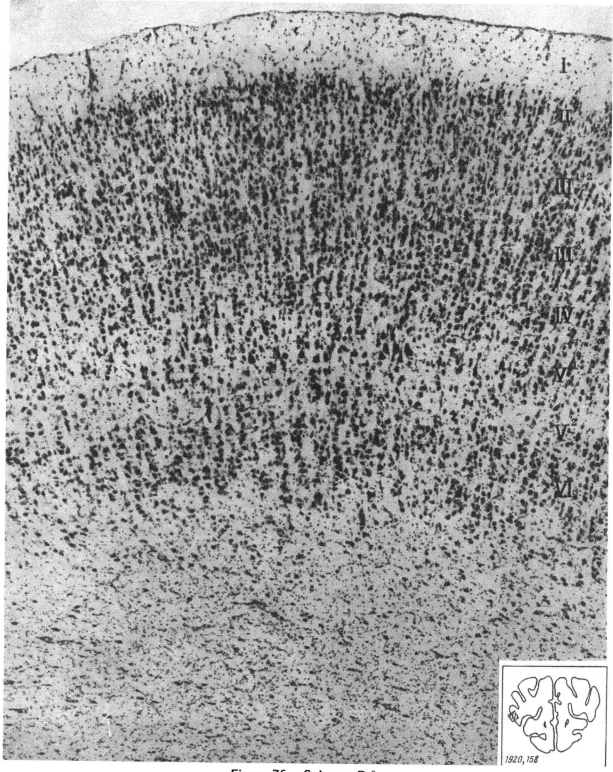

Figure 76 – Subarea *Pc*^s₄

Subarea Pc$^i_4$ (*Subarea Postcoronalis Quarta Inferior*) (Fig. 77)

The following are characteristic for both subarea Pc$^i_4$ and subarea Pc$^s_4$: The cortex is of medium width (1.75 mm), the form of the cellular elements is similar, there is a large number of cells in the upper layers, striae of translucence are in layer *V*, and there is an abrupt transition into white matter.

In contrast to subarea Pc$^s_4$, there is an absence of large cells in layers *III* and *V* in subarea Pc$^i_4$. The radial striations as well as the subdivisions of the cortex into layers are less distinct.

Layer *I* is of medium width and consists of small and medium-sized cells of various forms.

Layer *II* is narrow and is composed of small cells, mostly of triangular form. It is poorly separated from layer *III*.

Layer *III* is of medium width and is divided into two sublayers: Sublayer *III^{1+2}* has fewer cells than sublayer *III^3*; the cells of sublayer *III^3* are larger than those in sublayer *III^{1+2}*.

Layer *IV* is narrow and is composed of small cells of a rounded form. It is penetrated by cells of layers *III* and *V*.

Layer *V* is of medium width and has few cells, mostly medium sized; occasionally there are single large cells of a pyramidal form.

Layer *VI* is relatively wide, and the upper portion is rich in cells of various forms. The lower portion contains a smaller number of cells.

Area Pc$_4$ differs from the adjacent area Pc$_3$ in that it has a more distinct radial striation, more cells in the upper layers, smaller cells in layers *III* and *V*, and a wider layer *VI* (Fig. 80).

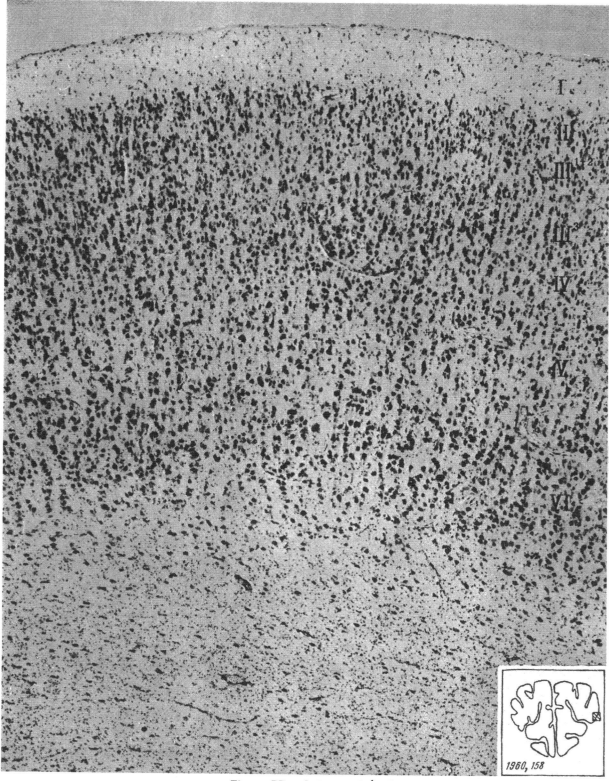

Figure 77 – Subarea Pc^j_4

Area TPc (Area Temporopostcoronalis) (Fig. 78)

Area *TPc* lies in the anterior section of the ectosylvian gyrus (Fig. 50 and 51). Its superior boundary extends along the anterior portion of the suprasylvian sulcus which delimits *area TPc* and areas Pc_2 and Pc_1. The posterior boundary (with area T_3) passes partly across the processus acominis of the ectosylvian sulcus and partly across the free surface of the ectosylvian gyrus at the transition of its anterior middle sections. The inferior boundary passes in the depth of the anterior portion of the ectosylvian sulcus, which separates areas *TPc* and Pl_2. The anterior boundary (with area Pc_4) runs across the free surface of the anterior portion of the ectosylvian gyrus.

Area *TPc* represents a gradual transition from the areas of the temporal region to the areas of the postcoronal region but is, according to its structure, closer to the latter.

Area *TPc* has a cortex of medium width (1.9 mm). The upper levels are narrower than the lower, and richer in cells; in layer *V* one finds very large cells. The differentiation of the cortex into layers is well expressed. Radial striations extend distinctly across the entire width.

Layer *I* is of medium width and is composed of small cells of rounded form.

Layer *II* is narrow and very rich in cells which are mostly of a triangular shape. The boundary with layer *I* is undulant. Layer *II* is well isolated from layer *III*.

Layer *III* is narrow and is divided into two sublayers: Sublayer III^{1+2} has few cells; in sublayer III^3 there are single large cells of a pyramidal form together with small, widely scattered cells.

Layer *IV* does not form a compact layer. In places, it is diffusely penetrated by cells of layers *III* and *V*.

Layer *V* is wide and is clearly divided into two sublayers: Sublayer V^1 is rich in cells; in it, one finds single, very large cells of a pyramidal form. Sublayer V^2 is poor in cells and contains a wide stria of translucence.

Layer *VI* is wide and has few cells; these are mostly small, oval, elongated, and arranged in thin radial raws.

Toward the back, area *TPc* changes into area T_3. It differs from the latter in that it has a narrower cortex, better isolation of layer *II* from layer *III*, very large cells of a pyramidal form in sublayer V^1, and a distinct stria of translucence in sublayer V^2. Area *TPc*, in comparison with area Pc_4, is much poorer in cells and shows a better radial striation of the lower portion.

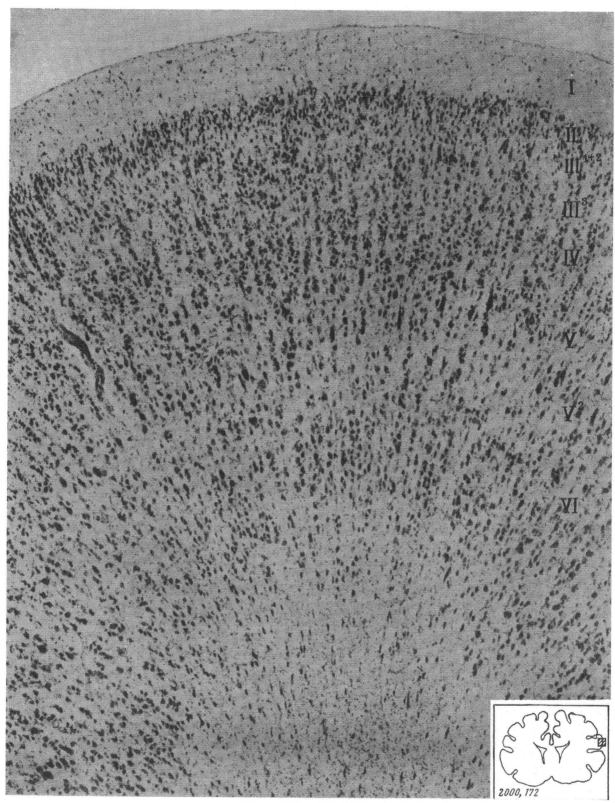

Figure 78 – Area *TPc*

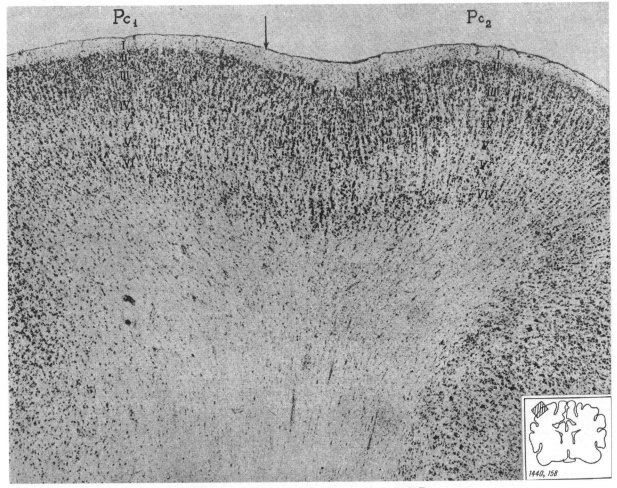

Figure 79 – The border of area Pc_1 and Pc_2.

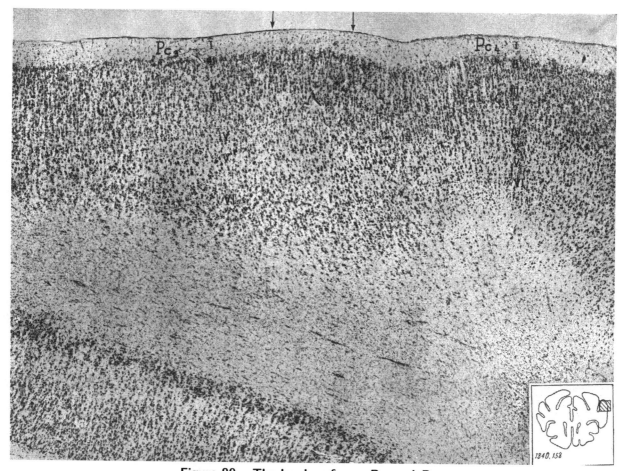

Figure 80 – The border of area Pc_3 and Pc_4.

Area Prc₁ (Area Praecoronalis Prima) (Fig. 81)

Area Prc_1 lies on the external and medial surfaces of the hemispheres occupying a small portion of the anterior and almost all of the posterior portion of the sigmoid gyrus (Fig. 50 and 51). In front it is bounded (from area Prc_2) by the cruciate sulcus. Below (from areas Pc_2 and Pc_3) it is bounded by the coronary sulcus; at the back, the boundary with area Pc extends across the free surface of the marginal gyms. On the medial surface of the hemisphere the anterior section of the splenial sulcus separates area Prc_1 from the anterior limbic area L_2.

Area Prc_1 is characterized by a rather narrow cortex (the width is 1.5 mm), an abundance of cells in the upper portion where there are mostly small and medium sized cells of a triangular form, a large number of gigantic pyramidal cells of Betz in layer V, the absence of layer IV, and an indistinct radial striation of the upper layers of the cortex. The boundary with white matter is distinct.

Layer I is of medium width and is rich in cells.

Layer II is narrow, very rich in small cells, and clearly separated from layer III.

Layer III is rather wide and rich in cells, which increase in size deeper in the layer. In the center of this layer, there is an area of translucence. All this makes it possible to divide layer III into three sublayers: Sublayer III^1 is composed of small cells; sublayer III^2 contains fewer cells than sublayer III^1, some of these being single, rather large cells of pyramidal form; sublayer III^3 is rich in cells, mostly of medium size.

Layer IV is missing.

Layer V consists of two sublayers. The upper sublayer V^1 contains intensively stained gigantic cells of Betz, lying usually in nests of 2 or 3 cells, less frequently singly. The lower sublayer V^2 has few cells; sometimes there are in it single cells of Betz.

Layer VI is of medium width; it consists of cells of irregular form, and is distinctly separated from layer V.

The basic difference between area Prc_1 and the adjacent areas Pc_1, Pc_2, and Pc_3 is the absence of layer IV and the presence in layer V of a great number of gigantic pyramidal cells, some of especially large dimensions.

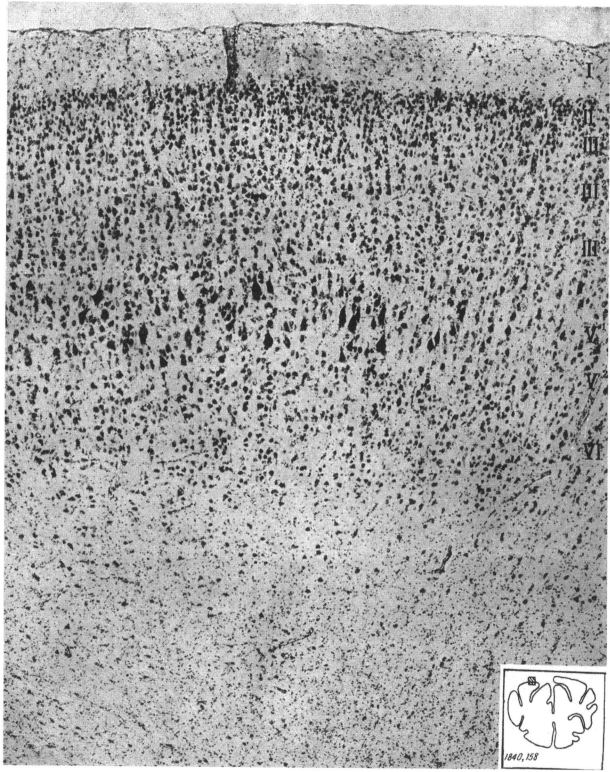

Figure 81 – Area *Prc₁*.

Area *Prc₂* (Area *Praecoronalis Secunda*) (Fig. 82)

Area Prc_2 is located on the external and medial surface of the hemisphere. It occupies the anterior section of the sigmoid gyrus, the posterior section of gyrus proreus, and also descends toward the back of the presylvian sulcus, in the form of a narrow stria (Fig. 50, 51). The posterior boundary of area Prc_2 passes from the top downward, at first along the floor of the cruciate sulcus, and then across the free surface of the sigmoid, coronal, and ectosylvian gyri, parallel to the presylvian sulcus, separating area Prc_2 from areas Prc_1, Pc_3, and Pc_4. The anterior boundary of area Prc_2 extends over the free surface of gyrus proreus and descends into the depth of the presylvian sulcus, separating area Prc_2 from areas F_2, F_1, and I_2. On the medial surface of the hemisphere, the inferior boundary of area Prc_2 extends across the free surface of the sigmoid gyrus, dividing area Prc_2 and the transitional area Prc_2-L_2.

The cortex of area Prc_2 is of medium width (1.8 mm). The upper layers are richer in cells than the lower. The cortex is basically composed of cells of medium and rather large size, of an irregular form. The radial striation is indistinct. The transition into white matter is gradual.

Layer *I* is of medium width, rich in cells of a rounded form of small and medium size.

Layer *II* is very rich in medium sized cells. One finds in it more frequently than in other layers cells of irregular and also triangular form.

Layer *III* is relatively wide and can be subdivided into sublayer III^{1+2}, composed of small cells, and sublayer III^3, consisting of large cells of irregular form. The boundary with layer *V* is indistinct.

Layer *IV* is missing.

Layer *V* has few cells, mostly large. There are two sublayers: The upper sublayer (V^1) is richer in cells than the lower (V^2); the latter contains a stria of translucence.

Layer *VI* is of medium width. It contains a greater number of cells than layer *V*. The cells are of medium size and are arranged in radial rows.

Area Prc_2 differs from area Prc_1 in that it has no gigantic cells of Betz (which makes the structure of area Prc_2 more isomorphous). It has a wider cortex, and the transition into white matter is gradual.

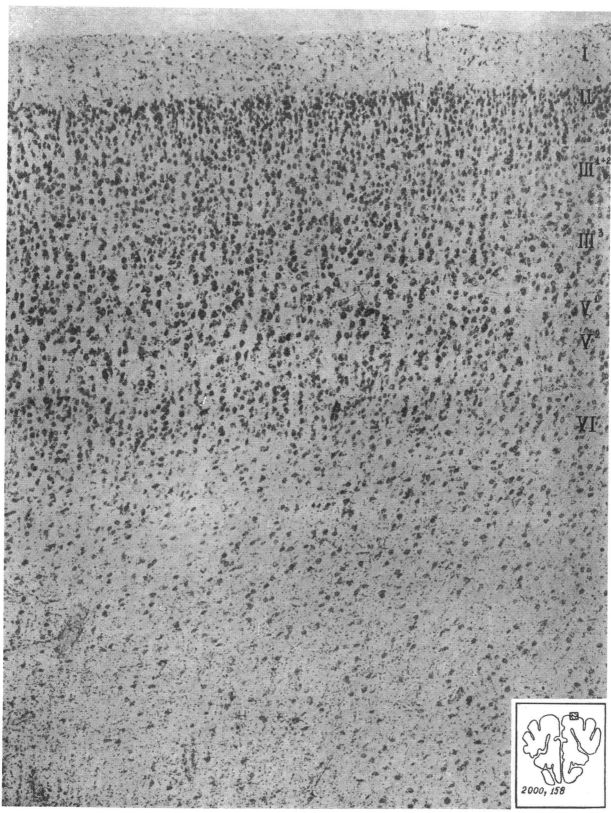

Figure 82 – Area *Prc₂*.

Subarea Prc_2-L_2 (*Subarea Praecoronalis Limbica*) (Fig. 83)

Subarea Prc_2-L_2 (subarea praecoronalis secunda limbica) can be distinguished on the medial surface of the hemisphere, at the point of transition of area Prc_2 into area L_2. It is located in the inferior section of the anterior portion of the sigmoid gyrus (Fig. 50 and 51). Area Prc_2 gradually changes its structure at the point of transition into the limbic area. Its cortex becomes slightly wider (the width is 2 mm) mainly on account of the upper layers. The radial striation is more distinct. Layer VI is richer in cells. The cells of subarea Prc_2-L_2 are slightly smaller than the cells of area Prc_2.

Layer I is of medium size and contains fewer cells, which are smaller than those in area Prc_2.

Layer II is narrow and rich in cells of medium size and of triangular and irregular form.

Layer III is wide and can be divided into two sublayers: Sublayer III^{1+2} is composed of cells of mostly triangular form, arranged in radial rows; in sublayer III^3 the cells are slightly larger, less intensively stained, and mostly polyangular or irregular.

Layer IV does not appear.

Layer V is rarefied and poorly separated from layer III. It divides into two sublayers: Sublayer V^1 contains medium sized cells of various forms, larger than the cells in layer III but smaller than the corresponding cells of area Prc_2; sublayer V^2 contains a stria of translucence.

Layer VI is wide and rich in cells of an oval, irregular form.

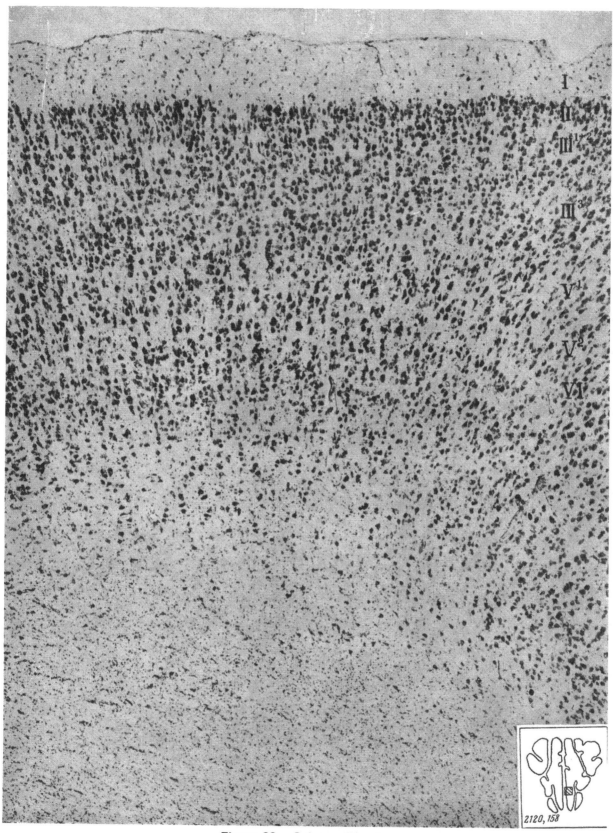

Figure 83 – Subarea *Prc₂-L₂*.

Area F_1 (Area Frontalis Prima) (Fig. 84)

Area F_1 lies on the external surface of the hemisphere in the inferior portion of the gyrus proreus (Fig. 50 and 51). From below, it is bounded by the anterior rhinal sulcus. From above the boundary extends along the free surface of the gyrus proreus separating area F_1 from area F_2. From the back, the boundary passes partly along the sylvian sulcus where area F_1 adjoins area Prc_2, and partly along the free surface, separating area F_1 and I_2.

The cortex of area F_1 is of medium width (2 mm) and has fewer cells than the other areas of the frontal region. The division into layers is indistinct. The upper portion is wider than the lower because of the wide layer III. The boundary with white matter is distinct.

Layer I is rather wide and has few cells.

Layer II has few cells. It consists of small cells of a triangular form and is poorly separated from layer III.

Layer III is wide. The size of the cells increases slightly as one penetrates deep into the layer, thus permitting layer III to be divided into sublayers. Sublayer III^{1+2} has few cells; these are small and medium sized. Sublayer III^3 is richer in cells. One finds in it single, larger cells. Layer III is poorly separated from the layer which lies underneath it.

Layer IV does not show.

Layer V is subdivided into two sublayers: Sublayer V^1 is rich in large cells, mostly of a rounded and irregular form; sublayer V^2 has faw cells and forms a thin, translucent stria.

Layer VI is of medium width. It is composed of cells of diverse form and size.

Area F_1 differs from the adjoining area I_2 in that the cortex is narrower, layer II is not clearly separated from layer III, layer III is wide, the stria of translucence in layer V is less distinct, and there is an abrupt boundary with white matter which lies underneath.

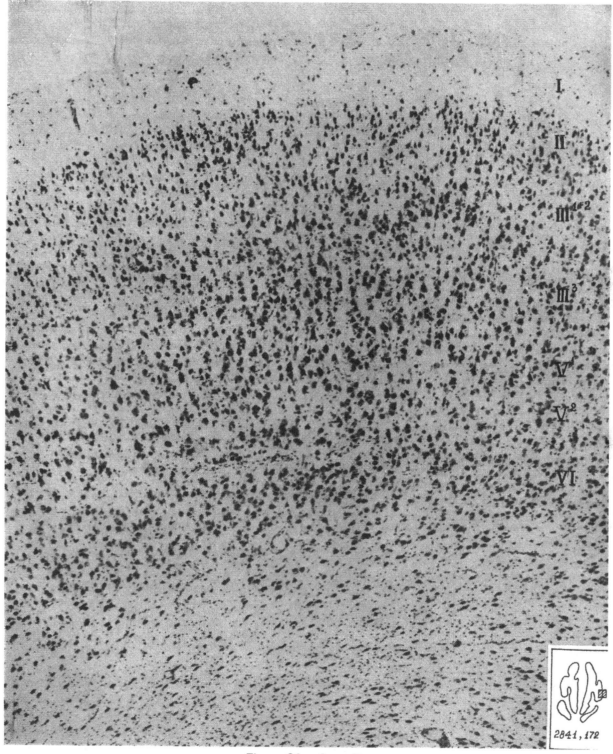

Figure 84 – Area *F₁*.

Area F_2 (*Area Frontalis Secunda*) (Fig. 85)

Area F_2 occupies the superior portion of gyrus proreus lying on both the external and medial surfaces of the hemisphere (Fig. 50 and 51). The inferior boundary (with area F_1) and superior boundary (with area F_3) of the area extend across the free surface of the gyrus proreus; the posterior boundary passes in the depth of the presylvian sulcus, where area F_2 adjoins area Prc_2.

Characteristic of area F_2 is a slightly narrower cortex (the width is 1.5 mm), a great number of cells, and a very distinct radial striation, especially in the upper portion. The upper portion is wider than the lower, mainly on account of layer *III*. The boundary with white matter is distinct.

Layer *I* is of medium width and has few cells, predominantly of small size.

Layer *II* is narrow and rich in cells of a pyramidal form. The boundary with layer *III* is unclear.

Layer *III* is wide and rich in cells. It divides into two sublayers: Sublayer III^{1+2} is composed predominantly of small cells of a pyramidal form; sublayer III^3 is richer in cells and consists of larger cells of a rounded and irregular form.

Layer *IV* does not show.

Layer *V* is rather narrow. It is rich in cells of medium size, basically of pyramidal form. It subdivides into sublayer V^1, richer in cells, and sublayer V^2 which is less rich in cells.

Layer *VI* is of medium width and is composed of a large number of multipolar cells, diverse in size, but smaller than the cells of layer *V*.

Area F_2 differs from area F_1 in that it has more cells, a more distinct separation between layer *II* and layer *III*, and a more distinct radial striation.

In contrast to area Prc_2, area F_2 is composed of smaller cells and shows an abrupt transition into white matter.

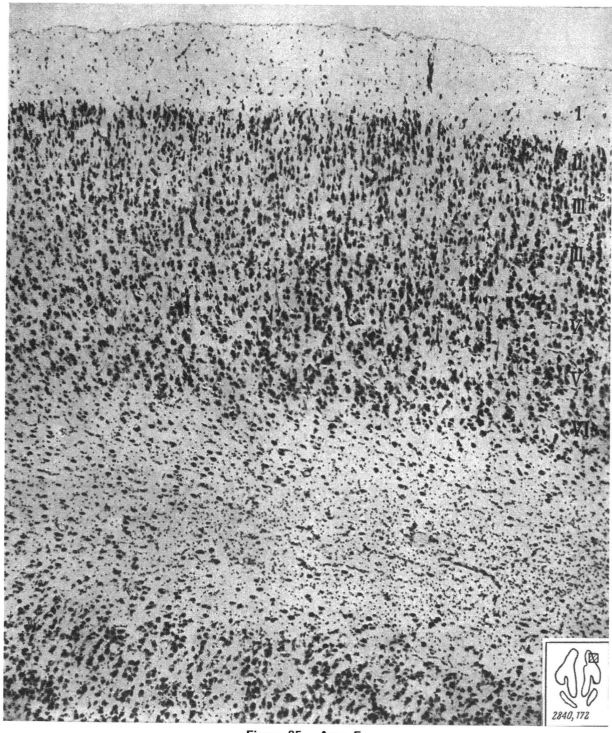

Figure 85 – Area *F₂*.

Area F_3 (*Area Frontalis Tertia*) (Fig. 86)

Area F_3 lies on the medial surface of the hemisphere, and occupies the superior section of gyrus proreus (Fig. 50 and 51). In front, area F_3 borders areas F_2 and F_4. In the back, it borders subareas Prc_2-L_2 and F-L_2. From above it borders areas Prc_2 and F_2.

The cortex of area F_3 is of medium width (1.9 mm) and is rich in cells. The upper portion is only slightly wider than the lower. The division into layers is rather clear and the boundary with white matter is distinct.

Layer I is wide and has few cells.

Layer II is narrow and contains a great number of small cells, mostly of triangular form.

Layer III is wide and divides into two sublayers: Sublayer III^{1+2} contains fewer cells than sublayer III^3; its cells are somewhat smaller and there is a predominance of triangular cells. Sublayer III^3 is composed mostly of cells of a rounded or irregular form and they are less intensively stained than the cells of sublayer III^{1+2}.

Layer IV does not show.

Layer V is divided into two oublayers: Sublayer V^1 contains a great number of large cells of a pyramidal form and intensively stained; sublayer V^2 has few cells mostly of medium size and irregular form.

Layer VI is rather wide and is composed of medium-sized cells of a rounded and irregular form. It is well separated from layer V. The boundary with white matter is distinct.

In contrast to area F_2, area F_3 has a very wide cortex because of the lower portion, which widens considerably, and there are large cells in layer V.

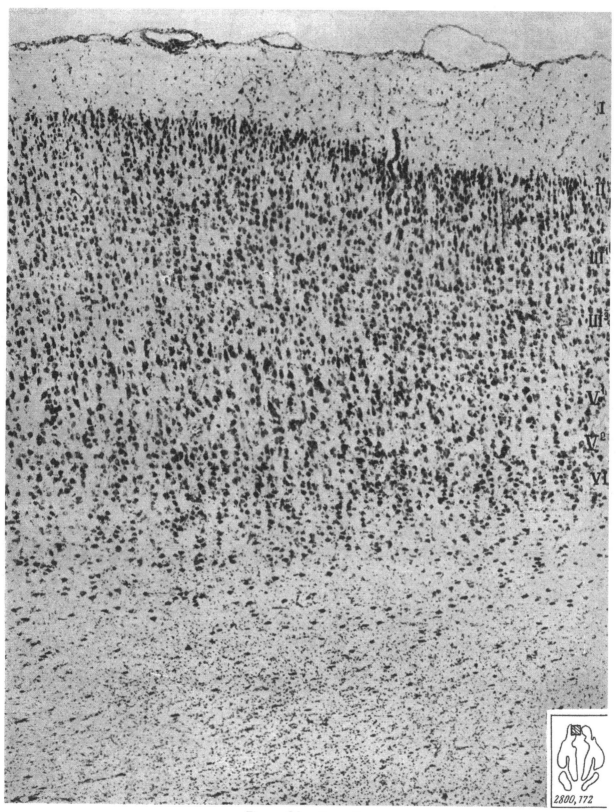

Figure 86 – Area *F₃*.

Area F_4 (*Area Frontalis Quarta*) (Fig. 87, 88)

Area F_4 lies on the medial surface of the hemisphere and occupies the lower portion of gyrus proreus (Fig. 50 and 51). Above, it adjoins area F_3; at the back it borders on subarea F-L_2 and below on area *ta*.

Area F_4 has a narrow cortex, rich in cells (the width of the cortex is 1.4 mm). The upper portion is wider than the lower, because of a wide layer *III*. The basic mass of cells are of small and medium size; this area contains fewer large cells than the other areas of the frontal region. It is characterized by a rather clear radial striation and an abrupt boundary with white matter.

Layer *I* is wide and has few cells.

Layer *II* is narrow and rich in small cells which are mostly of triangular form. It is well separated from layer *III*. In places, the cells are gathered into groups.

Layer *III* is wide and is subdivided distinctly into two sublayers. Sublayer III^{1+2} is composed of deeply stained cells of triangular form. Sublayer III^3 is composed of larger cells of a polyangular and irregular form and less deeply stained. It is richer in cells than sublayer III^{1+2}.

Layer *IV* does not show.

Layer *V* is narrow and is divided into two sublayers. Sublayer V^1 is rich in cells of irregular form, irregularly oriented toward the surface of the cortex. Sublayer V^2 has few cells.

Layer *VI* is narrow and rich in small, flattened cells.

At the place of transition of area F_4 from the medial to the lower surface of the hemisphere one can observe minor structural changes (Fig. 88), such as an increase in the number of cells in the upper layers and a gradual narrowing of the cortex.

In comparison with area F_3, area F_4 has a thinner cortical diameter, mainly the result of a narrowing of the lower layers. There are no large cells in layer *V*.

The structure of the areas of the frontal region is variable. Fig. 88 shows the structural form in the vicinity of the frontal pole.

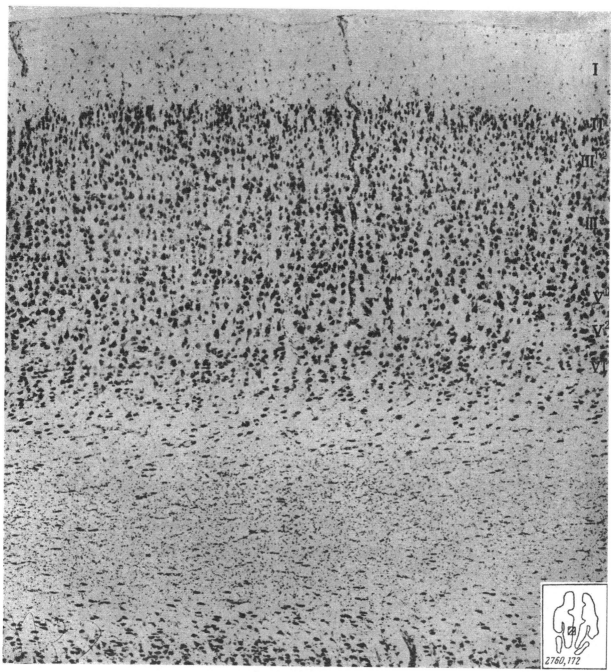

Figure 87 – Area *F₄*.

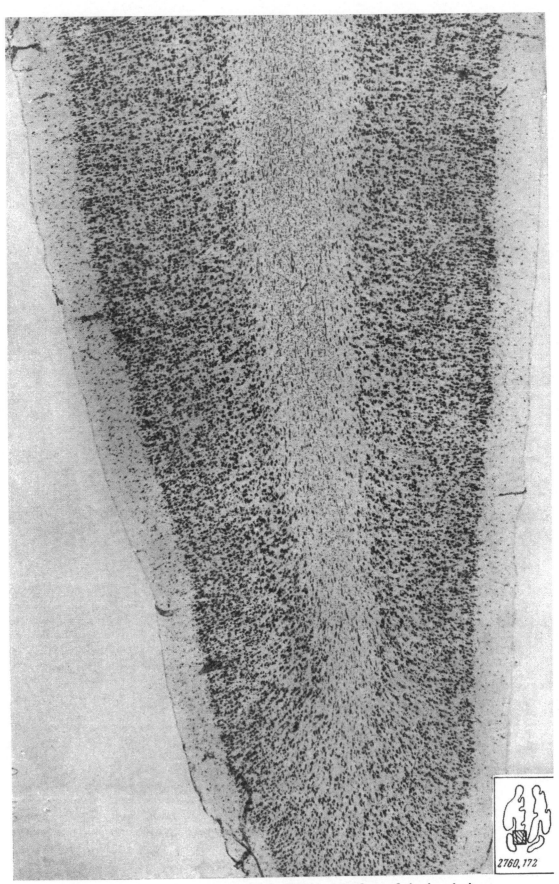

2760, 172

Figure 88 – Area F_4 on the medial and lateral surface of the hemisphere.

Subarea F-L₂ (*Subarea Fronto-Limbica*) (Fig. 89)

In its posterior portion area F_4 merges into the limbic area, gradually changing its structure and forming subarea F-L_2 (Fig. 50 and 51).

Subarea F-L_2 lies in the anterior section of the fornicate gyrus. In structure, it resembles area F_4.

The cortex of subarea F-L_2 is wider (width 1.95 mm) than that of area F_4.

The cortex is rich in small and medium sized cells. In the upper levels, one can see radial striations. The boundary with white matter is distinct.

Layer *I* is wide and consists of small rounded cells.

Layer *II* is narrow and rich in small and medium sized cells, mostly of triangular form. It is distinctly separated from the layer *III*.

Layer *III* is relatively wide and is divided into two sublayers: Sublayer III^{1+2} is composed of small cells, mostly triangular, which are more intensely stained than the cells of sublayer III^3. Sublayer III^3 consists of somewhat larger cells of irregular form and lightly stained.

Layer *IV* is not present.

Layer *V* consists of cells of medium size and various forms, and is divided into two sublayers. Sublayer V^1 is rich in cells; sublayer V^2 has fewer cells.

Layer *VI* is wider and richer in cells here than in area F_4, and consists of small and medium sized cells of a rounded and spindle-shaped form, extending in a horizontal direction.

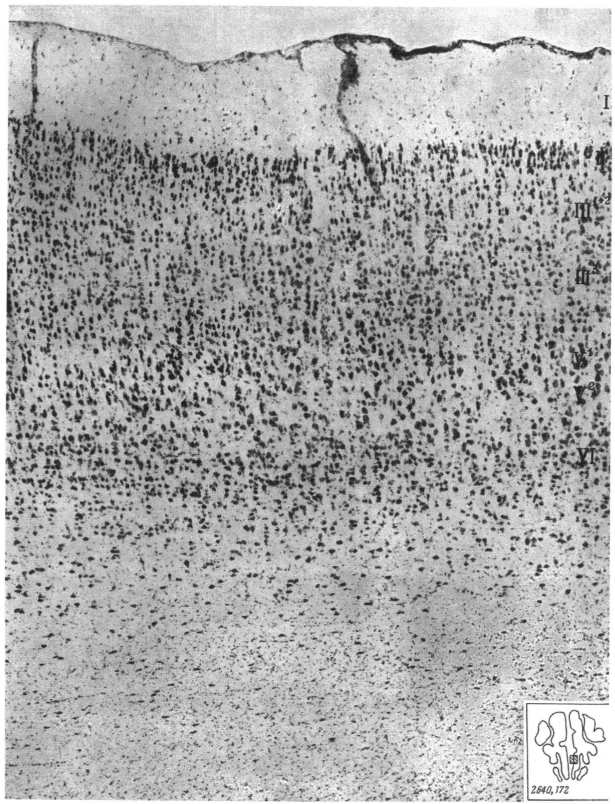

Figure 89 – Subarea *F-L₂*.

Area L_1 (*Area Limbica Prima*) (Fig. 90)

Area L_1 lies in the posterior section of the limbic gyrus (Fig. 50 and 51). It is separated from areas O_1, O_2, OP, P, Pc_1 in the back and above by the retrosplenial and splenial sulci. Below, the boundary extends partly within the sulcus of the corpus callosum and partly along the free surface of the limbic gyrus.

Area L_1 has a rather narrow cortex rich in cells. The upper portion is wider and richer in cells than the lower. The differentiation of layers is comparatively distinct. Layer IV is very distinct. The boundary with white matter is abrupt. The thickness of the cortex averages 1.4 mm.

Layer *I* is of medium width and consists of small rounded cells.

Layer *II* is narrow and has a great number of small triangular cells vertically directed. It is poorly separated from layer *III*.

Layer *III* is rich in cells, among which are many of a pyramidal form. These gradually increase in size as one penetrates deep into the layer, thus making it possible to divide layer *III* into two sublayers. Sublayer *III^{1+2} consists of small cells; sublayer III^3 consists of larger cells.*

Layer *IV* stands out clearly and is composed of a great number of rounded cells, among which there are single small cells, similar in form to the pyramidal cells.

Layer *V* is of medium width and is divided into two sublayers. Sublayer V^1 consists of cells of pyramidal form, of medium and large size. Sublayer V^2 has few cells and forms a stria of translucence.

Layer *VI* is rich in cells of medium size, and rounded and polyangular form.

Area L_1 is not homogeneous in its structure as it changes into area L_2 (Fig. 94), but the differences in structure are not significant enough to warrant a further division of the area in question.

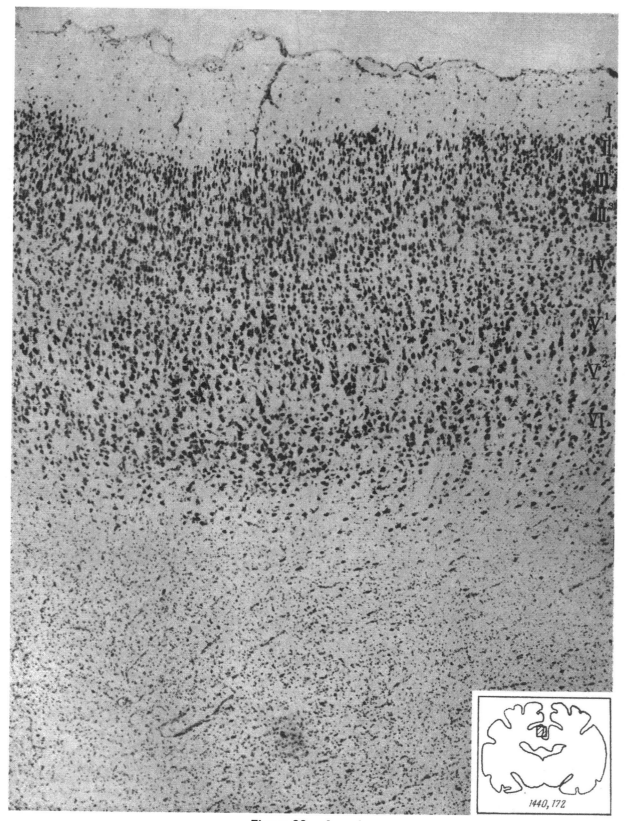

Figure 90 – Area *L₁*.

Area L₂ (Area Limbica Secunda) (Fig. 91)

Area L_2 lies in the anterior section of the limbic gyrus (Fig. 50 and 51). The superior and anterior boundaries (with areas Prc_2-L_2 and F-L_2) pass partly over the free surface of the limbic gyrus and partly within the genual sulcus. The inferior boundary passes within the sulcus of the corpus callosum (with area Pt_3) and over the free surface of the limbic gyrus (with area ta of the archeocortex).

Area L_2 has a narrow cortex poor in cells (its width is 1.1 mm). The cortex is clearly subdivided into an upper and lower portion on the basis of the form and size of the cells. In the upper portion the cells are smaller and of a rounded form. In the lower portion, there is a predominance of larger cells of irregular form. The radial striation extends up to layer *II*. The boundary with white matter is distinct.

Layer *I* is of medium width and is rich in mmall cells of rounded form.

Layer *II* is rich in cells of medium size of a rounded and partly triangular form. It changes gradually into layer *III*.

Layer *III* is of medium width and contains fewer cells than layer *II*. One finds in it irregularly distributed nests of translucence.

Layer *IV* is not evident.

Layer *V* is formed of medium sized cells and is somewhat translucent in the lower portion.

Layer *VI* is of medium width and is divided into two sublayers. Sublayer VII consists of email and medium sized cells of various forms. Sublayer VI2 contains a small number of cells of predominantly triangular form.

In comparison with area L_1, area L_2 has a narrower cortex, layer *IV* is missing, there are fewer cellular elements and the layers are not as clearly differentiated.

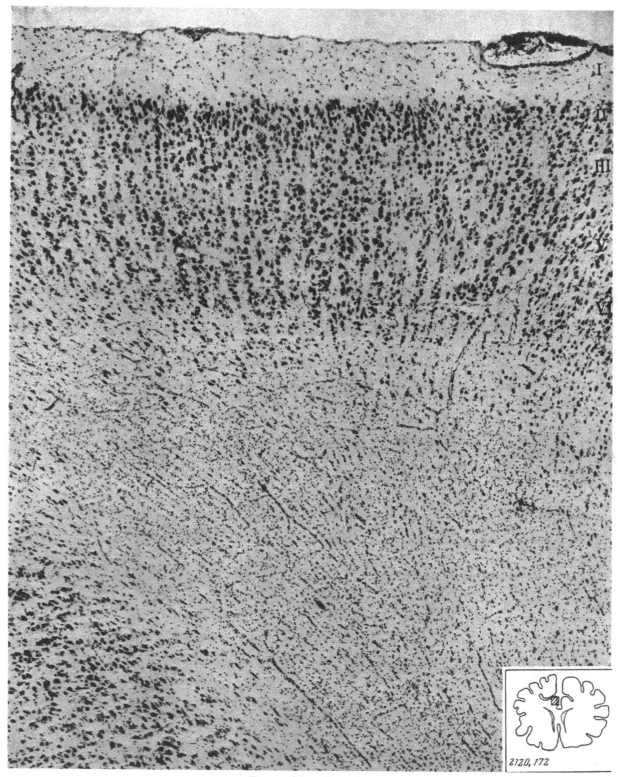

Figure 91 – Area L₂.

Area *Pt₁* (*Area Peritectalis Prima*) and *Pt₂* (*Area Peritectalis Secunda*) (Fig. 92)

Area Pt_1 lies in the posterior half of the limbic gyrus, occupying the medial portion of the superior part of the sulcus of the corpus callosum. Characteristic of this area is a narrow cortex, poorly differentiated into layers, with a predominance in the entire width of small cells of a rounded or irregular form. The boundary with white matter is distinct.

Layer *I* is of medium width.

Layer *II* and *III* represent a single complex which becomes cuneiform in the direction toward the corpus callosum.

Layer *IV* is formed of small cells.

Layer *V* consists of cells of mostly oblong and triangular form, larger in size than the cells of layer *III*. The layer is wide and is divided into two sublayers. One finds in sublayer V^1 separate large cells, similar in form to the pyramidal cells. Sublayer V^2 is translucent.

Layer *VI* is relatively wide and has a few small cells of polymorphous character. The layer is wide and is composed of triangular and spindle shaped cells.

Area Pt_2 is located laterally from area Pt_1. It occupies the superior part of the sulcus of the corpus callosum and emerges, partly, on the free surface of the limbic gyrus.

In this area, the cortex is wider than in area Pt_1. The radial striation stands out clearly and extends over the entire thickness. The lower portion of the cortex is wider than the upper. The boundary with white matter is distinct.

In contrast to area Pt_1, area Pt_2 has a wide cortex, a radial striation over its entire thickness, and large pyramidal cells in layer *V*.

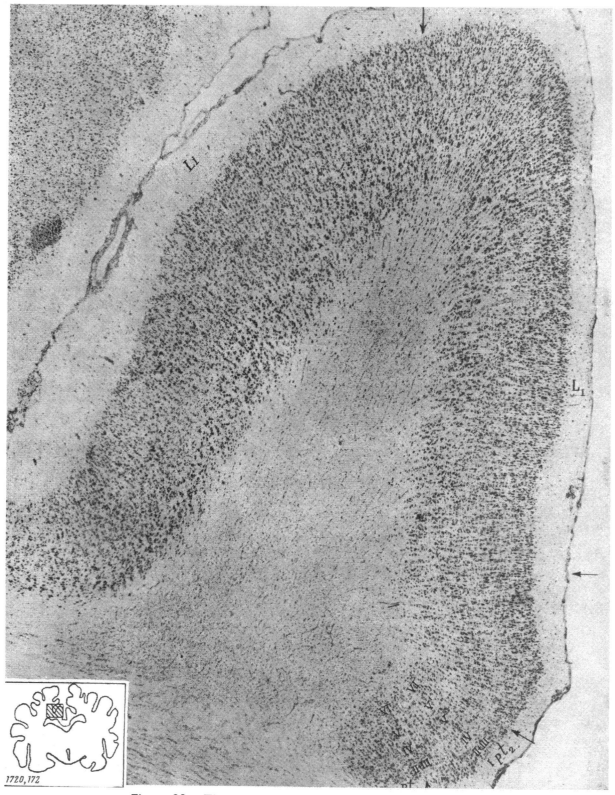

Figure 92 – The structure of the cortex of the limbic gyrus.

Area Pt₃ (*Area Peritectalis Tertia*) (Fig. 93)

Area Pt_3 lies in the anterior section of the limbic gyrus, occupying the superior part of the sulcus of the corpus callosum.   It is characterized by a narrow cortex, poor differentiation of layers, and predominance in the entire thickness of cells of a rounded and irregular form.

Layer *I* is wide.

Layers *II* and *III* form a single complex. Layer *IV* is not evident.

The cells of layer V are somewhat larger than the cells of layer *III*. The boundary between layers *III* and *V* is indistinct.

Layer *VI* is composed of small cells. It is divided into sublayer V^1, rich in cells, and aublayer V^2 with fewer cells.

The basic difference between area Pt_3 and areas Pt_1 and Pt_2 is the absence of layer *IV* and a rather weak differentiation of the thickness of the cortex.

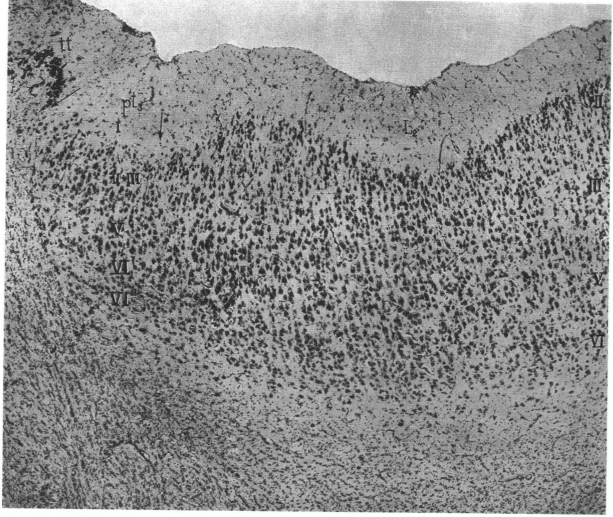

Figure 93 – Area *Pt₃*.

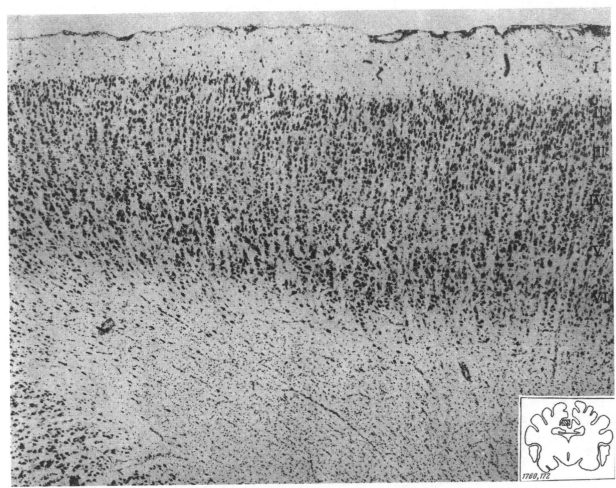

Figure 94 – The transition of area *L₁* into *L₂*.

The Paleocortex, Archicortex, and Intermediate Cortexi (*Paleocortex, Archicortex Et Cortex Intermedius*)

The cortex of the large hemispheres includes the neocortex, which possesses all the formations described above, as well as the paleocortex, the archicortex and the intermediate cortex.   There are few data on the function of these three cortices (Poniatovskiy [1128]; Bekhterev [2]; Zavadskiy [1149]; Allen [1091]; Filimonov [715]; Savich [1137]; Langutina, Rozhanskiy, and Urmanicheyeva [1121]).   In descriptive anatomy these regions are often united under the concept of an "olfactory brain" (rhinencephalon).   Properly, however, this term should refer only to a small part of the so-called olfactory brain; that is, the olfactory tubercle and especially the prepyriform region.   The greater part of the regions belonging to the olfactory brain are only remotely connected with olfaction and represent a substratum of "nonolfactory" functions.   So far, the character of these functions has not yet been determined.   Judging by the polymorphous structure of the regions of the "olfactory brain," one has to assume that their functions are multiform, although less complicated than the function of the neocortex.

The paleocortex, which appears very early in phylogeny is characterized by an incomplete separation from the subcortical cellular accumulation and very primitively constructed cortical lamina located underneath (*striatum, nucleus septi, amygdala, substantia innominata, claustrum inferius*).

The archicortex, which appears in phylogeny later than the paleocortex but earlier than the neocortex, is very well developed in reptiles.   It has a cortical lamina which is completely separated (as in the neocortex in contrast to the paleocortex) from the subcortical cellular accumulations.   However, the cortical lamina of the archicortex differs sharply from the cortical lamina of the neocortex, in its morphogenesis, as well as in a much less complicated stratification.

The archi- and paleocortex are separated from the neocortex by the intermediate cortex.

The paleocortex includes the olfactory tubercle, the diagonal region, the septum pellucidum, the periamygdalar region, and the prepyriform region.

The olfactory tubercle (*tuberculum olfactorium, TO,* Fig. 50), which occupies the anterior section of the anterior perforated substance, lies between the lateral and medial olfactory gyrus.   From the back and inside, it borders on the diagonal region.   It divides into two areas: area TO^1, lying toward the medial, and area TO^2, lying posteriorly.   Area TO^2 (Fig. 95) is characterized by a rather disproportionate zonal layer, as to width, and a very gyrose cortical lamina, with occasional nests of microcellular accumulations.   Area TO^1 has a less complex but equally gyrose cortical layer; the zonal layer is just as disproportionate but somewhat narrower.[1]

The diagonal region (*regio diagonalis, D,* Fig. 50) lies anteriorly on the medial part of the hemisphere, adjoining the lamina terminalis, and then merges with the base, where it occupies the posterior section of the anterior perforated space.   Almost the entire expanse of the diagonal region is represented by area D^2, characterized by a moderately wide zonal layer and a cortical lamina with large, angular, heavily stained cells penetrating into it from substantia innominata.   Area D^1, which occupies only the very last part of the posterior section of the region (at the boundary with the periamygdalar region), has a cortical lamina consisting of small, polymorphous cells.   Large, heavily stained cells exist only deep inside of the formation (Fig. 41 and 42).

The septum pellucidum (*septum pellucidum, s. massa septi pellucida, spt,* Fig. 50) is located on the medial part of the hemisphere.   Anteriorly it is between the corpus callosum and the diagonal region and posteriorly between the corpus callosum and the fornix.   The zonal layer is either barely visible or entirely missing.   The cortical lamina consists of polymorphous cells of medium size, somewhat rarefied and increasing in size in toward the ventricle (Fig. 42).

The periamygdalar region (*regio periamygdalaris, Pm,* Fig. 50) lies posteriorly from the diagonal region, medial to the prepyriform and entorhinal regions and toward the front of the entorhinal region (Fig. 36-40).   The basic areas are area *Pmm* and areas Pml^1, Pml^2, and *Pe*, lying lateral from it.   Area *Pmm* is characteristic for a cortical lamina consisting of small cells and occupies the anterior and medial sections of the region.   Area Pml^1 has a cortical lamina consisting of large cells.   It differs considerably from area Pml^2, where the cells are smaller and more compactly arranged.   Still more toward the outside, in the region of the semiangular sulcus, lies area *Pe*, which differs distinctly from area Pml^2 in the greater rarefaction of the cortical lamina.

The prepyriform region (*regio praepiriformis, Pp,* Fig. 50) occupies the lateral olfactory fissure.   The basic areas are the medial area Pp^2, adjoining the olfactory tubercle and the diagonal region, and the lateral area Pp^1, which enters the anterior rhinal sulcus, and borders, deep inside the latter, on the insular region (Fig. 37-43).

The region extends far beyond the limits of the posterior pole of the olfactory bulb.   Here the foremost section of the basic area Pp^1 forms area Pp_o^1 which has a strongly rarefied cortical lamina.   The foremost section of basic area Pp^2, area Pp^{oo} with a less rarefied cortical lamina of its own, and a narrow, heavily stained microcellular additional lamina, also merges into area Pp_o^1 and Pp^o.   Toward the back, areas Pp^o and Pp^{oo} change into areas Pp^1 and Pp^2, and area Pp^1 in turn divides into the lateral subarea ppie and the medial subarea Pp^1 i (Fig. 96).   In area ppli, the cortical lamina is more rarefied than in area Pp^1e.   Area Pp^2 has all along its length a

---

[1] After the materials of Filimonov [715], to whom the authors express their gratitude.

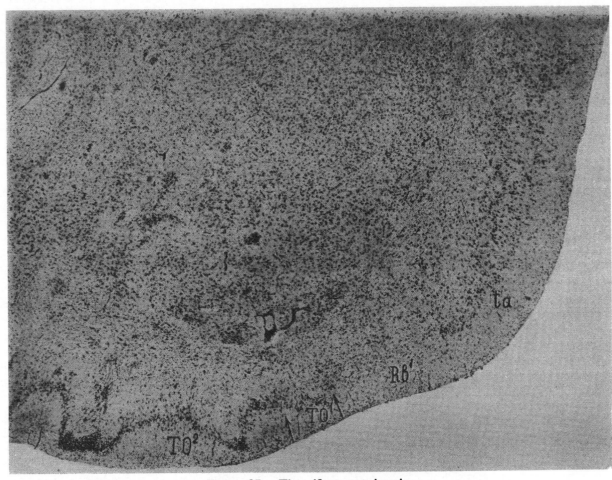

Figure 95 – The olfactory tubercle.

crudely gyrose complex cortical lamina and a heavily ex-panded zonal layer. Deep inside the sulcus, subarea ppie changes into area Pp^1a which shows a strong rarefaction Of the cortical lamina, and constitutes the transition into neocortex.

The archicortex includes the hippocampus, the den-tate fascia, and taenia tecta, the last area represent-ing only a considerably reduced continuation of the hip-pocampus (along the surface of the corpus callosum and further in front of the hippocampus).

The hippocampus (cornu Ammonis, CA, Fig. 50) oc-cupies the depth of the hippocampic fissure, and forms a voluminous torsion above the gplenium of the corpus callosum. Thus, one can distinguish here an inferior (temporal) section of the hippocampus (CAi), a superior (subcallosal) section (CAs), and connecting these a pos-terior section (CAp). Basically, the structure is similar in all sections, showing differences only in details. In Fig. 97 there is shown the superior or subcallosal section of the hippocampus. The outermost areas form the subiculum (sub), with a wide, moderately compact cortical lamina in the superior layer and a rarefied cortical lamina in the inferior portion, consisting of small cells. Then follows area h^1, with a narrower and much more compact external layer composed of pyramidal cells of medium size, and a wide internal layer composed of cells of the same type but more thinly spread. The following area, h^2, has a corti-cal lamina composed of large, radially directed, pyramidal cells, arranged in 3 or 4 rows. The cells are more com-pact than in area h^1. The rarefied deep layer is missing here. Area h^3 has a distended cortical lamina consisting of large but diffusely located cells. Areas h^4 and h^5 en-ter completely into the cavity of the sac formed by the extremely firm cortical lamina of the dentate fascia. In area h^4 the cells are smaller in size and their arrangement is less compact than in the area h^3, and especially in area h^2. Area h^5 consists of small, very thinly spread cells.

The dentate fascia (fascia dentata, FD) has the same elements as the hippocampus. It is characterized by an extremely compact, brightly stained microcellular corti-cal lamina, which forms the so-called fascial capsule into which enter areas h^4 and h^5 of the hippocampus (Fig. 97).

As pointed out before, taenia tecta (tt, Fig. 97) represents the foremost continuation of the hippocam-pus greatly reduced. It consists of several sections: the supracallosal section, covering the superior surface of the corpus callosum, the subcallosal section, covering the in-ferior surface of the genu of the corpus callosum, and the precallosal section, extending downward and forward to the olfactory bulb (the internal olfactory gyrus). In the supracallosal section, the taenia tecta is greatly reduced and is represented by a series of small rarefied and brightly stained polymorphous cells. In the anterior part of the supracallosal section the cortical lamina widens (3 or 4 rows of cells). The size of the cells increases slightly and the cortical lamina retains the same character as the sub-callosal section. The precallosal section is represented, along its entire length, by area ta. In the back, area ta is characterized by a narrower cortical lamina, which widens toward the front. The cortical lamina is rarefied and is formed mostly of pyramidal cells of medium size (Fig. 95).

The intermediate cortex separates the neocortex from the paleocortex and archicortex. The intermediate cor-tex is the peripaleocortex (peripalaeocortex) and is repre-sented essentially by area Pp^1a, already described above. The intermediate cortex, separating the archicortex from neocortex, is the periarchicortex. It is differentiated in a more complex manner. Its basic regions are the pre-subicular region, adjoining the hippocampal region, and the entorhinal region located between the presubicular re-gion and the neocortex (Fig. 46).

In both the presubicular and entorhinal regions, there stand out three basic layers: external, medial, and in-ternal. The internal layer, representing the immediate continuation of the archicortical or hippocampal lamina, is often separated from the superior layer by a light layer, poor in cells - the dissecant layer ($Diss^2$).

The presubicular region (praesubicularis s. prae-subiculum, Psb) divides into the internal area Psb^1 and the external area Psb^2. In both areas, the superior and the medial layers are of the microcellular type. In area Psb^1, the cortical lamina is much narrower, because of stenosis of the medial layer, and area $Diss^2$ is wider and lighter than area Psb^2 (Fig. 99).

The entorhinal region (regio entorhinalis, E, Fig. 50) is characterized by a more complex striation. In most cases, the external layer differs distinctly from the me-dial. In addition to $Diss^2$, in a number of formations there also stands out a $Diss^1$ layer within the limits of the internal layer. According to the way the dissecants are exposed and the character of the layers in the entorhinal region, three basic regions stand out: posterior (ep), me-dial or particular (epr), and anterior (ea), as well as three transitional subregions - the posterior (etp), lateral (etl), and anterior (eta), which bring about the transition of the entorhinal regions into the formations of the neocortex. Most differentiated is the particular entorhinal subregion, which divides into a number of areas (epr^o, epr^1, epr^1e, epr^{1a}, epr^{1am}).

In Fig. 98 is illustrated the posterior subregion. In area ep, there is a macrocellular intermittent external layer, with occasional clearly visible mammillaries. In ad-dition, there is a wide medial layer consisting of medium sized cells, the clearly visible $Diss^1$, and the microcellu-lar internal layer. Medially from area ep can be seen area epr^o, representing the transition from the posterior entorhinal subregion to the medial subregion.

The external layer here is also macrocellular; the me-dial layer is wider, and consists of cells of smaller size. $Diss^1$ is missing, but one can notice $Diss^2$, located at a greater depth.

Fig. 99 represents the medial and anterior entorhinal regions and the anterior section of the presubicular region. Above on a portion of the hippocampal fissure lie the anterior presubicular areas Psb^1 and Psb^2 with a micro- and polycellular layer and medial layer and a very distinct $Diss^2$, and with the internal layer constituting the immediate continuation of the archicortex (Sub). At the base is area epr^1, which is characteristic for the medial entorhinal subregion, with an external layer consisting of large cells which form occasional mammillaries. The medial layer is slightly less macrocellular. $Diss^2$ is distinctly visible. The internal layer is compact and consists of cells of medium size. In areas epr^1 and epr^{1am} the cortex is narrower because of the narrowing of $Diss^2$, which here too remains very distinct. Area ea belongs to the anterior entorhinal subregion. Its basic peculiarity is a marked rarefaction of the deep floor of the medial layer. This results in the formation of $Diss^1$, merging with $Diss^2$ into one single wide and light dissecant ($Diss^{1+2}$).

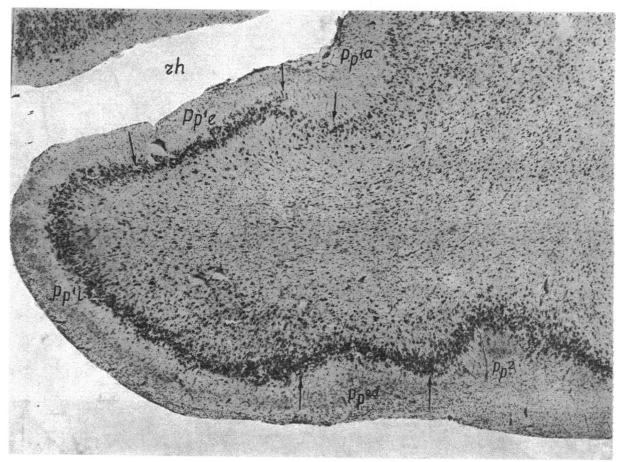

Figure 96 – Prepyriform region.

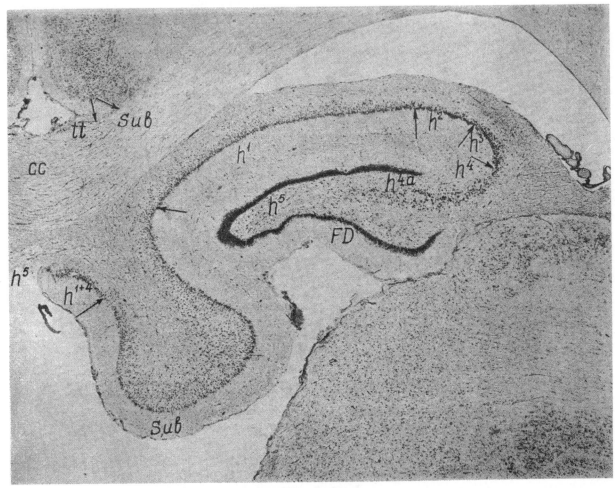

Figure 97 – Archicortex.

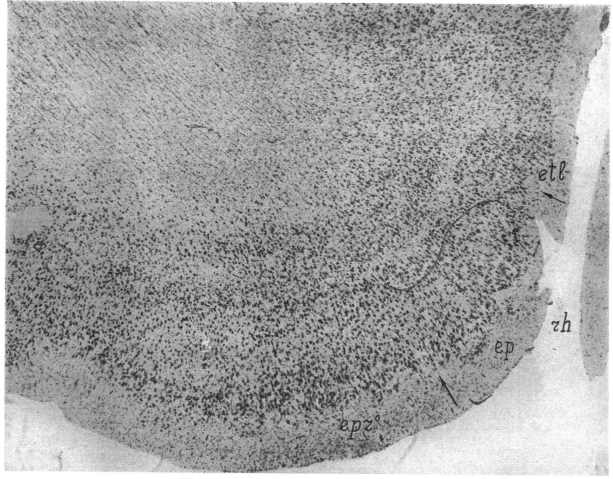

Figure 98 – Posterior entorhinal subregion.

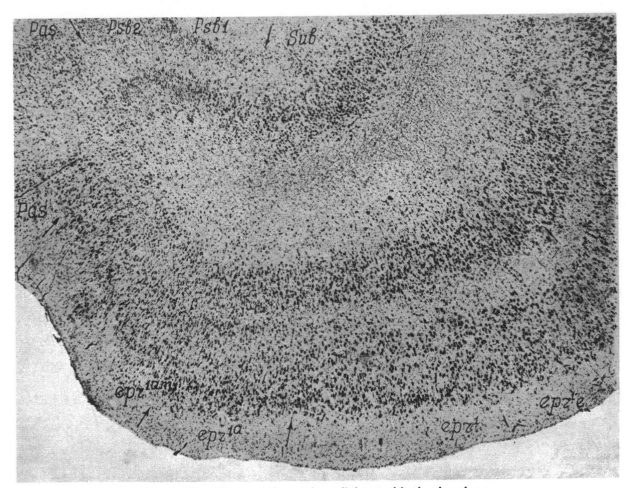

Figure 99 – The anterior and medial entorhinal subregions.

THE TOPOLOGY OF THE SUBCORTICAL FORMATIONS AND THEIR PROJECTION UPON THE CRANIUM

There is a lack of specific information in the literature which would permit location of various subcortical formations in the dog, in their relationship to external landmarks on the cranium. Such information is absolutely necessary in order to expose these or other subcortical nuclei without disturbing the integrity of the more superficial formations. The research on the brain of the monkey (Clark and Henderson [10]; Olszewsky [577]), of the cat (Clark and Henderson [9]; Hess [27]; Jiménez-Castellanos [539]; Johnson [269]; Jasper and Ajmone-Marsan [536]; Reinoso [347]), of the rabbit (Sawyer, Everett and Green [601]), and the rat (Kreig, 1946 [*Editors' note: The Kreig reference could not be found in the bibliography. We assume that the authors' made a mistake. Consequently, we made a substitution.*]) are well known.

For the canine brain, however, there exist corresponding data only on the nuclei of the hypothalamus (Knott and Shipton, 1956). (Editor's note: See also "Stereotaxic Atlas of the Dog's Brain" by Lim *et al.*, C.C. Thomas, Springfield, Illinois 1960.)

This chapter presents data on the location of subcortical formations in relation to selected external landmarks on the cranium. This makes it possible to do the work without a stereotaxic apparatus, as well as reference to the three reciprocally perpendicular planes (horizontal, frontal and sagittal) which are universally adopted in the work with stereotaxic apparatus. We have worked out the data for animals of different sizes, so that the experimenter during the operation can choose the scale closest to the cranial size in the animal operated on.

The following measurements of the head were determined: (1) length from the posterior point of the inion to the post-superior edge of the orbit (see Fig. 110, ill. 2); (2) width between the internal auditory canals; (3) height between the two planes extending horizontally through the lateral auditory canals and the superior surface of the cranium; (4) length of the inion on its inferior surface, from its hindmost point to the base.

A comparison of the length of the heads of different sizes shows that the variability of this length depends, basically, on the difference in the size of the facial part of the cranium. However, the cerebral part of the cranium changes comparatively little, and for this reason, even in the case of a considerable difference in head sizes, this change does not exceed 3-4 cm. Thus, for example, the length of the head of the smallest of all measured dogs (the Bolognese) equals from the inion to the tip of the snout 11 cm. and to the posterior edge of the orbit 6 cm. In the largest dog (German shepherd) these measurements are respectively 21.7 cm. and 10 cm. In other words, the overall length of the head differs more than 10 cm., whereas the length of the cerebral part of the cranium differs only 4 cm. However, if one takes for comparison the heads of dogs of average size, then the difference in absolute size of the cerebral part of the cranium, and correspondingly, of the same parts of the head, is considerably smaller and remains within the limits of 1 cm. or less frequently 2 cm. If one takes into consideration that in different dogs the size of the inion varies, and if one measures the length of the cerebral part of the head not from the posterior point of the inion, but from its base, then this dimension differs still less among different dogs of medium size.

The material that follows here is divided into two parts:

The first part is concerned with procedures carried out without the stereo-toxic apparatus. This material includes the frontal series of slices through the cranium in animals of various sizes, the numeral scale compiled on the basis of these series, and the projections of the most important subcortical formations upon the superior surface of the cranium. The work is based on calculations from the following orientors: (1) the pole of the inion, (2) the sagittal plane, and (3) the superior surface of the cranium.

The frontal series of cranial sections (Fig. 101-108) were prepared as follows: After taking the measurements of the head, the carotid arteries were filled with 10% formalin solution. Then the skin and muscles were removed and the cranium with the brain was sawed into slices 4 mm thick in a perpendicular direction, toward the superior surface of the cranium. One mm of brain tissue was lost in the sawing. The slices were fixed, according to the method of Talalayev [64], in permanent lamellar preparations, from which the photographs in the atlas were made. There are two figures for each head, since each series of slices was photographed from both sides. In every instance, the first figure shows the posterior surface of the slice; the second figure shows the anterior surface. The Roman numerals on the figures give the serial number of the section, counting from the back to the front, from the pole of the inion. The Arabic number under each slide indicates the distance in millimeters of the section from the pole of the inion.

When referring to the frontal series of sections, the numbered figure and the projection of the subcortex upon the cranium, one should remember that the electrode has to be directed, under all circumstances, into the planes of the slices, i.e., perpendicularly to the superior surface of the cranium. Work should begin with the section from our figures of a head of approximately the same size as the head of the dog in the experiment. (The length of the cranium in our measurements corresponds approximately to the length of the dog's head, since measuring proceeds from the posterior edge of the orbit to the posterior point of the inion. Thus, the thickness of the skin does not substantially affect the given measurements.) One should also take into account possible variability in the length of the inion (within the limits of 1 to 7 mm) in dogs. Even though the length of the head of the dog in the experiment and the length of the head selected from the figures are similar, one must subtract the size of the inion from the length of both heads.

The calculation of the distance of the subcortical formation from the external orientors indicated by us can be carried out immediately on one series of frontal slices. In order to do this, one locates a section on which there is the nucleus which is of interest. The distance from the superior surface of the cranium and the midline to the nucleus can be determined by simply measuring with a ruler. The number under the section indicates the distance in millimeters between this nucleus and the posterior end of the inion (from the pole). However, it is obvious that this last measurement will be correct for the dog in the experiment only when the length of the inion in the dog in the experiment and the comparable dog in the atlas are the same. When these sizes are different, it will be necessary to subtract this difference in the calculation. Keeping this in mind, when using the measurements of the dog in the atlas and comparing it with the dog in the experiment, one should consider the distance of the nucleus in question, not from the pole but from the base of the inion (by way of subtracting the length of the inion from the length of the dog's head). One should add to the figure so arrived at the length of the inion of the dog in the experiment and 2 to 3 mm for the thickness of the skin, since in our series the calculations were carried out on the cranium.

The calculations of the distance of the subcortical nucleus from the pole of the inion can be represented in a formula:

$$L = L_1 + 2 + I$$

where L is the distance of the formation sought from the pole of the inion of the dog in the experiment, L_1 is the distance from the base of the inion of the dog selected from the atlas and I is the length of the inion of the dog in the experiment.

Following is an example of the use of the frontal series of sections. Let us assume that we have to insert an electrode into the anterior commissure of the brain in a dog with a head length of 82 mm. The length of the inion is 5 mm. The length of the head of the dog without the inion, i.e., from the base of the inion, will be 77 mm. This is exactly the length of the head without the inion in dog No. 17 (Fig. 105 and 106), the entire length being 78 mm, and the length of the inion 1 mm. Therefore, the experimentor should measure the coordinates of the anterior commissure in No. 17. The anterior comisaure can be seen on the posterior surface of Section 10 and on the anterior surface of sections 9 and 10. It stands out best on the posterior surface of section 10, from the end of the inion at a distance of 46 mm, or else from the base of the inion at 45 mm. One calculates the distance from the end of the inion which will locate this formation in the dog in the experiment, where the length of the inion is entirely different, 5 mm. Applying the formula given above, L = 45 mm + 5 mm (the length of the inion in the dog in the experiment) + 2 mm for the thickness of the skin = 52 mm. Consequently, in order to reach the anterior commissure of the cerebrum of the dog in the experiment, one has to insert the electrode into the brain at a distance of 52 mm, in front of the pole of the inion. The distances from the midline and the superior surface of the cranium are measured on the section with a ruler. In dog No. 17, these are respectively 3.5 and 38 mm. This will be true for the dog in the experiment as well. [*Editor's note: Because it was necessary to deduce the size of the Atlas in this English translation, the reader should note the enlargement and if not 1:1, correct for this accordingly. For example, it is 0.75:1 for Fig. 105.*]

For the convenience of the experimentor we have also supplied a chart giving the distances of some of the most important subcortical nuclei from the external orientors adopted by us. In the upper part of the chart there are data on the measurements of the canine cranium. Further, the distances are given of the medial points of the most important subcortical formations from the pole of the inion, from the base of the inion, from the superior surface of the cranium, from the sagittal plane, and from the coronal suture.

When working with the numbered chart, one must first select a head similar in size, as described above. Then one must take the number of the selected head in order to determine the distance from the sagittal plane and from the superior surface of the cranium. The distance from the posterior end of the pole of the inion is calculated according to the same formula as for the frontal series of the slices.

Here is an example of how to use the chart: Let us assume that we have to reach the medial geniculate body in the brain of a dog with a head length of 86 mm and an inion length of 4 mm, making the length of the head without the inion 82 mm. The size of the head of the dog in the experiment is closest to that of Nos. 9, 10, and 15 on the numbered chart. In Nos. 9 and 10, the length of the cranium without the inion equals 80 mm; in No. 15 it is 83 mm. We look on the chart for the coordinates of the medial geniculate body in these three dogs.

The distance from the end of the inion in No. 15 is 35 mm, in Nos. 10 - 30 mm, and in No. 9 - 35 mm; i.e., there seems to be great variability. However, if one subtracts from these figures the length of the inion, i.e., if one takes the distance from the base of the inion, then these figures will appear to be almost the same: for No. 15 - 31 mm, No. 9 - 29 mm, and No. 10 - 30 mm. Let us take the mean value, 30 mm, add to it 3 mm for the thickness of the skin, and 4 mm for the length of the inion of the dog in the experiment, and the result is 37 mm. The numbers which show in the chart, the distance of the numbers from the sagittal plane and from the superior surface of the cranium also fit, essentially, the head of the dog in the experiment. Thus, the electrode should be inserted perpendicularly to the superior surface of the cranium, 33 mm to the front of the base of the inion or else 37 mm to the front of the pole of the inion, 32 mm into the depth of the superior surface of the cranium and 9 mm lateral to the sagittal plane.

For better orientation of the experimentor, we made projections of the hemispheres of the cerebrum, of the basic sulci and subcortical formation, upon the superior surface of the cranium (Fig. 109-114), in the same animals which appear on the numbered Chart and in Figs. 101 to 108. In making the projections, the measurements of the hemispheres as well as of the most important subcortical formations (length and diameter), which were arrived at by making measurements on each section, were transferred upon the photograph with the lines of the sections plotted on it in Roman numerals. In the process, and in conformity with the method of plotting projections, some formations with a narrow diameter but lying in the brain not vertically but on a slant appeared on the projection somewhat wider.

The second portion of the material presented by us is intended to be used while working with a stereotaxic apparatus. This includes the series of sagittal sections through the cranium in three dogs of different size, and the series of frontal projections of the brain of one dog. This material permits the calculation of three reciprocally perpendicular planes: the horizontal, leading through the middle of the external auditory canal and the inferior edge of the orbit; the frontal, leading perpendicularly to the horizontal plane, through the centers of both auditory canals; and the sagittal, leading at an angle to two other planes along the midline of the head. One can see in the illustration how all these planes pass through the head of the dog. The entire right half of the cranium was removed, together with the corresponding hemisphere of the brain, in such a way that the medial surface of the left hemisphere can be seen with a wire threaded through it 10 mm higher than the horizontal plane and parallel to it. The level of passage of the horizontal plane is also visible, since there remained the bone part of the right orbit and part of the temporal bone with the internal auditory canal. The vertical white line indicates the frontal plane (Fig. 101).

In the preparation of the sagittal series of sections, the head with the brain was fixed the same way as described for the frontal series.

In order to obtain a horizontal plane, the cranium with the brain was placed in the solution in such a way that its surface passed through the middle of the auditory canals and the lower edges of the orbit. The level of the liquid was marked by a line on the cranium. After that, another line was drawn perpendicularly to the first line through the middle of the auditory canals making the frontal plane. The cranium with the brain was then sawed in the direction of the sagittal plane, into slices of an average thickness of 4 mm. About 1 mm of the brain was lost in the process. In dogs Nos. 5 and 18, the first section was carried out along the midline, and in No. 19 it deviated 3 mm from the midline. There remained the marks of the horizontal and frontal planes previously drawn on the lateral bone parts of the section.

After combining these marks we obtained, on the plane of every slice, two reciprocally perpendicular lines marking the horizontal and frontal planes. From these sagittal series, there were also made according to the method of Talalayev [64] permanent lamellar preparations, the photographs of which are shown in the figures.

The sagittal series of slices include two figures for each animal (Figs. 115 - 120), the first showing the medial surface of the sections and the second the lateral surface. The Roman numerals signify the ordinal number of the section counting from the sagittal plane; the Arabic numbers give the distance in millimeters from the surface of the section to the sagittal plane. The sagittal and frontal planes are marked on the sections with white lines. The place of their intersection is the zero point from which one should begin to count.

In the work with the sagittal series of the sections, one should select a head similar in size to the head of the animal in the experiment, described for the frontal series, i.e., subtracting the variability of the length of the inion.

In Figs. 121-131 of the atlas there are a series of projections of the frontal sections of the brain of the dog of medium size, enlarged 8-10:1 (the length of the head is 78 mm, the length of the inion, 1 mm). On these projections, it is easy to determine the distance of a particular subcortical nucleus from all three basic planes: the frontal, horizontal, and sagittal. The number in the lower left corner of each projection refers to the distance in mil-

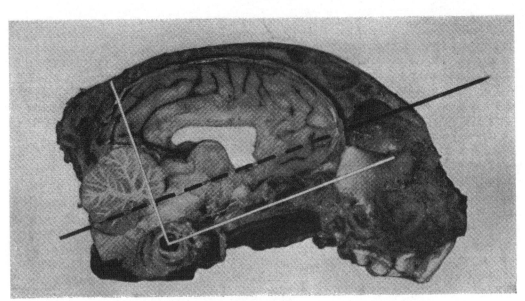

Figure 100.

limeters from the frontal plane. The zero line transacting every projection horizontally is parallel to the horizontal plane and is drawn 8 mm higher than the latter. The chart beginning at the zero line makes it easy to determine the distance of a particular formation from this line. The distance from the sagittal plane is shown on the chart, drawn along the lower edge of the projection.

The series of projections was prepared in the following manner. With the help of the stereotaxic apparatus, two 1 mm steel wires were passed through the head of the dog, from the back toward the front in planes parallel to the horizontal plane and 8 mm higher than the latter. The wires were passed through both hemispheres and 3 mm lateral from the midline. Then there were passed from both sides two more vertical wires 12 mm lateral from the midline in a plane parallel to the frontal, but 34 mm to the front of the latter. After that, the upper part of the cranium was removed and the head with the brain and the wires in it was subsequently fixed in 5% and 10% formalin solution for several days. The brain was then cut vertically along the planes of the vertical wires which had been inserted into the brain, making it possible to make a later section of the brain in a plane parallel to the frontal plane, and also to calculate the distance of each section from this plane (since it was known that the first section was at a distance of 34 mm anteriorly from the frontal plane).

A number of measurements were carried out on the brain after removal from the cranium. These included measurement of the height, width, and length of the brain, in order to determine the shrinkage of the brain in different directions and different parts, in the process of subsequent work on it involving the usual method in the preparing of serial cytoarchitectural sections. Repeated measurements of the same regions of the brain were carried out on the series of preparations stained according

to the method of Nissl. It turned out that the linear coefficient of shrinkage in all parts equals approximately 1.4 mm, which almost coincides with the coefficient established by Sarkissow [62] for the human brain (1.2-1.24 mm). Proceeding from here, in drawing the projections of the slices we enlarged the figures 11.6 times, which thus equals a 10 fold enlargement of the fresh brain.

However, in comparing the lengthwise measurements of the brain, which should bring out not only the compression of the brain but also the loss of brain mass during the process of cutting, it turned out that each 20-micron slice of the prepared series corresponds to 30 microns of unprepared tissue. This varied in different parts of the brain from 29 to 30 microns. This coincides with the data of Rose (30 microns) for the brain of the rat and slightly more than the figure supplied by Sarkisov for the human brain (28 microns). Knowing how many microns of unprepared tissue corresponded to a 20 micron slice prepared for our series, we were now able to calculate the distance from the frontal plane of corresponding segments of unprepared tissue. The hole remaining in each section, from the wire which penetrated the brain parallel to the horizontal plane and 8 mm above it, permits one to draw a zero line and thus to calculate the distance of any subcortical nucleus from the horizontal plane.

The material mentioned in this chapter perhaps requires further discussion. First of all, it is evident from the table that the coronal suture is not a sufficiently exact orientor for operations on the subcortical formations, since in different dogs there may be different locations of subcortical nuclei from this suture. Thus, in dogs Nos. 18 and 19, the suture is pushed out in front, and in dogs Nos. 6 and 11, it is further back as compared with the subcortical formations lying underneath.

Our material also shows that the distance of every cortical formation from the base of the inion and from the frontal plane is different in dogs with different head sizes, approximately in proportion to the difference in the length of the head without the inion. The same can be said of differences in the distances of the subcortical formations from the horizontal plane. The depth of the location of the subcortical formations does not always change proportionally, if one measures from the superior surface of the cranium; here the difference in thickness of the cranial bones is a factor. Thus, the greatest deviation occurs in dog No. 19, in which the thickness of the cranial bones is almost twice the thickness of the bones in other dogs.

In dog No. 17 there can be noted a slight deviation of the subcortical formations located in the anterior part of the cerebrum. The reason for this is a considerable thickening of the bones in the anterior part of the cranium.

[Editor's note: The reader is again cautioned in using the figures in this chapter to note the enlargements, which vary considerably from the original in this translation because of reasons of economy in publication. If this inconvenience is accepted, the figures can be used to obtain exact measurements of location of various subcortical structures without too much difficulty.]

		Dog No. 8	Dog No. 15	Dog No. 10	Dog No. 9	Dog No. 17	Dog No. 11
Distance to each formation	from the tip of the inion to the posterior edge of the orbit	97	87	81	85	78	74
	the length of the inion	7	4	1	5	1	1
	from the tip of the inion to the coronal suture	62	52	50	54	48	44
	the height of the cranium	52	44	43	50	43	42
	the width of the cranium	62	52	57	56	65	57
Size of the Cranium		52					

Name of the Subcortical Formation	Distance to each					Distance to each					Distance to each					Distance to each					Distance to each					Distance to each				
	from the tip of the inion	from the base of the inion	from the superior surface of the cranium	from the sagittal plane	from the coronal suture	from the tip of the inion	from the base of the inion	from the superior surface of the cranium	from the sagittal plane	from the coronal suture	from the tip of the inion	from the base of the inion	from the superior surface of the cranium	from the sagittal plane	from the coronal suture	from the tip of the inion	from the base of the inion	from the superior surface of the cranium	from the sagittal plane	from the coronal suture	from the tip of the inion	from the base of the inion	from the superior surface of the cranium	from the sagittal plane	from the coronal suture	from the tip of the inion	from the base of the inion	from the superior surface of the cranium	from the sagittal plane	from the coronal suture
Fastigial Nucleus	22	15	35	2	40	18	14	31	2	34	15	14	32	2	35	18	13	34	2	35	12	11	31	2	36	12	11	30	1	32
Dentate Nucleus	22	15	31	6	40	18	14	29	6	34	15	14	30	6	35	18	13	30	6	35	12	11	30	6	36	12	11	26	4	32
Olive, Superior	28	21	45	4	34	23	19	43	4	29	20	19	43	4	30	22	17	43	4	30	17	16	42	4	31	15	14	40	4	29
Posterior Corpus Bigeminum	30	23	35	6	32	27	23	31	5	25	23	22	31	6	27	27	22	23	5	27	22	21	32	5	26	20	19	31	5	24
Anterior Corpus Bigeminum	33	26	36	3	29	30	26	31	3	22	27	26	31	3	23	31	26	33	6	23	26	25	33	2	22	24	23	31	2	20
Medial Geniculate Body	38	31	36	9	24	35	31	32	9	17	30	29	32	9	20	35	30	33	9	20	30	29	35	9	18	29	28	32	2	15
Lateral Geniculate Body	39	32	31	9	23	36	32	27	9	16	31	30	27	9	19	36	31	33	9	19	31	30	30	9	17	30	29	27	9	14
Pulvinar of the Optic Thalamus	-	-	-	-	-	39	35	26	5	13	34	33	26	5	16	38	33	27	5	16	33	32	29	5	15	31	30	28	5	13
Medial Nucleus of the Optic Thalamus	45	38	33	2	17	42	38	32	2	10	36	35	32	2	14	40	35	31	2	14	35	34	33	2	13	34	33	31	2	10
Lateral Nucleus of the Optic Thalamus	45	38	30	7	17	42	38	30	7	10	36	35	30	6	14	40	35	29	6	14	35	34	32	6	13	34	33	28	6	10
Ventral Nucleus of the Optic Thalamus	45	38	36	3	17	42	38	34	3	10	36	35	35	3	14	40	35	34	3	14	35	34	37	3	13	34	33	34	3	10
Anterior Nucleus of the Optic Thalamus	51	44	31	3	11	47	43	31	3	5	42	41	28	3	8	45	40	28	3	8	40	39	30	3	8	38	37	28	2	6
Red Nucleus	40	33	42	2	22	36	32	40	3	16	31	30	37	3	16	35	30	39	3	19	30	29	40	2	18	29	28	37	2	15
Substantia Nigra	40	33	42	5	22	36	32	40	5	16	31	30	39	5	16	35	30	40	5	19	30	29	42	5	18	29	28	39	3	15
Septum	57	50	27	12	5	53	49	25	14	-1	48	47	24	12	-1	52	47	24	12	2	46	45	26	13	2	45	44	24	11	-1
Body of the Caudate Nucleus	51	44	25	7	11	47	43	24	8	5	42	41	23	7	5	46	41	23	7	8	40	39	26	8	8	39	38	24	6	5
Head of the Caudate Nucleus	57	50	27	6	5	53	49	28	6	-1	48	47	25	5	-1	52	47	25	5	2	46	45	28	6	2	45	44	25	5	1
Globus Pallidus (the external Member)	56	49	36	8	6	52	48	32	8	0	46	45	31	7	0	49	44	31	8	5	43	42	33	9	5	41	40	31	8	3
Putamen	56	49	32	10	6	52	48	30	10	0	46	45	29	10	0	49	44	29	11	4	43	42	31	12	5	41	40	30	10	3
Amygdala	49	42	38	14	13	46	42	38	13	6	40	39	35	13	6	46	41	35	12	10	40	39	39	13	8	38	37	35	11	6

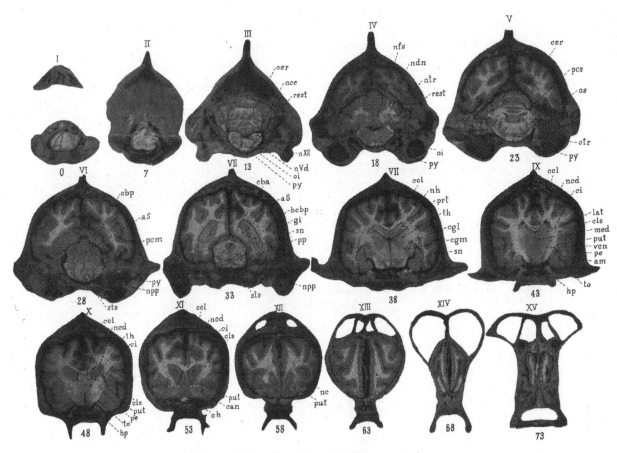

Figure 101 — Dog No. 15. The posterior

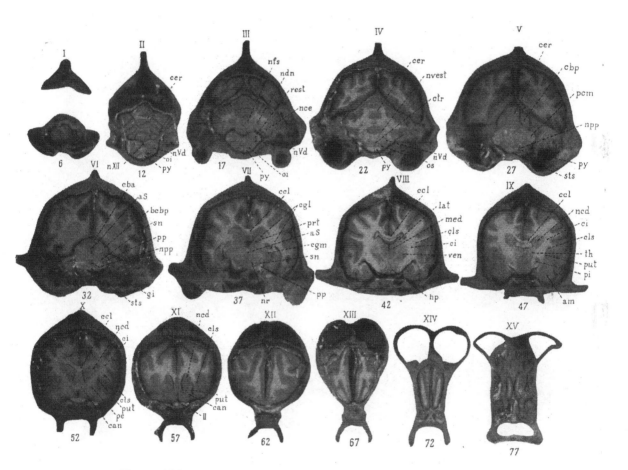

Figure 102 – Dog No. 15. The anterior surface of the sections.

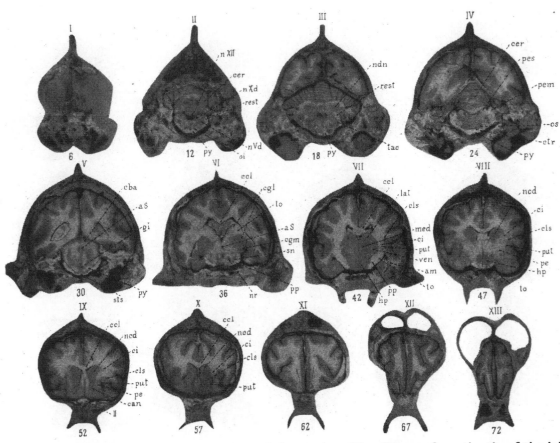

Figure 103 – Dog No. 9. The posterior surface of the section. The distance from the tip of the inion to the posterior edge of the orbit is 85 mm. The length of the inion is 5 mm.

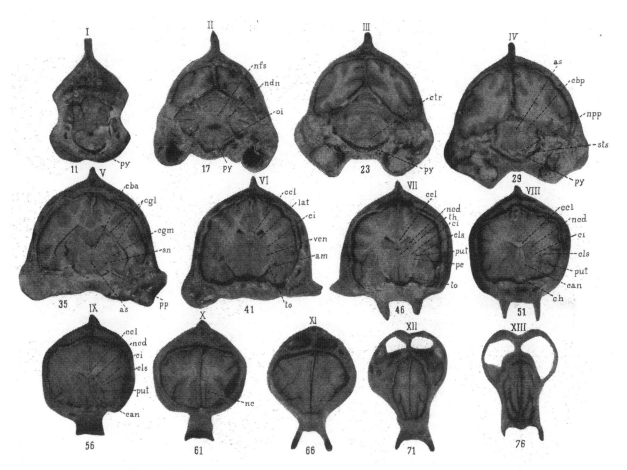

Figure 104 – Dog No. 9. The anterior surface of the sections.

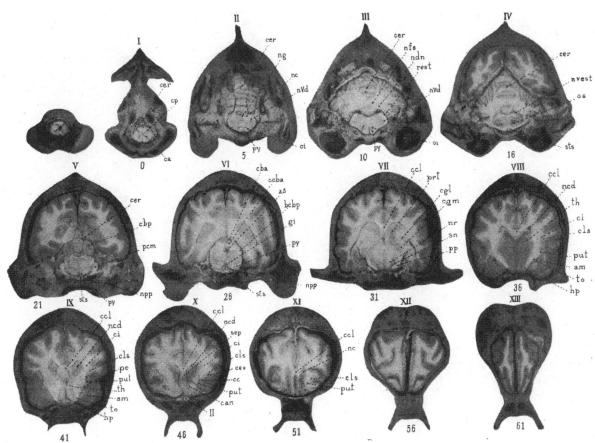

Figure 105 – Dog No. 17. The posterior surface of the section. The distance from the tip of the inion to the posterior edge of the orbit is 78 mm. The length of the inion is 1 mm.

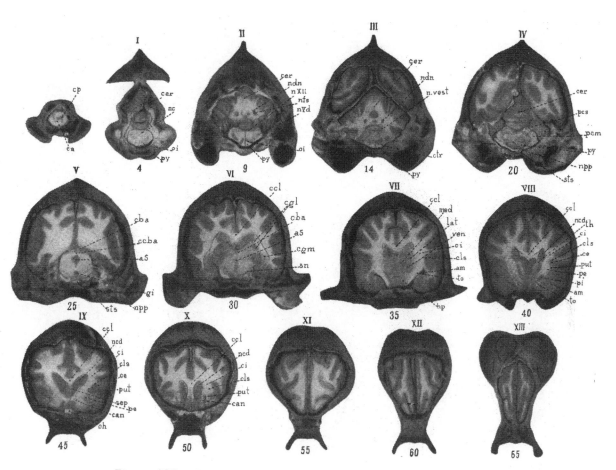

Figure 106 – Dog No. 17. The anterior surface of the sections.

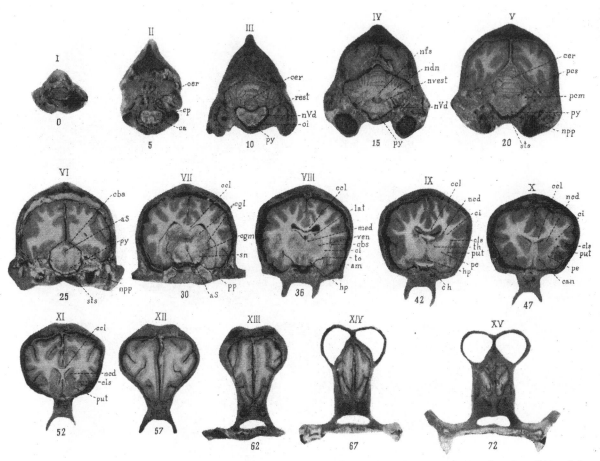

Figure 107 – Dog No. 10. The posterior surface of the section. The distance from the tip of the inion to the posterior edge of the orbit is 81 mm. The length of the inion is 1 mm.

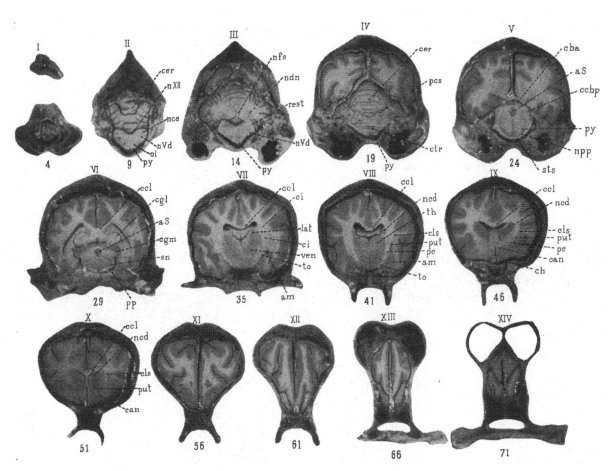

Figure 108 – Dog No. 10. The anterior surface of the sections.

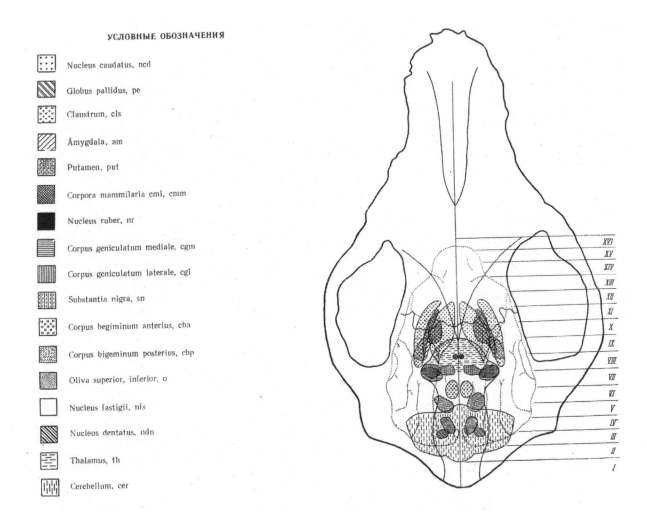

УСЛОВНЫЕ ОБОЗНАЧЕНИЯ

Nucleus caudatus, ncd

Globus pallidus, pe

Claustrum, cls

Amygdala, am

Putamen, put

Corpora mammilaria cml, cmm

Nucleus ruber, nr

Corpus geniculatum mediale, cgm

Corpus geniculatum laterale, cgl

Substantia nigra, sn

Corpus begiminum anterius, cba

Corpus bigeminum posterius, cbp

Oliva superior, inferior, o

Nucleus fastigii, nfs

Nucleus dentatus, ndn

Thalamus, th

Cerebellum, cer

Figure 109 – Dog No. 15. The projections on the cranium of the hemispheres and the subcortical formations.

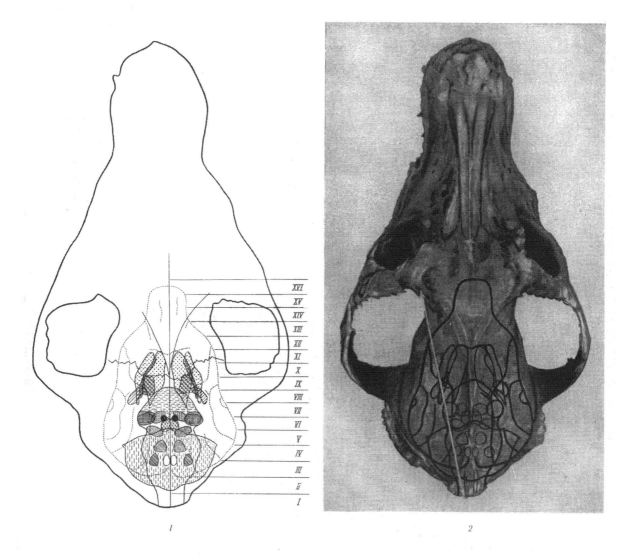

1   *2*

Figure 110 – Dog No. 9. The projections on the cranium of the hemispheres and the subcortical formations (ill. 1 and 2).

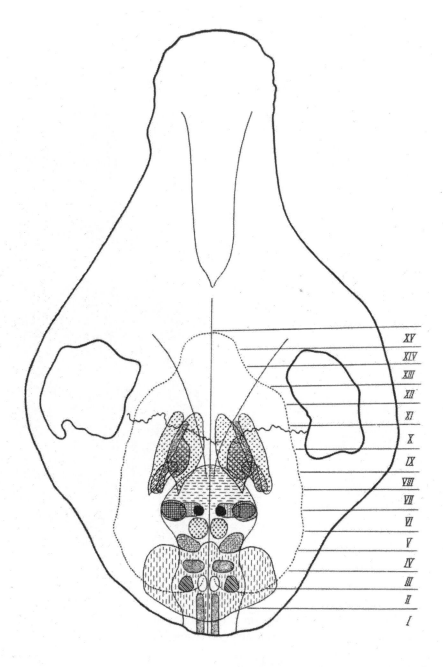

Figure 111 – Dog No. 17. Projections upon the cranium of the hemispheres and the subcortical formations.

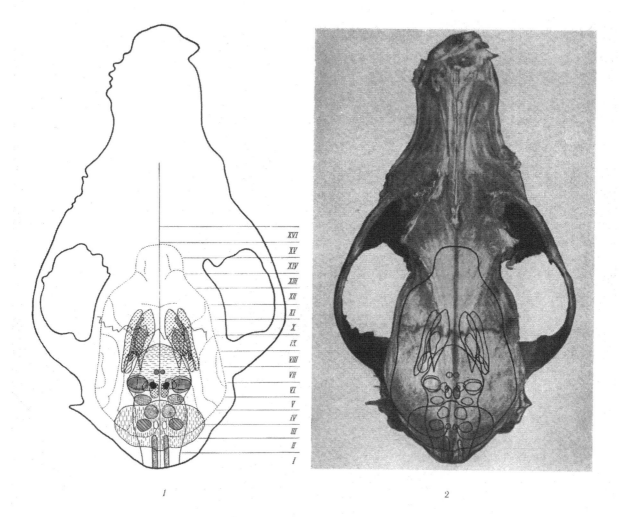

1   *2*

Figure 112 – Dog No. 10. Projections upon the cranium of the hemispheres and the subcortical formations (ill. 1 and 2).

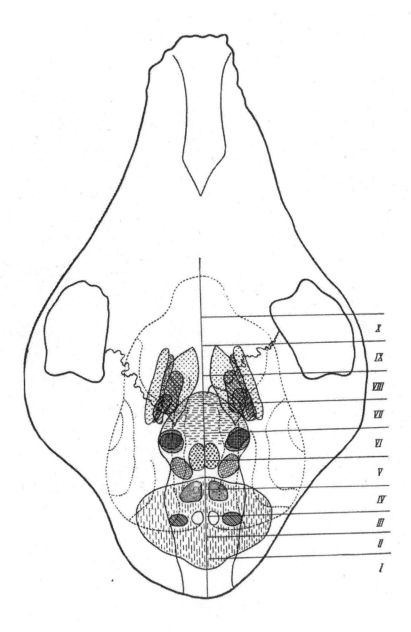

Figure 113 – Dog No. 6. Projections upon the cranium of the hemispheres and the subcortical formations.

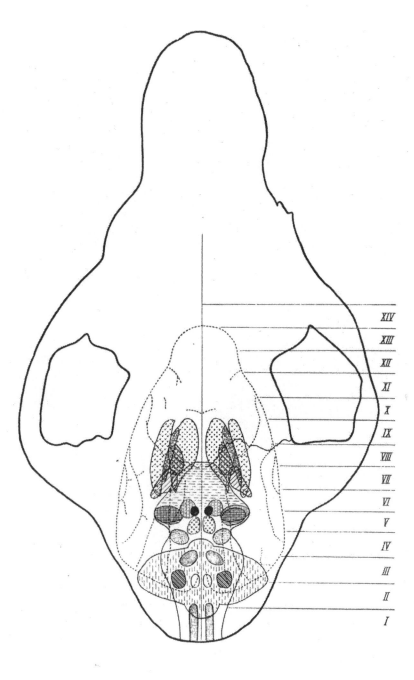

Figure 114 – Dog No. 11. Projections upon the cranium of the hemispheres and the subcortical formations.

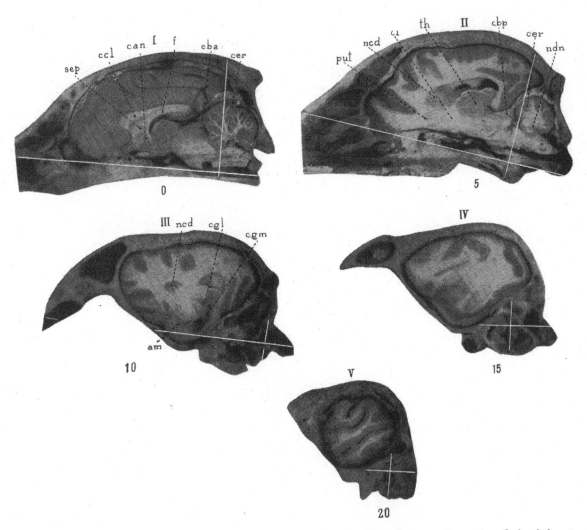

Figure 115 – Dog No. 5. The internal surface of the sections. The distance from tip of the inion to the posterior edge of the orbit is 73 mm. The length of the inion is 1 mm.

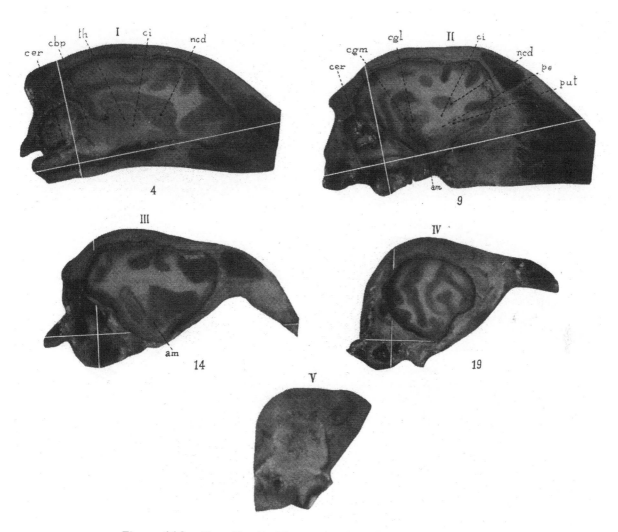

Figure 116 – Dog No. 5. The external surface of the sections.

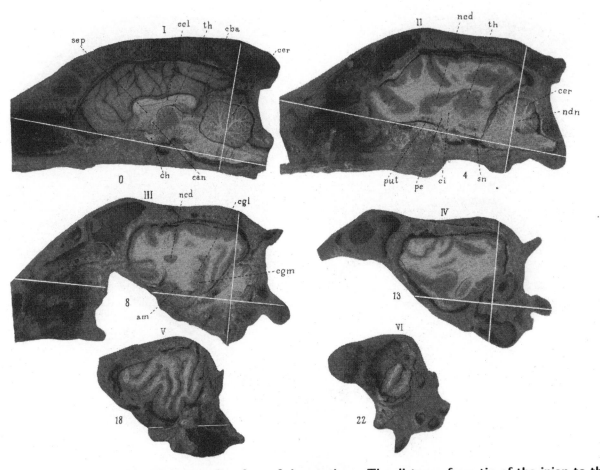

Figure 117 – Dog No. 18. The internal surface of the sections. The distance from tip of the inion to the posterior edge of the orbit is 93 mm. The length of the inion is 7 mm.

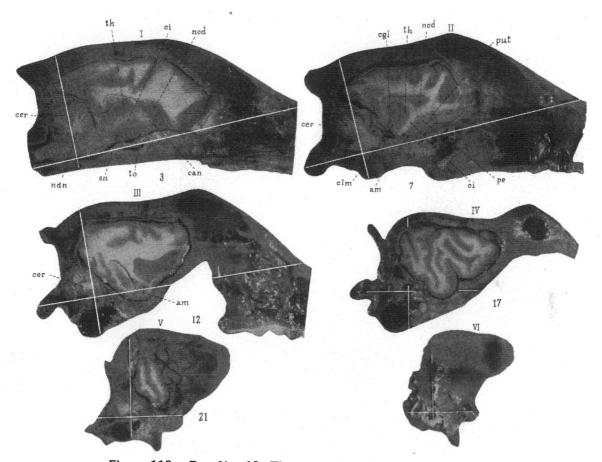

Figure 118 – Dog No. 18. The external surface of the sections.

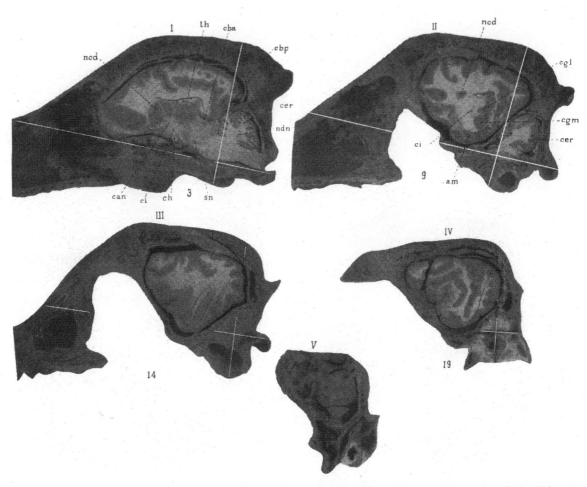

Figure 119 – Dog No. 19. The internal surface of the sections. The distance from tip of the inion to the posterior edge of the orbit is 91 mm. The length of the inion is 7 mm.

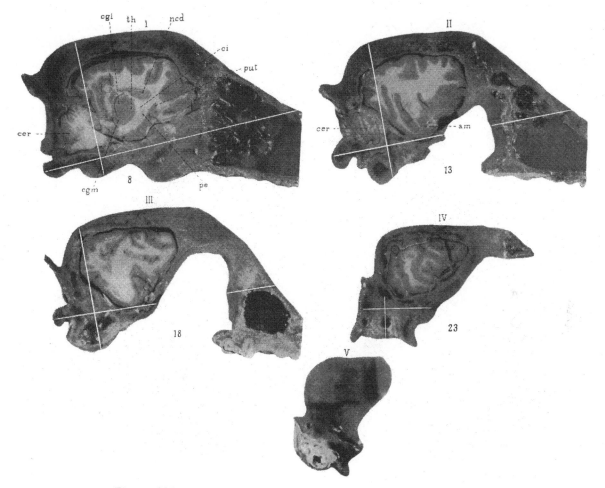

Figure 120 – Dog No. 19. The external surface of the sections.

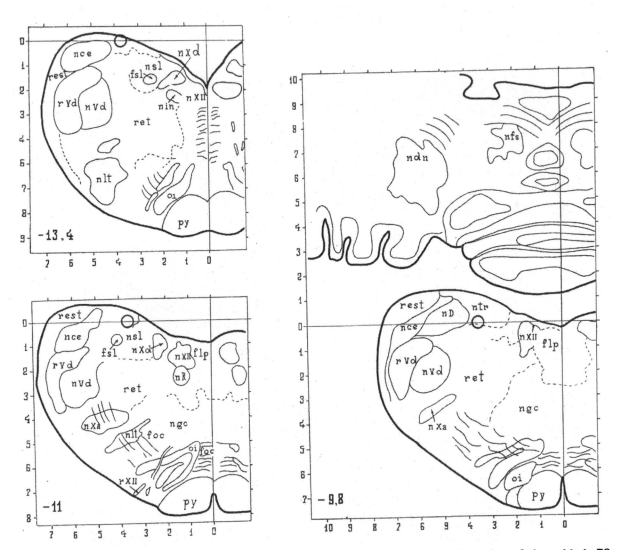

Figure 121 – Dog No. 303. The distance from tip of the inion to the posterior edge of the orbit is 78 mm. The length of the inion is 1 mm.

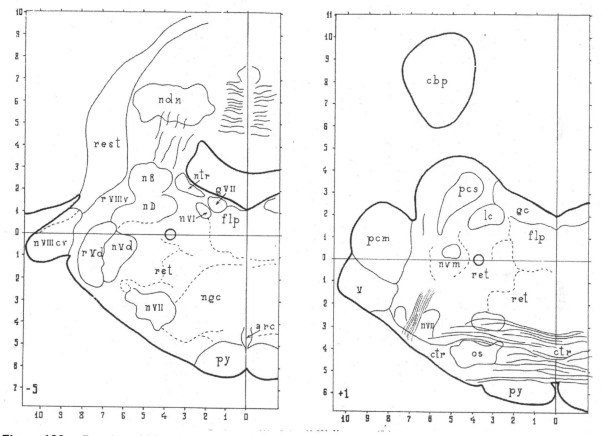

Figure 122 – Dog No. 303. The distance from tip of the inion to the posterior edge of the orbit is 78 mm. The length of the inion is 1 mm.

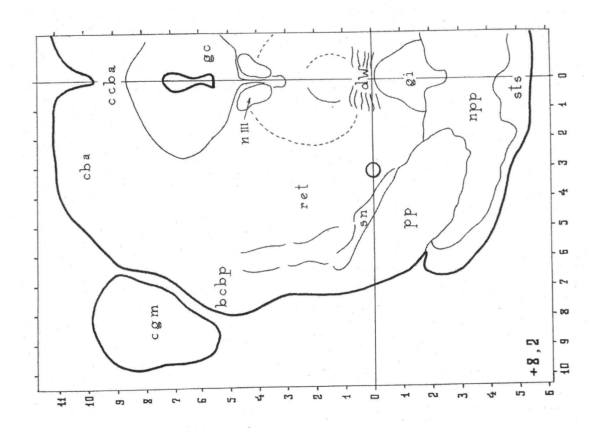

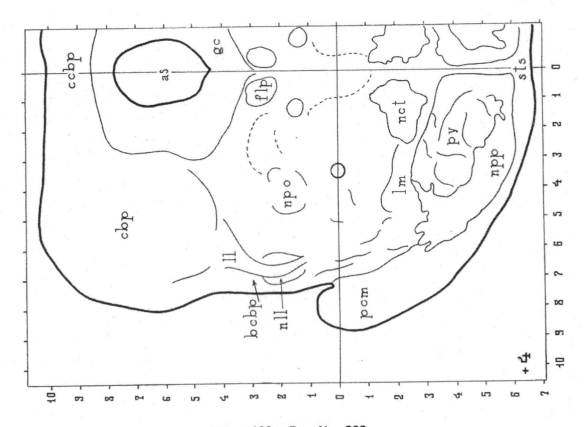

Figure 123 – Dog No. 303.

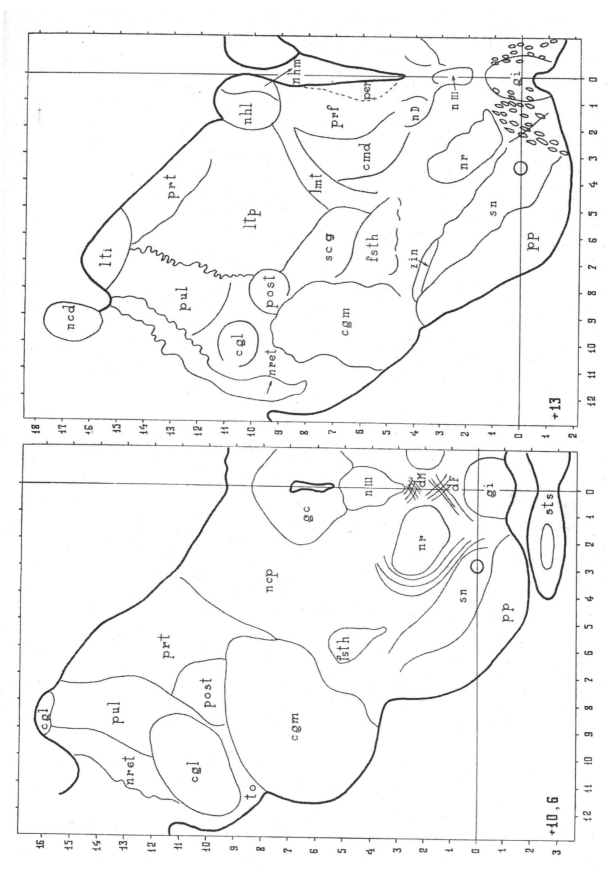

Figure 124 – Dog No. 303.

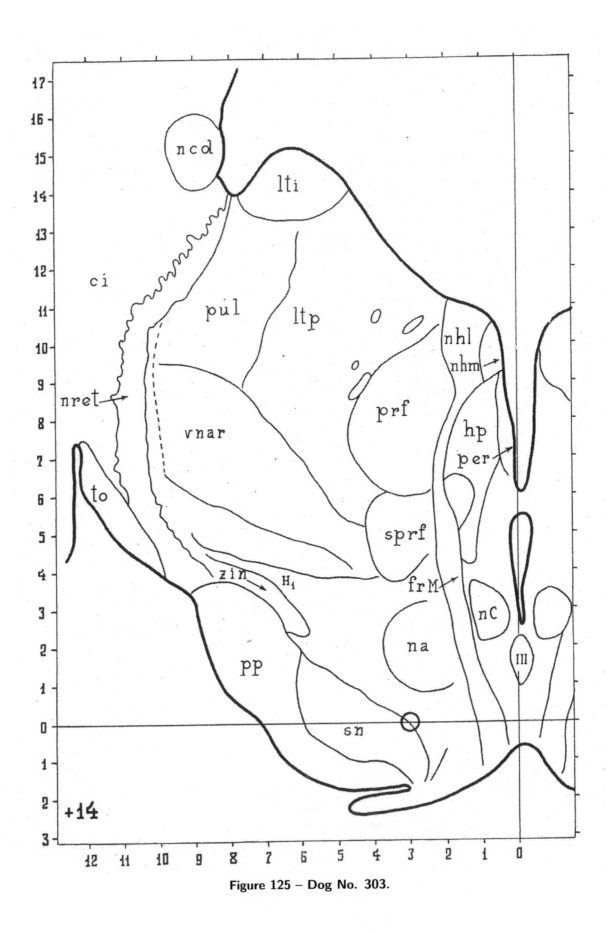

Figure 125 – Dog No. 303.

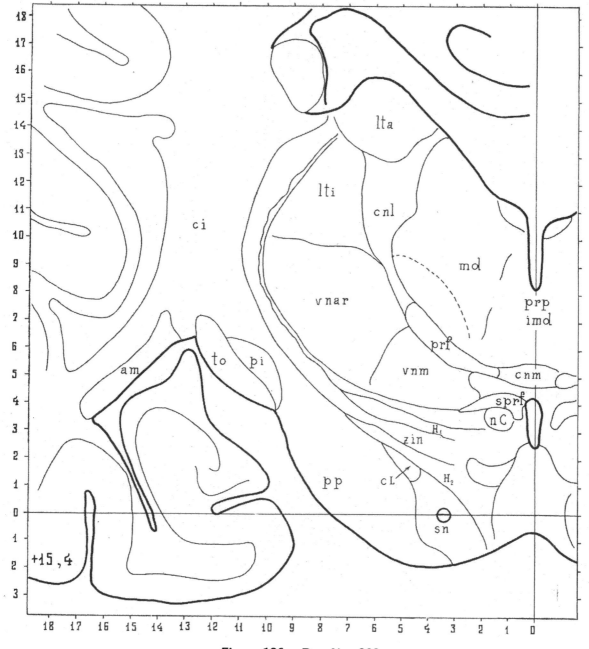

Figure 126 – Dog No. 303.

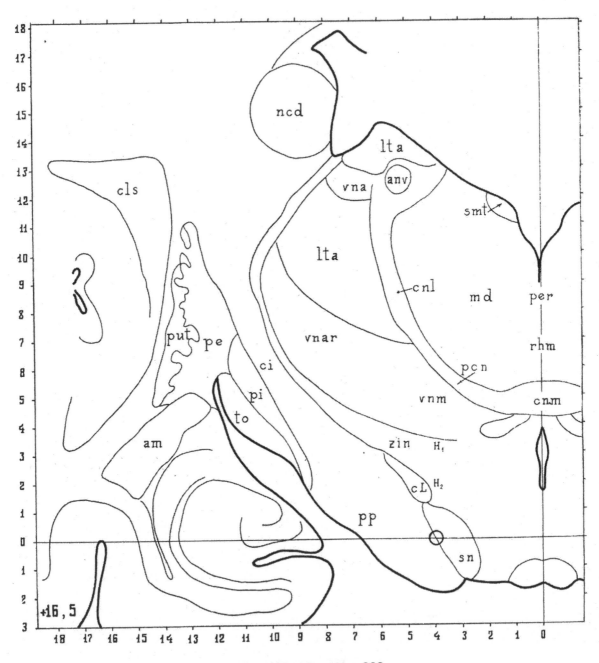

Figure 127 – Dog No. 303.

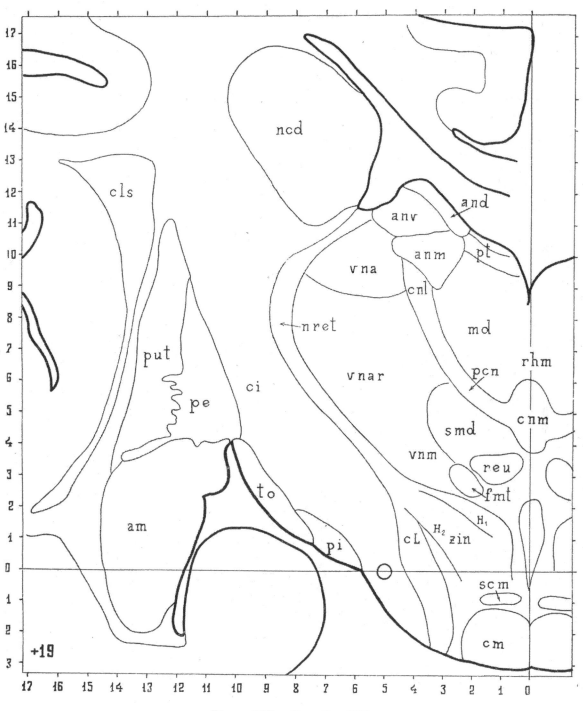

Figure 128 – Dog No. 303.

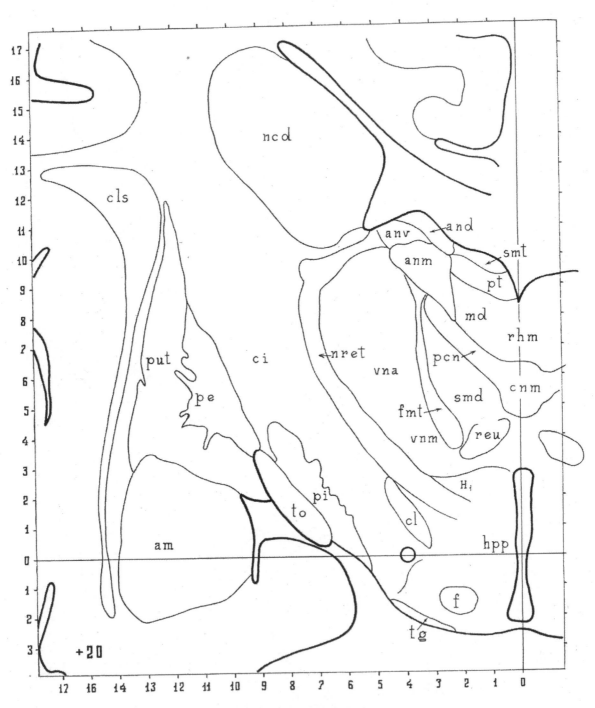

Figure 129 – Dog No. 303.

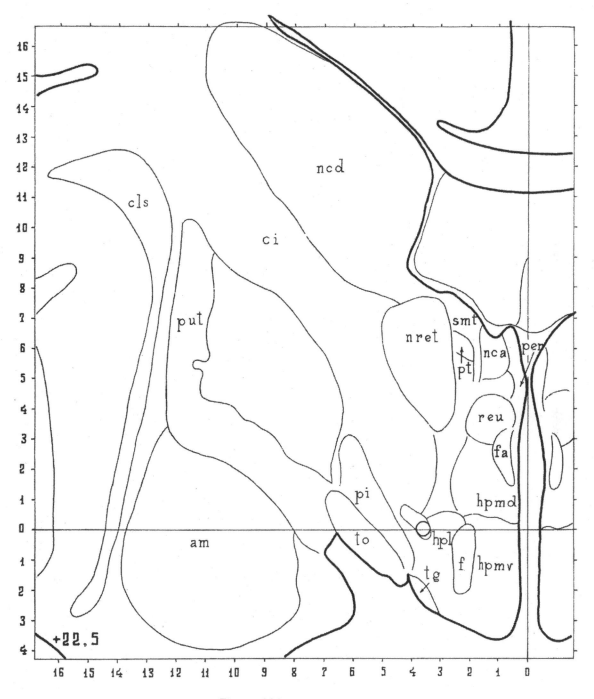

Figure 130 – Dog No. 303.

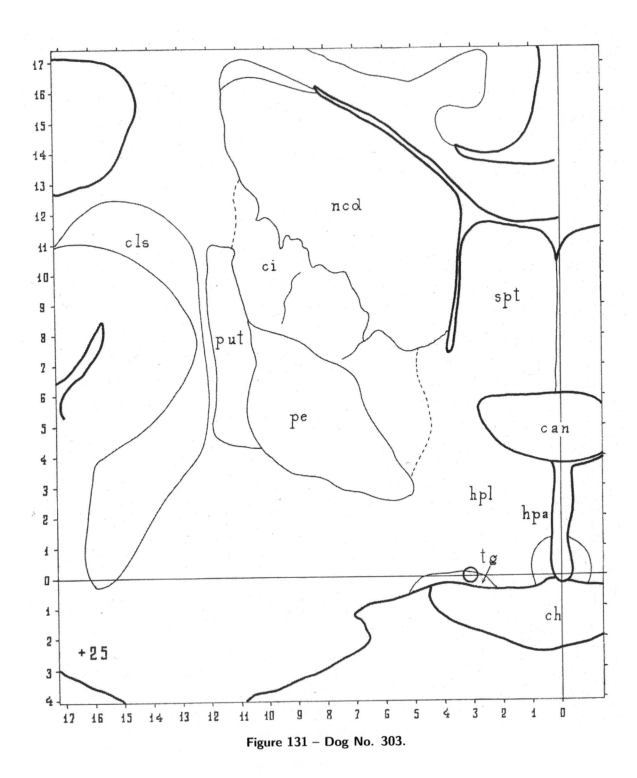

Figure 131 – Dog No. 303.

BIBLIOGRAPHY

Research concerning all areas of the central nervous system

[1] BEKHTEREV, V. Conducting tracts of the spinal cord and the cerebrum. *Part I, SPB, 1896; p. II, SPB.* (1898).

[2] BEKHTEREV, V. The basis of the teaching about the functions of the brain. *SPB, ed. I-VII.* (1905-1907).

[3] BLUMENAU, L. The human brain. *L-M.* (1925).

[4] BOGOLIUBSKIY, S. On the analogous symptoms in the canine cranium. *Russian Zoological Journal, VIII, 3, 7.* (1928).

[5] BROUWER, B. Anatomical, phylogenetical and clinical studies of the central nervous system. *Baltimore.* (1927).

[6] BRÜHL, C. Carnivorengehirn. *Zootomie der Tierklassen. Wien.* (1896).

[7] BUCHANAN, A. Functional neuroanatomy. *London.* (1948).

[8] CAJAL, S. Histologie du systeme nerveux de l'homme et des vertébrés. *V. 1-2, Paris.* (1909-1911).

[9] CLARK, R., AND HENDERSON, E. Atlas of photographs of sections of the frozen cranium and brain of the cat (felis domestica), j. psychol. a. *Neurol. 18, 3, 391.* (1911).

[10] CLARK, R., AND HENDERSON, E. Investigation of the central nervous system. *Johns Hopkins Hospital report, Special volume, I, 1.* (1920).

[11] CORDER, R., AND LATIMER, H. The prenatal growth of the brain and of its parts and of the spinal cord in the dog. *J. Comp. Neurol., 90, 193.* (1949).

[12] DEITERS, O. Untersuchungen über gehirn und rückenmark des menschen und der säugetiere. *Braunschweig.* (1865).

[13] DEKANOSIDZE, T. The structural and some functional changes in the nervous system in the ontogenesis, in the dog. *Autoessay of the dissertation. Tblishi.* (1955).

[14] DELL, P., AND OLSON, R. Projections thalamiques, corticales et cerebelleuse des afférences viscérales vagales. *C. r. Soc. biol., 145, 108.* (1951).

[15] DELMAS, P. La topomètre encèphalique l'homme. *La Presse med. 60 degree année, 25 dec., 82, 1784.* (1952).

[16] DOLGO-SABUROV, B. New teachings on the interneuronal relations in the brain. *Journal on Superior Nervous Activity, IV, 6, 903.* (1954).

[17] EDINGER, L. Der hund und hein gehirn. *Stuttgart.* (1910).

[18] EDINGER, L. Vorlesungen über den bau der nervösen zentralorgane des menschen und der tiere. *Leipzig.* (1911).

[19] ELLENBERGER, W., AND BAUM, H. Systematische und topographische anatomie des hundes. *Berlin.* (1891).

[20] ELLENBERGER, W., AND BAUM, H. Handbuch der vergleichenden anatomie der haustiere. *Berlin.* (1932).

[21] FELICIANGELI, G. Experimenteller beitrag zur kenntnis der funktionen des hundehirns. *Folia neurobiol., 4, 449.* (1910).

[22] FERRIER, D. The functions of the brain. *London.* (1876).

[23] FLATAU, E., AND JACOBSOHN, L. Handbuch der anatomie und vergleichende anatomic d. zentralnervensystems säugetiere. *Berlin-Leipzig.* (1899).

[24] FULTON, J. Physiology of the nervous system. *London-New York.* (1943).

[25] GILLILAN, L., AND TNCKARD, J. Correlation of certain neurological disfunctions with congenital anatomical abnormalities of the central nervous system of five cats. *Anat. Rec., 118, 302.* (1954).

[26] GRUNSTEIN, A. The tracts and centers of the nervous system. *M.* (1946).

[27] HESS, W. Die methodik der lokalisierten reizung und ausschaltung subkortikaler hirnabschnitte. *Beitr. z. Physiol. d. Hirnstammes. I. Teil, Leipzig.* (1932).

[28] HORANYI, B. Bedeutung der struktur der zentralnervensystems im lichte der pawlowschen physiologie. *Acta physiol. Hungar., Suppl., 4, 18.* (1953).

[29] HUSCHE, E. Schädel, hirn und seele des menschen und der tiere. *Jena.* (1854).

[30] IVANOV-SMOLENSKIY, A. The basic problems of the patho-physiology of the superior nervous activity. *M.* (1933).

[31] JAKOB, C., AND ONELLI, C. Vom tierhirn zum menschenhirn (atlas). *München.* (1911).

[32] KALISCHER, O. Experimentelle physiologic des grosshirns. *B. kh.: Handbuch d. Neurologie. M. Lewandowsky hrsgb., Berlin, 1, 365.* (1910).

[33] KAPPERS, A., HUBER, G., AND CROSBY, E. The comparative anatomy of the nervous system of vertebrates including man. *Vol. 1-2, New York.* (1936).

[34] KARPLUS, J. Zur kenntnis des wariabilitat und vererbung am zns des menschen und einiger saugetiere. *Leipzig-Wien.* (1921).

[35] KASTANYAN, E. Teaching on the conducting tracts and centers. *Rostov on the Don.* (1902).

[36] KIKIN, A. A brief zootomy or manual to the perception of the structure of the bodies of domestic animals. *Vols. I and II.* (1837).

[37] KLATT, B. Nocheinmal: Hirngrösse und korpergrosse. *Zool. Anz., 155, 9-10, 215.* (1955).

[38] KONONOVA, E. Atlas of the brainstem of man and animal. *M.* (1947).

[39] KUHLENBECK, H. Vorlesungen liber das zentralnervensystem der wierbeltiere. *Jena.* (1927).

[40] LANDAU, E. Beitrag zur kenntnis des katzenhirns. *Morphol. Jahrb., 38, 1-2, 1.* (1908).

[41] LANGLEY, J. The structure of the dog's brain. *J. Physiol., IV, 248.* (1884).

[42] LATIMER, H. The weights of the brain and of its parts, of the spinal cord and of the eyeballs in the adult cat. *J. comp. Neurol., 68, 395.* (1938).

[43] LATIMER, H. The weights of the brain and of its parts and the weight and length of the spinal cord in the dog. *Growth, 6, 39.* (1942).

[44] LAVDOVSKIY, M., AND OVSIANIKOV, F. Foundations for the study of the microscopic anatomy of man and animals. *SPB.* (1887-1888).

[45] LEONTOVICH, T., AND MERING, T. Data on the topography of the subcortical formations of the canine brain, conformably to the experimental interference on them. *Bulletin of Experimental Biology and Medicine, 42, 8, 71.* (1956).

[46] LEWANDOWSKY, M. Untersuchungen iaber die leitungsbahnen des trunkus cerebri und ihren zusammenhang mit denen der medulla spinalis und des cortex cerebri. *Jena.* (1904).

[47] LINDSLEY, D., SCHREINER, L., KNOWLES, W., AND MAGOUN, H. Behavioral and eeg changes following chronic brain stem lesions in the cat. *EEG clin. Neurophysiol., 2, 4, 403.* (1950).

[48] LISSAK, K. Die bedeutung zentralnervösen strukturen in der pawlowschen physiologie. *Acta physiol. Hungar. Suppl., 4, 16.* (1953).

[49] LORENTO DE NO, R. A study of nerve physiology. *New York.* (1947).

[50] LÖWENTHAL, N. Neuer experimental anatomischer beitrag zur kenntnis einiger bahnen in gebirn und ruckenmark. *Intern. Mschr. f. Anat. u. Physiol., 5-7.* (1893).

[51] MEYNERT, T. Vom gehirn des saugetiere. *In S. Stricker's Handbuch der Lehre von den Geweben des Menschen und der Tiere. Leipzig.* (1871).

[52] MONAKOW, C. Die lokalisation im grosshirn. *Wiesbaden.* (1914).

[53] MONNIER, M. Topographische tafeln des hirnstammes der katze fdr experimental physiologische untersuchungen. *Helv. Physiol. Acta. 1, 437.* (1943).

[54] MONNIER, M. A short atlas of the brain stem of the cat and rhesus monkey for experimental research. *Wien.* (1949).

[55] MORAWSKI, J. Gehirnuntersuchungen bei katzen- und hundefamilien (mit berlack-sichtigung des geschlechtes und der entwicklung). *Jahrb. f. Psych. u. Neurol. 33, 306.* (1912).

[56] MORRISON, L. Anatomical studies of the central nervous system of dogs without forebrain or cerebellum. *Haarlem.* (1929).

[57] MUKHIN, N. On the structure of the central gray matter of the cerebrum. *Neurological Herald, IX, 2, 121.* (1901).

[58] MUNK, H. Ober die funktionen von hirn und ruckenmark. *Berlin.* (1909).

[59] PAPEZ, J. The comparative neurology. *New York.* (1929).

[60] ROSE, M. Quotation from sarkissow, s.a. *J. f. Psychol. u. Neurol., 41, 1-2, 76.* (1930).

[61] ROZHANSKIY, N. Outlines of the physiology of the nervous system. *M.* (1957).

[62] SARKISSOW, S. On the shrinking of the brain when submerged in paraffin. *Yearb. for Psychology and Neurology. 41, 1 and 2, 76.* (1930).

[63] SEPP, E. History of the development of the nervous system from the cranium - less to human. *M.* (1949).

[64] TALALAYEV, V. Lamellar pathologo-anatomic preparations, and their production. *In the book: V.T. Talalayev. Selected Works. M.* (1953).

[65] WINKLER, C., AND POTTER, A. An anatomical guide to experimental researches on the rabbit's brain. *Atlas. Amsterdam.* (1911).

[66] WINKLER, C., AND POTTER, A. An anatomical guide to experimental researches on the cat's brain. *Atlas. Amsterdam.* (1914).

[67] ZURABASHVILI, A. To the architectonic of the cerebrum and the spinal cord of cerebellarless dogs. *Works of the Institute of Physiology in the name of I.P. Pavlov. M-L, 3, 101.* (1949).

The Spinal Cord

[68] ALLEN, W. Location in spinal cord of pathways which conduct impulses from cerebrum and superior colliculus, affecting respiration. *J. comp. Neurol., 36, 451.* (1927).

[69] AMASSIAN, V. Fiber groups and spinal pathways of cortically represented visceral afferents. *J. Neurophysiol., 14, 445.* (1951).

[70] APTER, I. The significance of posterior columns of the spinal cord in the conducting of reflexes. *Ukranian Visnik, eksp. pedogogies of reflexology. 3-4, 249.* (1927).

[71] ASKEROV, V. The change of the functions of the kidneys as the result of the hemisection of the spinal cord in the dog. *Dissertation, M.* (1956).

[72] ASRATIAN, E. The sequels of the diametrical section of the posterior half of the spinal cord in the dog. *Collected volume dedicated to the memory of the acad. P.P. Lazarev. M.* (1955).

[73] ASRATIAN, E. The dynamic specialization and location of the functions in the spinal cord. *In the book: V.M. Bekhterev and the contemporary psych-neurology. Theses of lectures. L.* (1957).

[74] BARRINGTON, F. The location of the paths subserving micturition in the spinal cord of the cat. *Brain, 56, 126.* (1933).

[75] BARSEGIAN, P. Peculiarities of the conditional-reflectory activity in whelps after damage of the anterior half of the spinal cord. *Report 2. Conditional reflexes of whelps after cross-cutting of the front half of the spinal column. Problems of superior nervous activity and compensatory adaptations. Erevan.* (1957).

[76] BARSEGIAN, R. On the physiology of the split spinal cord. *Journal of Physiology, SSSR, 24, 6, 1043.* (1938).

[77] BAZILEVSKIY, A. Investigations according to the method of marchi of early descending palingenesis in the spinal cord, after the unilateral section of the posterior cerebellar peduncle. *A review of psychiatry, neurology, 6, 430.* (1896).

[78] BEKHTEREV, V. On the relative development and different positions of the pyramidal fasciculus in man and in animals. *Medical review, 34, 13-14, 108.* (1890).

[79] BERITOV, I. Neuro-sawing of the spinal cord and its physiological aspect. *Journal of Physiology, SSSR, XXIV, 1-2.* (1938).

[80] BOHM, E. An electro-physiological study of the ascending spinal anterolateral fiber system connected to course cutaneous afferents. *A spinobulbo-cerebellar system. Acta Physiol. Scand., 29, Suppl. 106.* (1953).

[81] BOROVIKOV. The role of the posterior columns of the spinal cord in the conducting of muscular sensitivity. *Diss. SPB.* (1900).

[82] BRODAL, A., AND KAADA, B. Exteroceptive and proprioceptive ascending impulses in pyramidal tract of cat. *J. Neurophysiol. 16, 6, 567.* (1953).

[83] BRODAL, A., AND REXED, B. Spinal afferents to the lateral cervical nucleus in the cat. *J. comp. Neurol., 98, 2, 179.* (1953).

[84] BRODAL, A., AND WALBERG, F. Ascending fibers in pyramidal tract of cat. *Arch. Neurol. and Psychiat., 68, 755.* (1952).

[85] BRODAL, A., WALBERG, F., AND BLACKSTAD, T. Termination of spinal afferents to inferior olive in cat. *J. Neurophysiol. 13, 431.* (1950).

[86] CARDIN, A. Attivith locomotrice nel cane spinalizzato cronico. *Boll. Soc. ital. biol. sperim., 29, 7, 1362.* (1953).

[87] CHIARUGI, E., ROSSI, G., AND ZANCHETTI, A. The spinal course of the corticofugal fibers arising in the motor cortex of the cat. *Confinia neurol., 15, 5, 304.* (1955).

[88] CHOLOKASHVILI, E. Quantitative distribution of the synapses on the cellular bodies and on the dendrite processes of the spinal cord. *Works of the Institute of Physiology, Tblisi, 9, 161.* (1953).

[89] DEESE, J., AND KELLOG, W. Some new data on the nature of spinal conditioning. *J. comp. Physiol. a. Psychol., 42, 3, 157.* (1949).

[90] DI BIAGIO, F., AND GRUNDFEST, H. Afferent relations of inferior olivary nucleus. *J. Neurophysiol., 18, 3, 299, 1955; 19, 1, 10.* (1956).

[91] DOBROTVORSKIY, O. On the secondary palingeneses in the spinal cord. *Psychiatric Review, 9, 671.* (1897).

[92] DURITSYN, F. On the study of the structure of the spinal cord in vertebrate animals. *The transactions of the V All-union convention of anatomists, histologists and embryologists. L., 474.* (1951).

[93] DURMISHYAN, M. On the reflectory activity of the injured spinal cord. *In the book: Disease, Treatment and Recovery. M., 415.* (1952).

[94] EWALD, I. Demonstration eines hundes dem ein 70 millim. *langes Stack der Hinterstrange des Rackenmarkes entfernt ist. Dtsch. med. Wschr., 30, 217.* (1898).

[95] FREEMAN, L. Return of function after complete transection of the spinal cord in rat, cat and dog. *Ann. Surg., 136, 193.* (1952).

[96] GAMBARIAN, L. Conditioned reflexes in the dog after a high section of the posterior columns of the spinal cord. *Erevan.* (1953).

[97] GETZ, B. The termination of spino-thalamic fibers in the cat as studied by the method of terminal degeneration. *Acta anat. (Basel), 16, 271.* (1952).

[98] GEYER, T. Materials on the question on the form and development of the protoplasmic processes of the nervous cells of the spinal cord. *Diss. M.* (1904).

[99] GLEES, P. The central pain tract (tractus spino-thalamicus). *Acta neuro-veget. 7, 1-4, 160.* (1953).

[100] GOLTZ, F., AND EWALD, I. Der hund mit verkurzten ruckenmarke. *Pflug. Arch. 63, 352.* (1896).

[101] GOLTZINGER, F. The sensory tracts in the spinal cord. *Diss. SPB.* (1896).

[102] GORIUN, G. On the morphological interrelations of the neurons in the gray substance of the spinal cord. *Diss. Roston on the Don.* (1952).

[103] GRUNDFEST, H., AND CAMPBELL, A. Origin, conduction and termination of impulses in dorsal spino-cerebellar tracts of cats. *J. Neurophysiol., 5, 275.* (1942).

[104] GRUNDFEST, H., AND GARTER, W. Afferent relations of inferior olivary nucleus. *J. Neurophysiol. 17, 72.* (1954).

[105] HECK, G. The cerebellar terminations of the spino-cerebellar fibers of the lower lumbar and sacral segments of the cat. *Brain, 50, 60.* (1927).

[106] IVANOVA, S. The disruption and restoration of the functions of the organism after a bilateral section, in half, of the cervical segments of the spinal cord in the dog. *Bulletin of Experimental Biology and Medicine. 7, 42.* (1950).

[107] KELL, J., AND HOFF, H. Descending spinal pathways mediating pressor responses of cerebral origin. *J. Neurophysiol., 15, 4, 299.* (1952).

[108] KENNARD, M. The course of ascending fibers in the spinal cord of the cat essential to the recognition of painful stimuli. *J. comp. Neurol., 100, 3, 511.* (1954).

[109] KRIEGER, H., AND GRUNDFEST, H. Afferent relations of inferior olivary nucleus. *III. Electrophysiological demonstration of a second relay in dorsal spino-olivary pathway in cat. J. Neurophysiol., 19, 1, 3.* (1956).

[110] KURU, AND MASURA. The spino-buibar tracts and the pelvic sensory vagus. *J. comp. Neurol. 104, 2, 207.* (1956).

[111] LANCE, J. Pyramidal tract in spinal cord of cat. *J. Neurophysiol., 17, 3, 253.* (1954).

[112] LANDAU, W. Autonomic responses mediated via the cortico-spinal tract. *J. Neurophysiol., 16, 299.* (1953).

[113] LAPINSKIY, M. A propos of spino-cerebral centers, assigned to the separate segments of the extremities and the muscular groups (in the dog). *M.* (1903).

[114] LAPINSKIY, M. The question of centripetal connections of the liver with the spinal cord. *Journal for the Improvement of Physicians. 4, 340.* (1927).

[115] LASSEK, A. A comparative volumetric study of the gray and white substance of the spinal cord. *J. comp. Neurol. 62, 361.* (1935).

[116] LASSEK, A. The pyramidal tract. *Springfield.* (1954).

[117] LEBEDEV, I. The course of the anterior fasciculi of the spinal cord in the cerebrum. *Diss. SPB.* (1873).

[118] LENHOSSEK, M. Über die pyramidenbahnen im ruckenmarke einiger saugetiere. *Anat. Ariz., 4, 208.* (1889).

[119] LESZLENYI, O. Vergleichend-anatomische studie caber die lissauersche randzone des hinterhorns. *Arb. a.d. Neurol. Inst. d. Wien. Univ., 19, 252.* (1911).

[120] LEWANDOWSKY, M. Experimentelle physiologic des ruckenmarks und des hirnstammes. *Hand. d. Neural. Hrsgb. von Lewandowsky, 1, 344.* (1910).

[121] LINOWIECKI, A. The comparative anatomy of the pyramidal tract. *J. comp. Neurol. 24, 509.* (1914).

[122] LIUBUSHIN, A. Some experimental data on the question of the endogenous fibers in the anterolateral columns of the spinal cord. *Diss. M.* (1903).

[123] LIUTOV, A. The efficiency of the spinal cord, depending on the level of its section. *Auto-essay of a dissertation, M.* (1955).

[124] LLOYD, D. Functional organization of the spinal cord. *Physiol. Rev., 24, 1.* (1944).

[125] MAFFRÉ, S. Étude physiologique et morphologique du faisceau pyramidal chez le chien d'après les consequence de son exclusion chronique. *Marseille, M. Léconte.* (1955).

[126] McCOUCH, G. Reflex development in the chronically spinal cat and dog. *J. Neurophysiol., X, 5, 425.* (1947).

[127] McCOUGH, G., DEERING, J., AND LING, T. Location of receptors for tonic neck reflexes. *J. Neurophysiol. 14, 3, 190.* (1951).

[128] McINTYRE, A. Spina-cerebellar pathways in the cat. *Proc. Univ. Otago Med. School, 2, 16.* (1951).

[129] MORIN, F. A new spinal pathway for cutaneous impulses. *Amer. J. Physiol., 183, 2, 245.* (1955).

[130] MORIN, F., AND CATALANO, J. Central connections of a cervical nucleus (nucleus cervicalis lateralis of the cat). *J. comp. Neurol. 103, 1, 17.* (1955).

[131] MORIN, F., CATALANO, J., AND LINDNER, D. Spina-cerebellar projections in the cat and monkey (macaca mulatta). *Anat. Rec., 115, 350.* (1953).

[132] MOTT, F. Microscopical examination of clarke's column in the man, the monkey and the dog. *J. Anat., 22, 479.* (1888).

[133] MÜNZER, E., AND WIENER, H. Experimentelle beiträge zur lehre von den endogenen fasersystemen des rückenmarkes. *Mschr. Psychiat. u. Neural., XXVIII, 1.* (1910).

[134] MURATOW, W. The secondary palingenesis after the destruction of the motor sphere of the cerebral cortex. *Arch. Anat. and Physiol., Anat. sect. 34.* (1893).

[135] NEMILOW, A. On the peripheric stratum of nerve cells and nerve fibers in the spinal cord of superior vertebrate animals. *Arch. of microsc. Anat. 77, 433.* (1911).

[136] NESMEYANOVA, T., AND SHAMARINA, N. On the character of the reflectory activity of the spinal cord, cut through. *Transact. Acad. Sciences of USSR, XCVII, 3, 547.* (1954).

[137] NIEMER, W., AND MAGOUN, H. Reticulo-spinal tracts influencing motor activity. *J. comp. Neurol. 87, 367.* (1947).

[138] NOVIKOVA, A., AND KHANUTINA, D. The question of the nature of the motor defensive conditioned reflexes in the dog with a half diametrical cut through the spinal cord. *Journal of Physiology SSSR, XXVI, 4, 346.* (1939).

[139] OBERSTEINER, H. Ueber clarke's posterior vesicular columns. *Arb. a.d. Neural. Inst. d. Wien, Univ. VIII, 2.* (1902).

[140] OSTROUMOV, N. About the regulation of respiratory motions. *The spinocerebral respiratory centers of mammals. In the book: The Works of the State Medical Institute of Kuibyshev. Kuibyshev, 2, 138.* (1948).

[141] PANKRATOV, M. Catatonia after cutting through the posterior columns of the spinal cord. *The works of the Institute of evolutional physiology and pathology of superior nervous activity, named after I.P. Pavlov. L., 1, 313.* (1947).

[142] PAPEZ, J. Reticulo-spinal tracts in the cat. *J. comp. Neurol., 31, 365.* (1926).

[143] PASS, J. Anatomic and functional relationship of the nucleus dorsalis (clarke's column) and of the dorsal spino-cerebellar tract (flechsig's). *Arch. Neural. a. Psychiatr. 30, 1025.* (1933).

[144] PAVLOV, I. About the vascular centers in the spinal cord. *Complete works. M.-L., I, 35.* (1951).

[145] PINES, L., AND GUTMAN, B. Palingenesis of the posterior columns of the spinal cord after cutting them at different levels. *The works of the Pavlov Institute of Physiology. M., L., II, 115.* (1947).

[146] POKROVSKIY, E. On the topography of the cat's spinal cord, its radicles and intervertebral ganglions. *Theses of the 4th Pavlov session of the students of the II Moscow Medical Institute. M., 15.* (1954).

[147] POPOV, N. The condition of the vegetative functions in the isolation of the central and peripheral nervous formations. *Journal of Physiology, SSSR, 17, 3.* (1934).

[148] RANSON, S., MUIR, J., AND ZEISS, F. Extensor tonus after spinal cord lesions in the cat. *J. comp. Neurol. 54, 13.* (1932).

[149] REICH, Z. Vom aufbau der mittelzone des rackenmarks. *Arb. a.d. Neural. inst. d. Wien. Univ., XVII, 314.* (1909).

[150] REXED, B. A cytoarchitectonic atlas of the spinal cord in the cat. *J. comp. Neurol. 100, 2, 297.* (1954).

[151] REXED, B., AND BRODAL, A. The nucleus cervicalis lateralis: a spino-cerebellar relay nucleus. *J. Neurophysiol. 14, 5, 399.* (1951).

[152] REXED, B., AND STROM, B. Afferent nervous connections of the lateral cervical nucleus. *Acta physiol. Scand. 25, 219.* (1952).

[153] ROTHMANN, AND M. Ueber die beziehungen des obersten halsmarkes zur kehlkopfinnervation. *Neurol. al., 5, 274.* (1912).

[154] ROTHMANN, M. Ueber die physiologische wertung der cortico-spinalen (pyramiden) hahn. *Arch. Anat. u. Physiol., Physiol. Abt. 3-4, 217.* (1907).

[155] RUSSKIKH, V. The synaptic apparatus of the cells of the spinal cord in the dog. *Nature 8, 39.* (1951).

[156] SCHIFFERDECKER, P. Ueber regeneration degeneration und architectur des racken-markes. *Virch. Arch., 67.* (1876).

[157] SCHILDER, P. Vergleichende histologische untersuchungen aber den nucleus sacralis stillingi. *Arb. a.d. Neurol. Inst., d. Wien. Univ. 18, 195.* (1910).

[158] SHERRINGTON, C., KRIG, R., DENNY-BROWN, D., IKKLS, G., AND LIDDELL, E. Reflectory activity of the spinal cord. *Bio. Med. Gis.* (1935).

[159] SOKOLOV, V. On the structure formatio reticularis of the spinal cord. *Theses of lectures of the scientific conference, dedicated to the 50 anniversary of the II Medical Institute in Moscow, M., 66.* (1957).

[160] SPITZKA, E. The comparative anatomy of the pyramidal tract. *J. comp. M.E.S., 7, 1.* (1885).

[161] SWANK, R. An abberrant pyramidal fascicle in the cat. *J. comp. Neurol., 60, 355.* (1934).

[162] SZENTAGOTHAI, J. Die ruckwirkung von funktioneller inanspruchnahme und inaktivitat auf morphologische merkmale der nervenelemente. *Acta physiol. Hungar., supra. 4, 17.* (1953).

[163] TAKAHASHI, D. Zur vergleichenden anatomie des seitenhorns im ruckenmark der vertebraten. *Arb. a.d. Neurol. Inst. d. Wien. Univ. 20, 62.* (1912).

[164] TITOVA, G. Skeletotopy of the spinal cord and the correlations of the nerves of the spinal cord and the sympathetic column in the dog. *Theses of lectures of the Ukranian conference of morphologists, II, 272.* (1956).

[165] TOWER, S. Function and structure in the chronically isolated lumbo-sacral spinal cord of the dog. *J. comp. Neurol. 67, 109.* (1937).

[166] TROSHIN, G. To the problem of the centripetal connections of the nuclei of the posterior columns. *Scientific reports of the University of Kazan for the year 1899. See all Neurol. Cbl., 19, 379.* (1900).

[167] TYSHETSKIY, A. On the excitability of the elements of the spinal cord through electric stimulation. *Diss. SPB.* (1870).

[168] URGANDZHIAN, T. The question of the conditioned reflex activity in the case of injury to the conducting tracts of the spinal cord. *The aspects of the superior nervous activity and compensatory adaptations. Erevan, II, 107.* (1957).

[169] VERHAART, W. The fiber structure of the cord in the cat. *Acta anat., 18, 2, 88.* (1953).

[170] VERHAART, W. The rubro-spinal tract in the cat, the monkey and the ape, its location and fiber content. *Mschr. Psychiatr. u. Neuxol., 129, 6, 487.* (1955).

[171] VERMEULEN, H. On the conus medullaris of the domestic animals. *Koninklijke Akad. van Wetènsch. appen. t. Amsterdam, XVIII, 4-5, 780.* (1915).

[172] VOROTYNSKIY. Materials for the study of the secondary palingeneses in the spinal cord, after its diametrical injuries. *Neurological News, V. 3, 53.* (1897).

[173] WALBERG, F., AND BRODAL, A. Spino-pontine fibers in the cat. *An experimental study. J. comp. Neurol., 99, 251.* (1953).

[174] YAKUBOVICH, N. Notes on the extremely thin structure of the cerebrum and the spinal cord. *Medico-military Journal. 70, 2, 2, 35.* (1857).

[175] ZURABASHVILI, A. The morphology of the sinaptic apparatus of the spinal cord. *Report Acad. of Sc. Georg. SSR 6, 644.* (1944).

[176] ZURABASHVILI, A., AND MEPISASHVILI, I. On the thin structure of the posterior horn of the spinal cord in animals. *The transactions of the Institute of Physiology named after I.S. Beritashvili. Tblisi, 4, 197.* (1941).

The Medulla Oblongata, Pons Varolii and the Mesencephalon

[177] ADELHEIM, K. The anatomy of the cerebrum. *On the nuclei of the tractus Peduncularis transversi (Guddeni). The works of the Physico-medical Society. M., 12, 4.* (1886).

[178] AFANASYEV, M. New data on the structure and functions of the lamina quadri-gemina in mammals. *Diss. M.* (1946).

[179] AIDAR ORLANDO, W., AND GEOHEGAN AND UNGEWITTER, L. Splanchnic afferent pathways in the central nervous system. *J. Neurophysiol., 15, 2, 131.* (1952).

[180] ALFEYEVSKIY, N. The study of the sensory and motor nuclei of the vagus nerve. *Diss. M.* (1907).

[181] ALLEN, W. Function of the cells in the motor root of the nervus trigeminus in the cat. *J. comp. Neurol., 38, 349.* (1925).

[182] ALLEN, W. Experimental-anatomical studies on the visceral bulbo-spinal pathway in the cat and guinea pig. *J. comp. Neurol., 42, 393.* (1927).

[183] ALLEN, W. Formatio reticularis and reticulo-spinal tracts, their visceral functions and possible relationship to tonicity and clonic contractions. *Wash. Acad. Sci., 22, 490.* (1932).

[184] ALLEN, W. Effects of sectioning pyramidal or extrapyramidal tracts on positive and negative conditioned reflexes in dogs. *Amer. J. physiol., 166, 1, 176.* (1951).

[185] APTER, J. Projection of the retina on superior colliculus of cats. *J. Neurophysiol., 8, 2, 123.* (1945).

[186] ARTYUKHINA, N. Comparative study of the red nucleus in mammals. *Autoessay of the dissertation. M.* (1952).

[187] BAGINSKY. Ueber den ursprung und den zentralen verlauf d.n. *Acusticus d. Kaninchens und d. Katze. Virch. Arch., 119, 91.* (1890).

[188] BARNARD, I. The hypoglossal complex of vertebrates. *J. comp. Neurol., 72, 489.* (1940).

[189] BARRON, D. A note on the course of the proprioceptor fibers from the tongue. *Anat. Rec., 66, 11.* (1936).

[190] BAUER, J. Ueber ein faserbündel der haube und dessen mögliche beziehung zum kauakt. *Anat. Anz., XXXIII, 6-7, 140.* (1908).

[191] BAUER, J. Die substantia nigra soemmeringii. *Arb. a.d. Neurol. inst. d. Wien, Univ., XVII, 435.* (1909).

[192] BEKHTEREV, V. On the so called, spasm center and on the center of locomotion of the body at the level of the pons varolii. *Neurological Herald, 4, 4, 97.* (1896).

[193] BEKHTEREV, V. On a specific nucleus of the reticular formation, at the level of the superior portions of the pons varolii. *Neurological Herald, 6, 2, 182.* (1898).

[194] BERITOV, I. Neuropil of the stem part of the cerebrum and its physiological role. *Journal of Physiology, SSSR, 22, 755.* (1937).

[195] BERRY, C., KARL, K., AND HINSEY, I. Course of the spinothalamic and medial lemniscus pathways in cat and rhesus monkey. *J. Neurophysiol., 13, 149.* (1950).

[196] BIRZIS, L., AND HEMINGWAY, A. Descending brain stem connections controlling shivering in cat. *J. Neurophysiol., 19, 37.* (1956).

[197] BLACKSTAD, T., BRODAL, A., AND WALBERG, F. Some observations on normal and degenerating terminal boutons in the inferior olive of the cat. *Acta anat., 11, 461.* (1951).

[198] BOHM, E., AND PETERSEN, I. Ipsilateral conduction in the medial lemniscus of the cat. *Acta physiol. Scand 29, Suppl., 106, 138.* (1953).

[199] BOLL, K. The topography of the nerve cells of the vagus and the origin of the ganglion jugulare and the ganglion nodosum in domestic animals. *Arch. of Veterin. Science, 42, 605.* (1912).

[200] BONVALLET, M., DELL, P., AND HUGELIN, A. Projections olfactives, gustatives, viscerales, visuelles et auditieves au niveau des formations griseés du cerveau anterieur du chat. *J. physiol., Paris, 44, 222.* (1952).

[201] BORISON, H., AND BRIZZEE, K. Morphology of emetic chemoreceptor trigger zone in cat medulla. *Proc. Soc. Exp. Biol. a. Med., 77, 38.* (1951).

[202] BOROWIECKI, S. Vergleichend-anatomische und experimentelle untersuchungen über das brückengrau und die wichtigsten verbindungen der brücke. *Arb. a. d. hirnanatom. Inst. in Zürich, V, 39.* (1911).

[203] BRIZZEE, K., AND BORISON, H. Studies on the localization and morphology of the chemoreceptor trigger (c. T.) zone in the area postrema of the cat. *Anat. rec., 112, 13.* (1952).

[204] BRIZZEE, K., AND NEAL, L. A reevaluation of the cellular morphology of the area postrema in view of recent evidence for a chemoreceptor function. *J. comp. Neurol., 100, 41.* (1954).

[205] BRODAL, A. Experimentelle untersuchungen über die olivo-cerebellare lokalisation. *Ztschr. ges. Neurol. u. Psychiatr., 169, 1.* (1940).

[206] BRODAL, A. Die verbindungen des nucleus cuneatus externus mit dem kleinhirn beim kaninchen und bei der katze. *Ztschr. ges. Neurol. u. Psychiatr., 171, 167.* (1941).

[207] BRODAL, A. Spinal afferents to the lateral reticular nucleus of the medulla oblongata in the cat. *An experimental study. J. comp. Neurol., 91, 259.* (1949).

[208] BRODAL, A. Experimental demonstrations of cerebellar connections from the peryhypoglossal nuclei (nucleus intercalatus, nucleus praepositus hypoglossi and nucleus of roller) in the cat. *J. Anat., 86, 110.* (1952).

[209] BRODAL, A. Reticulo-cerebellar connections in the cat. *An experimental study. J. comp. Neurol. 98, 113.* (1953).

[210] BRODAL, A., AND GOGSTAD, A. Rubro-cerebellar connections. *An experimental study in the cat. Anat. rec., 118, 3, 455.* (1954).

[211] BRODAL, A., AND JANSEN, J. The ponto-cerebellar projection in the rabbit and cat. *J. comp. Neurol., 84, 31.* (1946).

[212] BRODAL, A., AND ROSSI, G. Ascending fibers in brain stem reticular formation of cat. *Arch. Neurol. a. Psychiatr., 74, 1, 68.* (1955).

[213] BROWN, J. The nuclear pattern of the non-tectal portions of the midbrain and isthmus in the dog and cat. *J. comp. Neurol., 78, 365.* (1943).

[214] BROWN, J. Pigmentation of substantia nigra and locus coeruleus in certain carnivores. *J. comp. Neurol., 79, 393.* (1943).

[215] BRUESCH, S. The distribution of myelinated afferent fibers in the branches of the cats facial nerve. *J. comp. Neurol., 81, 169.* (1944).

[216] BUCHANAN, A. The course of the secondary vestibular fibers in the cat. *J. comp. Neurol., 67, 183.* (1937).

[217] BUCHER, V., AND BÜRGI, S. Untersuchungen über die faserverbindungen im zwischen- und mittelhirn der katze. *Confinia neurol., 6, 317.* (1945).

[218] BUCHER, V., AND BÜRGI, S. Some observations on the fiber connections of the di- and mesencephalon in the cat. *J. comp. Neurol., 93, 139, 1950; 96, 139.* (1952).

[219] BÜRGI, S. Ueber die zentralen haubenbahnen. *Studien an der Sammlung von W.R. Hess. Schweiz. med. Wschr., 2, 57.* (1954).

[220] BÜRGI, S. Über die verbindungen der kerne der hinteren commissur und die frage des vorhandenseins ascendieren der vestibularisbahnen. *Dtsch. Ztschr. Nervenheilk, 174, 235.* (1956).

[221] BÜRGI, S., AND MONNIER, M. Motorische erscheinungen bei reizung und ausschaltung der substantia reticularis pontis. *Helv. Physiol. acta, 1, 489.* (1943).

[222] BURKENKO, N., AND KLOSOVKIY, B. Bulbotomy, information i, the ceasing of hyperkinetic phenomena through cutting of the extrapyramidal tracts in the medulla oblongata. *Problems of Neurosurgery, I, 1, 5.* (1937).

[223] CAJAL, R. Beiträge zum studium der medulla oblongata des kleinhirns und des ursprungs der gehirnnerven. *Leipzig.* (1890).

[224] CHATFIELD, P. Salivation in response to localized stimulation of the medulla. *Amer. J. physiol., 133, 3, 637.* (1941).

[225] CLARK, W. The mammalian oculomotor nucleus. *J. Anat., 60, 426.* (1926).

[226] CLEES, P., LIVINGSTON, K., AND SALER, J. Der intraspinal verlauf und die endigungen der sensorischen wurzeln in den nucleus gracilis und cuneatus. *Arch f. Psychiatr., 187, 190.* (1951).

[227] CLEMENTE, C., AND VAN BREEMEN, V. Nerve fibers in the area postrema of cat, rabbit, guinea pig and rat. *Anat. rec., 123, 1, 65.* (1955).

[228] COLLIER, J., AND BUZZARD, F. Descending mesencephalic tracts in cat, monkey and man. *Brain, 24, 11, 177.* (1901).

[229] CORBIN, K. Probst's tract in the cat. *J. comp. Neurol., 77, 3, 455.* (1942).

[230] CRIGHEL, E., CHIVU, V., AND STERIADE, M. Cercetari asupra functiunii căii piramidale. *Studii şi cercetări de fisiologie şi neurologie, V, 1-2, 155.* (1954).

[231] DANIS, P. The functional organization of the third nerve nucleus in the cat. *Amer. J. Ophth., 31, 1122.* (1948).

[232] DARKSHEVICH, L. On the conducting of the light stimulus from the retina upon the oculomotor nerve. *Diss. M.* (1887).

[233] DARKSHEVICH, L. On the superior nuclei of the oculomotor nerve. *Arch. Anat. and Physiol., 107.* (1889).

[234] DARKSHEVICH, L., AND PRIBYTKOV, G. On the system of fibers on the floor of the third cerebral ventricle. *Neurol. News, 10, 47.* (1891).

[235] DAVENPORT, H., AND RANSON, S. The red nucleus and adjacent cell groups. *A topographic study in the cat and in the rabbit. Arch. Neurol. and Psychiatr. 24, 257.* (1930).

[236] DE NEEF, C. Recherches expérimentales sur les localisations motrices medullaires chez le chien et le lapin. *Le Nevraxe, 2, 69.* (1901).

[237] DELL, P., AND OLSON, R. Projections secondaires mésencéphaliques, diencéphaliques et amygdaliennes des afférences viscérales vagales. *C. r. Soc. biol., 145, 1088.* (1951).

[238] DU BOIS, F., AND FOLEY, I. Experimental studies on the vagus and spinal accessory nerves in the cat. *Anat. rec., 64, 283.* (1936).

[239] DUSSER DE BARENNE, J., AND MAGNUS, R. Beiträge zum problem der korperstellung. *III. Die Stellreflexe bei der grosshirnlosen Katze und dem grosshirnlosen Hunde. pflüg. Arch. ges. Physiol., 180, 75.* (1920).

[240] ECONOMO, C., AND KARPLUS, J. Zur physiologie und anatomic des mittelhirns. *Arch. f. Psychiatr., 46, 275 and 377.* (1910).

[241] ELDRED, E., AND SNIDER, R. Anatomical distribution on fast cerebellar-like activity within the brain stem. *Anat. rec., 106, 190.* (1950).

[242] ERIST, E. The descending connections of the optic thalami and the anterior corpus bigeminum. *Diss. St. P.* (1902).

[243] EVANS, B., AND INGRAM, W. The effects of combined red nucleus and pyramidal lesions in cats. *J. comp. Neurol., 70, 461.* (1939).

[244] FELDMAN, N. Ontogenesis of the anterior tuber of the lamina quadrigemina and the anterior geniculate bodies in dogs and guinea pigs. *Theses of lectures at the 33rd scientific session of the Astrakhan Medical Institute, Astrakhan, 66.* (1956).

[245] FERRARO, A., PACELLA, B., AND BARRERA, S. Effects of lesions of the medial vestibular nuclei. *J. comp. Neurol., 73, 7.* (1940).

[246] FLIEGELMAN, L. Ontogenesis and comparative-anatomical data on the development of the black substance. *In the book: Ontogenesis of the brain. L., 140.* (1949).

[247] FOX, C., AND SCHMITZ, I. The substantia nigra and the entopedunucular nucleus in the cat. *J. comp. Neurol., 80, 323.* (1941).

[248] FULTON, I., LIDDEL, E., AND BLOCH, D. The influence of unilateral destruction of the vestibular nuclei upon posture and the knee jerk. *Brain, 53, 327.* (1930).

[249] FURSTENBERG, A., AND MAGIELSKI, I. A motor pattern in the nucleus ambiguus. *Ann. Otol., 69, 788.* (1955).

[250] FUSE, G. Die innere abteilung des kleinhirnteils (meynert, i.a. *K.) und der Deitersche Kern. Arb. a.d. hirnanatom. inst. in Zürich, 6, 29.* (1912).

[251] FUSE, G. Ueber den abduzenskern der aäuger. *Arb. a.d. hirnanatom. Inst. in Zürich, 6, 401.* (1912).

[252] FUSE, G. Beiträdge zur anatomie des bodens des iv. *Ventrikels. Arb. a.d. Hirnanatom. Inst. in Zürich, 8, 213.* (1914).

[253] GEREBTZOFF, M. Contribution à l'étude des voies afférentes de l'olive inférieure. *J. Belge Neurol. et Psychiatr, 39, 719.* (1939).

[254] GERNANDT, B., AND THULIN, C. Vestibular connection of the brainstem. *Amer. J. Physiol., 171, lpl.* (1952).

[255] GERNANDT, B., AND THULIN, C. Effect of vestibular nerve section upon the spinal influence of the bulbar reticular formation. *Acta phisiol. Scand., 33, 120.* (1955).

[256] GORBATSEVICH, Z. To the question of interneuronal connections in the anterior tubers of the lamina quadrigemina. *Collections of works of the Kursk State Medical Institute. Kursk, II (X), 196.* (1955).

[257] GRAY, L. Some experimental evidence on the connections of the vestibular mechanism in the cat. *J. comp. Neurol., 41, 319.* (1926).

[258] GRUNDFEST, H., AND CARTER, W. Afferent relations of inferior olivary nucleus. *J. Neurophysiol., 17, 1, 72.* (1954).

[259] HATSCHEK, R. Zur vergleichenden anatomic des nucleus ruber. *Arb. a. d. neur. Inst. d. Wien. Univ., 15, 48.* (1907).

[260] HELD, H. Die zentralen bahnen des nervus acusticus bei der katze. *Arch. f. Anat. u. Physiol., Anat. Abt., 201.* (1891).

[261] HUBER, G., CROSBY, E., WOODBURNE, R., GILLILAN, L., DROWN, I., AND TAMTA, B. The mammalian midbrain and isthmus regions. *I. The nuclear pattern. J. comp. Neurol.*, 78, 129. (1943).

[262] HUKUHARA, T., NAKAYAMA, S., AND OKADA, H. Action potentials in the normal respiratory centers and its centrifugal pathways in the medulla oblongata and spinal cord. *Japan J. Physiol.*, 4, 2, 145. (1954).

[263] INGRAM, W., AND DAWKINS, E. The intramedullary course of the afferent fibers of the vagus nerve in the cat. *J. comp. Neurol.*, 82, 157. (1945).

[264] INGRAM, W., RANSON, S., AND BARRIS, R. The red nucleus, its reintion to postural tonus and righting reactions. *Arch. Neurol. a. Psychiatr.*, 31, 768. (1934).

[265] INGRAM, W., RANSON, S., HANNET, F., ZEISS, F., AND TERWILLIGER, E. Results of stimulation of the tegmentum with the horsley-clarke stereotaxic apparatus. *Arch. Neurol. a. Psychiatr.*, 28, 3, 513. (1932).

[266] JACOBSON, I. Collateral connections of the medial lemniscus in the brain stem of the cat. *S. Afr. J.M. Sci.*, 51, 8, 236. (1955).

[267] JASPER, H., AJMONE-MARSAN, C., AND STOLL, J. Corticofugal projections to the brain stem. *Arch. Neurol. a. Psychiatr.*, 67, 155. (1952).

[268] JERMULOWICZ, W. Untersuchungen über die kerne am boden der rautengrube (nucleus paramedianus, nucleus eminentiae teretis, nucleus praepositus hypoglossi, kappenkern der facialskniss). *Ztschr. f. Anat. u. Entwickl.*, 103, 3, 290. (1934).

[269] JOHNSON, F. An atlas of the brain stem reticular formation of the cat for use with the stereotaxic instrument. *Anat. rec.*, 115, 427. (1953).

[270] KANKELEIT, O. Zur vergleichenden morphologie der unteren säugetierolive (mit bemerkungen über kerne in der oliven peripherie). *Arch. f. Anat. u. Physiol., Anat. Abt.*, 1-3, 1. (1913).

[271] KELLER, A. Nervous control of respiration. *I. Observations on the localization of the respiratory mechanism in the isthmus, pons and upper medulla of the cat. Amer. J. Physiol.*, 89, 289. (1929).

[272] KELLER, A. Observations on the localization of the heat regulations mechanisms in the upper medulla and pons. *Amer. J. Physiol.*, 93, 665. (1930).

[273] KELLER, A. A cat and a dog exhibiting unilateral overflexion. *Amer. J. Physiol.*, 113, 77. (1935).

[274] KELLER, R. Ueber die folgen von verletzungen in der gegend der unteren olive bei der katze. *Arch. f. Anat. u. Physiol., Anat. Abt.*, 177. (1901).

[275] KIMMEL, D. Nigrostriatal fibers in the cat. *Anat. rec.*, 82, 425. (1942).

[276] KING, L. Cellular morphology in the area postrema. *J. comp. Neurol.*, 66, 1. (1937).

[277] KLIACHKIN, G. Materials to the study on the original and central passage of the v, vi, vii, ix, x, xi, and xii pairs of the cranial nerves. *Kazan.* (1897).

[278] KLOSOVKIY, B. On a, so far, not yet described group of cells in the infra-medullar part of the root of the nervus vestibularis in man and in some mammals. *Arch. Psychiatr. and nervous disord.*, 98, 255. (1932).

[279] KLOSOVKIY, B. The mechanism of the vestibular nystagmus and its participation in the cortical movements of the eye. *Diss. M.* (1939).

[280] KLOSOVKIY, B. The structure and functions of the mesencephalon. *1. On the straight conducting connections of the nucleus of the posterior corpus bigeminum with the red nucleus. Bulletin of Experimental Biology and Medicine, XXI*, 5, 3. (1946).

[281] KLOSOVSKIY, B., AND KOSMARSKAYA, E. On the regulation of the activity of the vasomotor center in the medulla oblongata. *Journal of Neuropathology and Psychiatry*, 53, 2, 130. (1953).

[282] KOHNSTAMM, O. Akustische reflexbahn. *Berl. Gesellschaft f. Psychiatr. u. Nervenheilk*, May 13. (1912).

[283] KOHNSTAMM, O. Der nucleus paralamniscalis inferior als akustischer reflexkern und als glied der centralen horleitung (nebst einer bemerkung über den bechterewschen kern und den nucleus lateralis pontis). *Arch. f. Ohrenheilk*, 89, 1, 59. (1912).

[284] KOSAKA, K. Ueber die vaguskerne des hundes. *Neurol. Cbl.*, 28, 406. (1909).

[285] KOSAKA, K. Zur frage der physiologischen natur der cerebralen trigeminuswurzel. *Fol. neuro-biol.*, 6, 1. (1912).

[286] KOSAKA, K., AND YAGITA, R. Ueber den ursprung des herzvagen. *Okayama-Igakkai-Zasshi*, 211. (1907).

[287] LEWY, F., AND KOBRAK, H. Neural projections of cochlear spirals on primary acoustic centers. *Arch. Neurol. a. Psychiatr.*, 35, 839. (1936).

[288] LIDDEL, E., AND PHILLIPS, C. Pyramidal section in the cat. *Brain, 67, 1.* (1944).

[289] LILJESTRAND, A. Respiratory reactions elicited from medulla oblongata of the cat. *B KH.: In honour of S. Ramon Cajal. Stockholm, 321.* (1953).

[290] LIM, R. Myelencephaletic sympathetic center and its relation to the hypothalamic sympathetic center. *Physiol. J., USSR, XXIV, 1-2, 236.* (1938).

[291] LINDSLEY, D., SCHREINER, L., KNOWLES, W., AND MAGOUN, H. Behavioral and eeg changes following chronic brain stem lesions in the cat. *EEG clin. Neurophysiol., 2, 483.* (1950).

[292] LISITSA, F. Olive-cerebellar connections. *Neuropathology and Psychiatry, IX, 11, 42.* (1940).

[293] LIVINGSTON, R., FRENCH, I., AND HERNANDEZ-PEON, R. Corticofugal projections to brain stem activating system. *Fed. Proc., 12, 89.* (1953).

[294] LORENTE DE NÓ, R. Anatomy of the eighth nerve. *The central projections of the nerve ending of the internal ear. Laryngoscope, 43, 1.* (1933).

[295] LUTHY, F. Lieber anatomische verbindungen zwischen unteren olive und kleinhirn. *Proc. Intern. Neur. Conf. Berne, 239.* (1931).

[296] MAGNUS, R. Körperstellung. *Berlin.* (1924).

[297] MAGOUN, H. Maintenance of the light reflex after destruction of the superior colliculus in the cat. *Amer. J. Physiol., 111, 91.* (1935).

[298] MAGOUN, H. Caudal and cephalic influences of the brainstem reticular formation. *Physiol. Review, 30, 459.* (1950).

[299] MAGOUN, H. An ascending reticular activating system in brain stem. *Arch. Neurol. a. Psychiatr., 67, 145.* (1952).

[300] MAGOUN, H., AND RANSON, S. The central path of the light reflex. *A study of the effect of lesions. Arch. Ophth., 13, 791.* (1935).

[301] MAGOUN, H., RANSON, S., AND MAYER, L. The pupillary light reflex after lesions of the posterior commissure in the cat. *Amer. J. Ophth., 18, 624.* (1935).

[302] MARBURG, O., AND WARNER, F. The pathways of the tectum (anterior colliculus) of the midbrain in cats. *J. Nerv. a. Ment. Dis., 106, 415.* (1947).

[303] MARSHALL, C. Experimental lesion of the pyramidal tract. *Arch. Neurol. a. Psychiatr., 32, 778.* (1934).

[304] MATZKE, H. The course of fibers arising from the nucleus gracilis and cuneatus of the cat. *J. comp. Neurol., 94, 439.* (1951).

[305] MCCOTTER, R. The nervus terminalis in the adult dog and cat. *J. comp. Neurol., 23, 2, 145.* (1913).

[306] MCKINLEY, W., AND MAGOUN, H. The bulbar projection of the trigeminal nerve. *Amer. J. Physiol., 137, 217.* (1942).

[307] MEDVEDEVA, N., AND SCHWABAUER, B. Material on the question of the influence of the substantia reticulatis on the chemistry of the blood. *Medico-biological Journal, 3, 238.* (1930).

[308] MINGAZZINI, G., AND POLIMANTI, O. Ueber die kortikalen und bulbären verbindungen des hypoglossus. *Mschr. f. Psychiatr. u. Neurol., XXVII, 187.* (1910).

[309] MISLAVSKIY, N. On the respiratory center. *Kazan, 1858; see also N.A. Mislavskiy, selected works. M., 21.* (1952).

[310] MOFFRE, D. The comparative anatomy of the nucleus intercalatus and adjacent structures. *Assen, van Gorcum a. Co.* (1942).

[311] MONAKOW, C. Der rote kern, die haube und die regio subthalamica bei einigen säugetieren und beim menschen. *Arb. a.d. hirnanat. Inst. in Zürich, 3, 59, 1909; 4, 107.* (1910).

[312] MORIN, F. Afferent projections to the midbrain tegmentum and their spinal course. *Amer. J. Physiol., 172, 483.* (1953).

[313] MORIN, G., BONNET, V., AND ZWIRN, P. Nature et évolution des troubles consécutifs à la section d'une pyramide bulbaire chez le chien. *C. r. Soc. biol., 143, 9-10, 710.* (1949).

[314] MORUZZI, G. The physiological properties of the brain stem reticular systems. *B KH.: Brain mechanisms and consciousness, Oxford, 21.* (1954).

[315] MUKHIN, N. The study of the histological structure of the medulla oblongata. *Archive of Psychiatry, Neurology and Legal Psychopathology, XIX, 2 and 3.* (1892).

[316] MUSKENS, L. An anatomo-physiological study of the posterior longitudinal bundle in its relation to forced movements. *Brain, XXXVI, 352.* (1913-1914).

[317] MUSKENS, L. Das supra-vestibuläre system bei den tieren und beim menschen. *Amsterdam.* (1934).

[318] MUSKENS, L. Experimentelle und klinische untersuchungen über die verbindungen der unteren
olive und ihre bedeutung fur die fallrichtung. *Arch.
Psychiatr., 102, 558.* (1934).

[319] NAKAMURA, T. Der rollersche kern. *Eine vergle-
ichend anatomische Untersuchung. Arb. a.d. neurol. Inst. d. Wien. Univ., 32, 61.* (1930).

[320] NEZLINA, N. Disruption and restoration of motor functions in dogs after a half-diametrical cut
through the brainstem at the level of the pons
varolii. *Transact. of the Acad. of Sciences USSR,
112, 6, 1153.* (1957).

[321] NIEMER, W., AND CHENG, S. The ascending
auditory system, a study of retrograde degeneration. *Anat. rec., 103, 490.* (1949).

[322] OGAVA, T. Myelogenetische studie über das corpus trapezoides und die oliva superior des menschen und einiger säugetiere. *Arb. a.d. anat. Inst.
d. kaiserlich. japan. Univ. zu Sendai, XVIII, 53.*
(1936).

[323] OGAWA, T. Experimentelle untersuchungen über
die mediale und zentrale haubenbahn bei der
katze. *Arch. f. Psychiatr., 110, 365.* (1939).

[324] OGAWA, T., AND MITOMO, S. Eine
experimentell-anatomische studie über zwei merk-
würkige faserbahnen im hirnstamm des hundes:
Tractus mesencephali-olivaris medians (economo
et karplus) und tractus tectocerebellaris. *Jap. J.
med. Sci. I. Anatomy, 7, 77.* (1938).

[325] ORLEY, V. Materials on the position of the centers of the medulla oblongata. *Theses of lectures
of the IX conference of physiologists of the South
of RSFSR. Rostov on the Don, 70.* (1949).

[326] OSIPOV, V. Further investigations in the field
of the central ends of a pair of cervical nerves.
Neurol. pathological Herald, VI, 2. (1898).

[327] OSIPOV, V. Investigations of the central beginning and ending of the accessory nerves (n. *accessorius Willisii). Neurol. pathological Herald, VI, 2.*
(1898).

[328] PANEGROSSI, G. Weiterer beitrag zum studium
der augenmuskelnervenkerne. *Mschr. f. Psychiatr.
u. Neurol., XVI, 268.* (1904).

[329] PAPEZ, J. Subdivisions of the facial nucleus. *J.
comp. Neurol., 43, 159.* (1927).

[330] PAPEZ, J. The superior olivary nucleus: its fiber
connections. *Arch. Neurol. a. Psychiatr., 24, 1.*
(1930).

[331] PAVLOVICH, E. Conducting structures of the
brainstem of the cat on horizontal slices. *Diss.
L.* (1949).

[332] PECHERKIN, A. The study of the nucleus of l.o.
Darkshevich. *Collection of scientific works, dedicated to the 100th anniversary of the first clinical
hospital in Perm. 119.* (1938).

[333] PITTS, R. The respiratory center and its descending pathways. *J. comp. Neurol., 72, 605.* (1940).

[334] PITTS, R., MAGOUN, H., AND RANSON, S. Localization of the medullary respiratory centers in
the cat. *Amer. J. Physiol., 126, 3, 673.* (1939).

[335] POLJAK, S. Untersuchungen am oktavussys-
tem der säugetiere und an dem mit diesem ko-
ordinierten motorischen apparat der hirnstamms.
J. Psychol. u. Neurol., 32, 170. (1926).

[336] POLJAK, S. Über die nervenendigungen in
den vestibularen sinnesedn. *stellen bei den
Säugetieren. Ztschr. f. Anat. u. Entwickl., 84, 131.*
(1927).

[337] PROBST, M. Ueber vom vierhügel von der brücke
und vom kleinhirn absteigende bahnen. *Dtsch.
Ztschr. f. Nervenheilk, 15, 192.* (1899).

[338] PROBST, M. Experimentelle untersuchungen
über die anatomie und physiologie des sehhügels.
Mschr. Psychiatr. u. Neurol., 7, 387. (1900).

[339] PROBST, M. Experimentelle untersuchungen
über die schleifenendigungen, die haubenbahn,
das dorsale längsbündel und die hintere commissur. *Arch. f. Psychiatr., 33, 1.* (1900).

[340] PROBST, M. Über die kommissur von gudden, meynert und ganser und über die folgen der
buibusatrophie auf die zentrale sehbahn. *Mschr.
Psychiatr., 17, 1.* (1905).

[341] RADEMARKER, G. Des stehen. *Berlin.* (1931).

[342] RANSON, S., AND MAGOUN, H. Respiratory and
pupillary reactions. *Arch. Neurol. a. Psychiatr.,
29, 6, 1179.* (1933).

[343] RASMUSSEN, A. An aberrant (recurrent) pyramidal bundle in the cat. *J. comp. Neurol., 51, 229.*
(1930).

[344] RASMUSSEN, A. Secondary vestibular tracts in
the cat. *J. comp. Neurol, 54, 143.* (1932).

[345] RASMUSSEN, A. Tractus tecto-spinalis in the cat.
J. comp. Neurol., 63, 501. (1936).

[346] RASMUSSEN, G. The olivary peduncle and other
fiber projections from the superior olivary complex.
J. comp. Neurol., 84, 141. (1946).

[347] REINOSO, F. Anatomisch-cartesianischer atlas zur anwendung bei experimentellen arbeiten am katzengehirn durch lakalisierungsmethoden von horsley-clark und hess. *B KH.: Anatomische Gesellschaft Verhandlungen. Jena.* (1954).

[348] ROLICH, G. The functional condition of the salivatory center in the dog after decerebration. *News, A. Sc. USSR. Series of biology. M.-L., 3, 120.* (1950).

[349] ROLLER, T. Ein kleinzelliger hypoglossuskern. *Arch. mikroskop. Anat., 19, 383.* (1881).

[350] ROMANOV, M. Zur frage von den zentralen verbindungen der motorischen hiernnerven. *Neurol. Cbl., XVII, 593.* (1898).

[351] ROSSI, G., AND BRODAL, A. Corticofugal fibers to the brain stem reticular formation. *An experimental study in the cat. J. Anat., 90, 1, 42.* (1956).

[352] ROZHANSKIY, N. Methods of studying the conduction in the subcortical stem part of the cerebrum. *Problems of Soviet physiology, biochemistry and pharmacology. M., I, 91.* (1949).

[353] RUSSEL, G. Some fiber connections in the brain stem of the cat. *Anat. rec., 115, 364.* (1953).

[354] RUSSEL, G. The dorsal trigemino-thaiamic tract in the cat reconsidered as a lateral reticulothalamic system of connections. *J. comp. Neurol., 101, 237.* (1954).

[355] RUSSEL, I. The origin and destination of certain afferent and efferent tracts in the medulla oblongata. *Brain, XX, 409.* (1897).

[356] SAGER, O. Cercetari asupra leratiilor nigrocorticale. *Com. Acad. Rep. Popul., Rom., 5, 3, 635.* (1955).

[357] SANO, T. Beitrag zur vergleichenden anatomie der substantia nigra, des corpus luysii und der zona incerta. *Mtschr. Psychiatr. u. Neurol., 27, 110, 28, 26.* (1910).

[358] SAVAS, A. Faseranalyse der fasciculus longitudinalis medians. *Acta anat., 21, 209.* (1954).

[359] SCHEIBEL, A. On detailed connections of the medullary and pontine reticular formation. *Anat. rec., 109, 345.* (1951).

[360] SCHNEIDER, A. The histology of the radix mesencephalica. *N. trigemini in the dog. Anat. rec., 38, 321.* (1928).

[361] SCHWABAUER, B., AND STRIGONOVA, A. Cytoarchitecture of the medulla oblongata and the vegetative nervous system. *Works of the medicobiological Institute of the Main Administr. of Scient. Instit., VI, 117.* (1929).

[362] SHEININ, I. Typing of the cells of the mesencephalis nucleus of the trigeminal nerve in the dog, based on nissl granule arrangement. *J. comp. Neurol., 50, 109.* (1930).

[363] SHEININ, I. Studies of the mesencephalic nucleus in the normal and experimental cat. *Anat. rec., 55, 36.* (1933).

[364] SHIMA, R. Zur vergleichenden anatomie des dorsalen vaguskern. *Arb. a. d. neurol. Inst., d. Wien, Univ., XVII, 190.* (1909).

[365] SNIDER, R., AND BARNARD, J. Electroanatomical studies of the afferent projection the inferior olive. *J. comp. Neurol., 91, 243.* (1949).

[366] SPILLER, W. Corticonuclear tracts for associated ocular movements. *Arch. Neurol. a. Psychiatr., 28, 2, 251.* (1932).

[367] STADERINI, R. Nucleus praepositus nervi hypoglossi, o nucleo intercalato? nota critica. *Anat. Anz., 87, 101.* (1938).

[368] STARZL, T., TAYLOR, C., AND MAGOUN, H. Collateral afferent excitation of reticular formation of brain stem. *J. Neurophysiol., 14, 479.* (1951).

[369] STOTLER, W. The projection of the cochlear nerve on the acoustic relay nuclei of the medulla. *Anat. rec., 103, 561.* (1949).

[370] STOTLER, W. An experimental study of the cells and connections of the superior olivary complex of the cat. *J. comp. Neurol., 98, 3, 401.* (1953).

[371] STOTLER, W. An experimental study of the origin, of the afferent fibers, of the inferior olivary nucleus, of the cat brain. *Anat. rec., 118, 359.* (1954).

[372] SZENTÁGOTHAI, J. Die lokalisation der kehlkopfmuskalatur in den vaguskernen. *Ztschr. f. Anat., 112, 704.* (1943).

[373] SZENTÁGOTHAI, J. The representation of facial and scalp muscles in the facial nucleus. *J. comp. Neurol., 88, 207.* (1948).

[374] SZENTÁGOTHAI, J. Functional representation in the motor trigeminal nucleus. *J. comp. Neurol., 90, 111.* (1949).

[375] SZENTÁGOTHAI, J. The general visceral efferent column of the brain stem. *Acta. morphol. Acad. Sci. Hungar, 11, 2, 313.* (1952).

[376] TAGAKI, I. Studien zur vergleichenden anatomie des nucleus vestibularis triangularis. *Der Nucleus intercalatus und der Nucleus praepositus hypoglossi. Arb. a.d. neurol. Inst. d. Wien. Univ., 27, 157, 235.* (1925).

[377] TANG, P. Localization of the pneumotaxic center in the cat. *Amer. J. Physiol., 172, 645.* (1953).

[378] TASIRO, S. Experimentell-anatomische untersuchungen über die efferenten bahnen aus den vierhügeln der katze. *Ztschr. f. mikr.-anat. Forsch., 47, 1.* (1940).

[379] TELIATNIK, F. On the endings of the glossopharyngeal nerve in the medulla oblongata. *Diss. St. P.* (1896).

[380] TRICOMI-ALLEGRA, G. Sulle connessioni bulbari del nervo vago. *Rivista di pathologia nervosa e mentale, 8, 2, 67.* (1903).

[381] TROSHIN, G. The loop, its beginning, ending, composition, connections and topography. *Scientific notes of the University of Kazan. Kazan, 101.* (1900).

[382] TROSHIN, G. The question of the motor connections of the anterior lamina quadrigemina. *Scientific notes of the University of Kazan. Kazan, 58, 5-6, 160.* (1900).

[383] TROSHIN, G. Central connections of sensory and motor cranial nerves. *Protocol of the scientific meeting of physicians of the clinic of nervous diseases of the Kazan University from April 26, 1900; see also Neurol. Mag., 21, 281.* (1902).

[384] TSURUJAMA, K. Untersuchungen über die medullären und gangliongren ursprünge des n. accessorius bei der katze. *J. Anat., VII, 1, I.* (1938).

[385] TURNER, R., AND GERMAN, W. Functional anatomy of the brachium pontis. *J. Neurophysiol., 4, 196.* (1941).

[386] VAN GEHUCHTEN, A. Connexions centrales du noyau de deiters et des masses grises voisines. *Le Névraxe, 6, 21.* (1904).

[387] VAN HÖEVELL, J. Remarks on the reticular cells of the oblongata in different vertebrates. *Proc. Acad. Sc. Amsterdam, 13, 1047.* (1911).

[388] VERHAART, W. Localisation of the medial lemniscus in the medulla and the pons. *Fol. psychiatr. neerl., 58, 35.* (1955).

[389] WALBERG, F. The lateral reticular nucleus of the medulla oblongata in mammals. *A comparative-anatomical study. J. comp. Neurol., 96, 283.* (1952).

[390] WALBERG, F. Ueber die sogenannte «zentrale haubenbahn». *Arch. f. Psychiatr., 193, 252.* (1955).

[391] WALBERG, F. Descending connections to the inferior olive. *An experimental study on the cat. J. comp. Neurol, 104, 1, 77.* (1956).

[392] WALLENBERG. Giebt es centrifugale bahnen aus dem sehhügel zum rückenmark. *Neurol. Cbl., 20, 2, 50.* (1901).

[393] WANG, S. Salivatory center in medulla of cat. *J. Neurophysiol., 6, 3, 195.* (1943).

[394] WILSON, W., AND MAGOUN, H. Functional significance of the inferior oliva in the cat. *J. comp. Neurol., 83, 69.* (1945).

[395] WINKLER, C. Experimenteller beitrag zur kenntnis der sekundären hörbahnen der katze. *Folio neuro-biol., 5, 8, 869.* (1911).

[396] WOODBURNE, R. A phylogenetic consideration of the primary and secondary centers and connections of the trigeminal complex in a series of vertebrates. *J. comp. Neurol., 65, 403.* (1936).

[397] WOOLARD, H., AND HARPMAN, J. The connection of the inferior colliculus and of the dorsal nucleus of the lateral lemniscus. *J. Anat., 74, 441.* (1940).

[398] YAGITA, K. Weitere untersuchungen über das speichelcentrum. *Anat. Anz., 35, 2-3, 70.* (1909).

[399] YAKUBOVICH, N. Microscopic investigation of the beginnings of the nerves in the spinal cord and the medulla oblongata. *Medico-military Journal, 68, 1, 9, 13.* (1856).

[400] YAMAMOTO, S. Studies on brain stem. II. *Comparative anatomical study of the facial nucleus of mammalia. Tohoku Exper. med., 56, 331.* (1952).

[401] YODA, S. Ueber die kerne in der medulla oblongata der katze. *Ztschr. f. mikr.- anat. Forsch., 48, 529.* (1940).

[402] YODA, S., AND KALAGIRI, J. Zur olivocerebellaren verbindungen der katze. *Ztschr. f. mikr.-anat. Forsch., 50, 256.* (1941).

[403] YURMAN, N. Anatomical and physiological investigations of the black substance of soemmering. *Diss. St. P.* (1900).

[404] ZHINKIN, I. The structure and interneuronal connections of the anterior corpus bigeminum in the cat. *Theses of lectures of the Ukranian conference of morphologists. Kharkov, II, 98.* (1956).

The Cerebellum

[405] ADRIAN, E. Afferent areas in the cerebellum connected with the limbs. *Brain 66, 289.* (1943).

[406] ALEKSANIAN, A. The functions of the cerebellum. *Ed. AMS, USSR.* (1948).

[407] ALLEN, W. Distribution of the fibers originating from the different basal cerebellar nuclei. *J. comp. Neurol., 36, 399.* (1924).

[408] ASRATIAN, E. The influence of the cerebellum and the cerebral cortex on the vegetative functions of the organism. *Neuropathology and Psychiatry, X, 3, 35.* (1941).

[409] BAZILEVSKIY, A. The descending systems of the cerebellum in the brainstem, according to the method of fresh palingenesis (marchi), diss. *St. P.* (1898).

[410] BENDER, L. Corticofugal and association fibers arising from the cortex of the vermis of the cerebellum. *Arch. Neurol. a. Psychiatr., 28, 1.* (1932).

[411] BESTA, C. Ueber die zerebro-zerebellaren bahnen. *Experiment. Untersuch., Arch. f. Psychiatr., 50, 323.* (1913).

[412] BOLK, L. Das cerebellum der säugetiere. *Harlem u. Jena.* (1906).

[413] BOTHMANN, M. Zur function des kleinhirns. *Neurol. Cbl., 29, 1205.* (1910).

[414] BRADLEY, O. On the development and homology of the mammalian cerebellar fissures. *J. Anat. a. Physiol, XXXVII, 221.* (1903).

[415] BRODAL, A. Experimentelle untersuchungen über retrograde zellveränderungen in der unteren olive nach läsionen des kleinchirns. *Ztschr. f.d. ges. Neurol., 166, 646.* (1939).

[416] BRODAL, A. The cerebellar connections of the nucleus reticularis lateralis (nucleus funiculi lateralis) in the rabbit and the cat. *Experim. investig. Acta Psychiatr. ct Neurol., 18, 171.* (1943).

[417] BRODAL, A. Les bases anatomiques des localisations cerebelleuses. *Acta Neurol. et Psychiat. belg., 53, 11, 657.* (1953).

[418] BRODAL, A., AND TORVIK, A. Cerebellar projection of paramedian reticular nucleus medulla oblongata in cat. *J. Neurophysiol., 17, 484.* (1954).

[419] BRUNNER, H. Die zentralen kleinhirnkerne bei den säugetieren. *Arb. a.d. Neur. Inst. a.d. Wien. Univ., 22, 200.* (1919).

[420] BÜRGI. Reizung und ausschaltung des brachium conjunctivum. *Helv. Physiol. acta. 1, 467.* (1943).

[421] CARREA, R., AND GRUNDFEST, H. Electrophysiological studies of cerebellar inflow. *1. Origin, conduction and termination of ventral spinocerebellar tract in monkey and cat. J. Neurophysiol., 17, 3, 208.* (1954).

[422] CHAMBERS, W., AND SPRAGUE, J. Functional localization in the cerebellum. *J. comp. Neurol., 103, 105, 1955; Arch. Neurol. a. Psychiatr., 74, 6, 653.* (1955).

[423] CHERNYSHEV, A. On the division of the cerebellum into paleo-neocerebellum. *Contemporary psychoneurology, VIII, 4-5, 297.* (1929).

[424] CLARK, R., AND HORSLEY, V. On the intrinsic fibers of the cerebellum its nuclei and its afferent tracts. *Brain, 28, 13.* (1905).

[425] DOW, R. The fiber connections of the posterior parts of the cerebellum in the rat and cat. *J. comp. Neurol., 63, 527.* (1936).

[426] FULTON, J., LIDELL, E., AND RIOCH, D. Relation of the cerebrum to the cerebellum. *Arch. Neurol. a. Psychiatr., 28, 3, 542.* (1932).

[427] GILMAN, I. The role of the cerebellum in the actualization of the cortical coordination of movements. *Autoreferat of a dissertation. M.* (1954).

[428] GREKER, R. Coordinatory motor functions of the cerebellar vermis. *Neurological Herald, 18, 1, 405.* (1911).

[429] GUREVICH, M. On the external appearance of the processes of the nervous cells of the cerebellar cortex in some superior animals, and on the connection between the function of the cells and the form of their dentrites. *Journal of Neuropathology and Psychiatry named for S.S. Korsakov, 4, 710.* (1903).

[430] HADDAD, B. Projection of afferent fibers from the knee joint to the cerebellum of the cat. *Amer. J. Physiol., 172: 511.* (1953).

[431] HAMSON, I. Relationship between cat cerebral and cerebellar cortices. *J. Neurophysiol., 12, 35.* (1949).

[432] HENNEMAN, E., COOKE, P., AND SNIDER, R. Cerebeliar projections to the cerebral cortex. *A.R.N.M.D. Patterns of Organization in the Central Nervous System, 30, 317.* (1950).

[433] HOHMAN, L. The efferent connections of the cerebellar cortex. *Research publications of Association for Research in Nervous and Mental Disease, Baltimore, XIV, 445.* (1929).

[434] INGVAR, S. Zur phyla- und ontogenese des kleinhirns nebst einem versuche zu einheitlicher erklärung der zerebellaren funktion und lokalisation. *Folia neuro-biol., 11, 205.* (1918).

[435] JANSEN, J., AND BRODAL, A. Experimental studies on the intrinsic fibers of the cerebellum. *II. The cortico-nuclear projection. J. comp. Neurol., 73, 267.* (1940).

[436] JANSEN, J., AND BRODAL, A. Aspects of cerebellar anatomy. *Oslo.* (1954).

[437] JANSEN, J., AND JANSEN, J. On the efferent fibers of the cerebellar nuclei in the cat. *J. comp. Neurol., 102, 3, 607.* (1955).

[438] JELGERSMAG. Drei fälle von cerebellar-atrophie bei der katze; nebst bemerkungen über das cerebro-cerebellare verbindung. *J. Psychol. u. Neural., 23, 105.* (1918).

[439] KARAMIAN, A. The evolution of cerebellar functions and the cerebral hemispheres. *L.* (1956).

[440] KLIMOV, P. The conducting tracts of the cerebellum. *Diss. Kazan.* (1897).

[441] KRASUSKIY, V. Conditioned reflexes in the dog after the operative injury of the cerebellum. *Autoreferat of dissertation. L.* (1955).

[442] KRESTOVNIKOV, M. The influence of the removal of a part of the cerebellum on some characteristics of the transversostriated musculature. *Russian Physiological Journal, XI.* (1928).

[443] KUNSTMAN, K., AND ORBELI, L. The question on the mechanism of motor disruption after the operative removal of the cerebellum, in dogs. *Physiological Journal, USSR, XV, 6, 549.* (1932).

[444] LARSELL, O. The cerebellum of the cat and monkey. *J. comp. Neurol., 99, 135.* (1953).

[445] LEWANDOWSKY, M. Experimentelle physiologie des kleinhirns. *Handb. d. Neurol., 1, 358.* (1910).

[446] LIFSHITZ, N. The influence of extirpation of the cerebellum upon the conditioned reflectory activity. *Works of the Physiological Institute named for I.P. Pavlov. M.-L., 2, 11.* (1947).

[447] LUCIANI, L. Das kleinhirn. *Leipzig.* (1893).

[448] MARBURG, O. Anatomie der nervus cochlearis, vestibularis und kleinhirn. *Hndb. d. Neurol. d. Ohres. Wien.* (1923).

[449] MCNALTY, A., AND HORSLEY, V. On the cervical spinobuibar and spinocerebellar tracts and on the question of topographical representation in the cerebellum. *Brain, 32, 237.* (1909).

[450] MEYEVSKIY, V. Proprioceptive reflexes in cerebellarless animals. *3rd Conference on physiological problems. M.-L., 82.* (1938).

[451] MNUKHINA, R. On the participation of the cerebellum in the processes of coordination of the reflexes of the brainstem. *Physiological Journal, USSR, XXXVII, 1, 52.* (1951).

[452] MORIN, F., AND HADDAD, B. Afferent projections to the cerebellum and the spinal pathways involved. *Amer. J. Physiol., 172, 497.* (1953).

[453] MORIN, F., AND LINDNER, D. Pathways for conduction of tactile impulses to the paramedian lobule of the cerebellum of the cat. *Amer. J. Physiol., 175, 247.* (1953).

[454] MORUZZI, G. Problems in cerebellar physiology. *Springfield, Illin.* (1950).

[455] MUSSEN, A. Experimental investigations on the cerebellum. *Brain, 50, 313.* (1927).

[456] ORBELI, L. On the functions of the cerebellum. *Physiological Journal, USSR, XIX, 1, 255.* (1935).

[457] ORBELI, L. New conceptions of the functions of the cerebellum. *Successes of contemporary biology, XIII, 2, 1.* (1940).

[458] PERELMAN, L. The question on the vegetative centers of the cerebellum. *Medico-biological Journal, 1, 37.* (1927).

[459] PINES, L., AND ZELIKIN, I. To the question on the connections of the cerebellum, in the dog. *Works of the Physiological Institute named for I.P. Pavlov. M.-L., 3, 88.* (1949).

[460] POPOV, N. Materials on the study of the functions of the cerebellum. *In the book: The Higher Nervous Activity. M., 1, 93.* (1929).

[461] PROBST, M. Zur anatomie und physiologie des kleinhirns. *Arch. f. Psychiatr., 35, 692.* (1902).

[462] RASMUSSEN, A. Origin and course of the fasciculus uncinatus (russell) in the cat with observations on other fiber tracts arising from the cerebellar nuclei. *J. comp. Neurol., 57, 165.* (1933).

[463] SHMELKIN, D. Materials to the question on the influence of extirpation of the cerebellum on the tonus of the skeletal musculature, in dogs. *Physiological Journal, USSR, XV, 1-2, 73.* (1932).

[464] SINNIEGE, I. Anatomische untersuchungen über verbindungen des kleinhirns des hundes. *Diss. Amsterdam.* (1938).

[465] SMIRNOV, A. A few remarks on the myeloid nerve fibers in the molecular stratum of the cerebellum in the grown dog. *Arch. microsc. Anat. and history of evolution, 52, 195.* (1898).

[466] SNIDER, R. Morphology of the cerebellar nuclei in the rabbit and cat. *J. comp. Neurol., 72, 399.* (1940).

[467] SNIDER, R. Recent contributions to the anatomy and physiology of the cerebellum. *Arch. Neurol. a. Psychiatr., 64, 196.* (1950).

[468] SNIDER, R., AND ELDRED, E. Electroanatomical studies on cerebro-cerebellar connections in the cat. *J. comp. Neurol., 95, 1.* (1951).

[469] SNIDER, R., McCULLOCH, W., AND MAGOUN, H. A cerebello-bulboreticular pathway for suppression. *J. Neurophysiol., 12, 325.* (1949).

[470] SNIDER, R., AND STOWELL, A. Receiving areas of the tactile, auditory and visual systems in the cerebellum. *J. Neurophysiol., 7, 331.* (1944).

[471] SPRAGUE, J., AND CHAMBERS, W. Regulation of posture in intact and decerebrate cat. *I. Cerebellum, reticular formation, vestibular nuclei. J. Neurophysiol., 16, 451.* (1953).

[472] STELLA, G., LATTI, P., AND SPERTI, L. Decerebrate rigidity in forelegs after deafferentation and spinal transection in dogs with chronic lesions in different parts of the cerebellum. *J. Physiol., 181, 2, 230.* (1955).

[473] STRAKH, I. The influence of partial removal of the cerebellum upon the working capacity of the neuromuscular apparatus. *Physiological Journal, USSR, XXX, 4, 523.* (1941).

[474] THOMAS, D., SPRAGUE, J., CHAMBERS, W., AND KAUFMAN, R. Terminal degeneration of the fastigiobulbar tracts in the cat, following partial and total unilateral destruction of the fastigial nucleus. *Anat. rec., 121, 374.* (1955).

[475] TORWIK, A., AND BRODAL, A. The cerebellar projection of the perihypoglossal nuclei (nucleus intercalatus, nucleus praepositus hypoglossi and nucleus of roller) in the cat. *J. Neuropath., 13, 515.* (1954).

[476] TURNER, R., AND GERMAN, W. Functional anatomy of the brachium pontis. *J. Neurophysiol., 4, 196.* (1941).

[477] VAN GEHUCHTEN, A. Le faisceau en crochet de russell ou faisceau cérébello-bulbaire. *Le Névraxe, VII, 2, 119.* (1906).

[478] VERZILOV, N. Secondary palingeneses after experimental injury to the cerebellum in animals. *Journal of Neuropathology and Psychiatry, S.S. Korsakov, 3, 417.* (1903).

[479] WHITESIDE, W., AND SNIDER, R. Relation of cerebellum to upper brainstem. *J. Neurophysiol., 16, 399.* (1953).

[480] ZELIKIN, I. On the cerebellofugal connections of the cerebellum, in dogs. *Works of the Physiological Institute named for I.P. Pavlov. M.-L., 4, 125.* (1949).

[481] ZIMKINA, A. The vegetative functions of the cerebellum. *Diss. M.* (1943).

[482] ZURABASHVILI, A. To the architecture of the cerebrum and the brain stem in cerebellarless dogs. *Works of the Physiological Instituted named for I.P. Pavlov. M.-L., 3, 101.* (1949).

The Midbrain

[483] ADES, H. Connections of the medial geniculate body in the cat. *Arch. Neurol. a. Psychiatr., 45, 138.* (1941).

[484] ADES, H., METTLER, F., AND CULLER, E. Effect of lesions in the medial geniculate bodies upon hearing in the cat. *Amer. J. Physiol., 125, 15.* (1939).

[485] ADLER, A. Zur topik des verlaufes des geschmackssinnfasern und anderer afferenten bahnen im thalamus. *Ztschr. ges. Neurol. u. Psychiatr., 149, 208.* (1934).

[486] ALLEN, W. Degeneration in the dog's mammillary body and ammon's horn following transection of the fornix. *J. comp. Neurol., 80, 283.* (1944).

[487] ANAND, B., AND DUA, S. Blood sugar changes induced by electrical stimulation of the hypothalamus in cat. *Indian J. Med. Research, 43, 123.* (1955).

[488] ANAND, B., DUA, S., AND SHOEUBERG, K. Hypothalamic control of food intake in cats and monkeys. *J. Physiol., 127, 143.* (1955).

[489] ANDERSSON, B., AND McCANN, S. The effect of hypothalamic lesions on the water intake of the dog. *Acta physiol. Scand., 35, 3-4, 312.* (1956).

[490] AUER, J. Terminal degeneration in the diencephalon after ablation of frontal cortex in the cat. *J. Anat., 90, 1, 30.* (1956).

[491] BACH, L., AND EWING, J. Degeneration studies discrete hypothalamic lesions. *Anat. rec., 106, 2, 171.* (1950).

[492] BARRIS, K., INGRAM, W., AND RANSON, S. Optic connections of the diencephalon and midbrain of the cat. *J. comp. Neurol., 62, 117.* (1935).

[493] BEATTIE, J., AND SHEEHAN, D. The effects of hypothalamic stimulation on gastric motility. *J. Physiol., 81, 2, 218.* (1934).

[494] BERQUIST, H. Mammillary bodies with related structures in vertebrate brain. *Lunds Univ. Arsskr., 3.* (1955).

[495] BISHOP, G., AND CLARE, M. Organization and distribution of fibers in the optic tract of the cat. *J. comp. Neurol., 103, 2, 269.* (1955).

[496] BISHOP, G., AND MARGALET, C. Radiation path from geniculate to optic cortex in cat. *J. Neurophysiol., 14, 6, 497.* (1951).

[497] BONVALLET, M., DELL, P., AND HIEBEL, I. Tonus sympathique et activitè électrique corticale. *EEG. a. clin. Neurophysiol., 6, 119.* (1954).

[498] BRÜGGER, M. Fresstrieb als hypothalamisches symptom. *Helv. Physiol. Acta, 1, 2, 183.* (1943).

[499] BUCHER, V., AND BÜRGI, S. Some observation on the fiber connections of the di- and mesencephalon in cat. *J. comp. Neurol., 98, 355; 99, 415.* (1953).

[500] BURACHEVSKIY, I. Materials on the study of the motor functions of the empty stomach in hypophysectomized animals, and in animals with an injury in the region of the tuber cinereum of the brain. *Problems of endocrinology, 1, 32.* (1936).

[501] BÜRGI, S. Die supraoptischen decussationen bei der katze. *Dtsch. Ztschr. f. Nervenheilk., 171, 220.* (1954).

[502] BÜRGI, S. Ueber zwei anteile der stria medullaris und die frage eines besonderen neuro-vegetativen mechanismus. *Arch. Neurol. a. Psychiatr., 192, 4, 301.* (1954).

[503] CHANG, H., AND KUCH, T. Spinal origin of the ventral supraoptic decussation (gudden's commissure). *J. Anat., 83, 1.* (1949).

[504] CLARK, W., MAGOUN, H., AND RANSON, S. Temperature regulation in cats with thalamic lesions. *J. Neurophysiol., 2, 202.* (1939).

[505] CLARK LE GROS, W. The homologies of the pulvinar in mammals. *Monit. Zool. ital., 41.* (1931).

[506] CLARK LE GROS, W. The structure and connections of the thalamus. *Brain, 55, 406.* (1932).

[507] CLARK LE GROS, W. Immediate problems of the anatomy of the thalamus. *IV congress neurologique international. Paris, I, 49.* (1949).

[508] CLARK LE GROS, W., BEATTIE, J., RIDDOCH, G., AND DOTT, N. The hypothalamus. *London.* (1938).

[509] CLARK LE GROS, W., AND MEYER, M. Anatomical relationships between cerebral cortex and hypothalamus. *Brit. med. Bull., 6, 341.* (1950).

[510] CROSBY, E., AND WOODBURNE, R. The comparative anatomy of the preoptic area and the hypothalamus. *Res. Publ. Ass. Nerv. a. Ment. Dis., 20, 52.* (1940).

[511] DEMPSEY, E., MORISON, R., AND MORISON, B. Some afferent diencephalic pathways related to cortical potentials in the cat. *Am. J. Physiol., 131, 718.* (1941).

[512] DERIABIN, V. The influence of injury of the thalami optici and the hypothalamic region on higher nervous activity. *Physiological Journal USSR, XXXII, 5, 533.* (1946).

[513] DROOGLEEVER-FORTUYN, J., AND STEFENS, R. On the anatomical relations of the intralaminar and midline cells of the thalamus. *EEG a. clin. Neurophysiol., 3, 393.* (1951).

[514] DUSSER DE BARENNE, J., AND SAGER, O. Über die sensiblen functionen des thalamus opticus der katze. *Ztschr. f. ges. Neurol. u. Psychiatr., 133, 231.* (1931).

[515] FOREL, A. Beitärge zur kenntnis des thalamus opticus und der ihn umgebenden gebilde bei den säugetieren. *A. Forel Gesammelte Hirnanatomische Abhandl. München, 17.* (1907).

[516] GASTAUT, H. The brain stem and cerebral electrogenesis in relation to consciousness. *Brain mechanisms and consciousness. Oxford, 249.* (1954).

[517] GAZE, R., AND GORDON, G. The representation of cutaneous sense in the thalamus of the cat and monkey. *Quart. J. exper. Physiol., 39, 4, 279.* (1954).

[518] GLEES, P. The contribution of the medial fillet and strio-hypothalamic fibers to the dorsal supraoptic decussation, with a note on the termination of the lateral fillet. *J. Anat., 78, 113.* (1944).

[519] GLORIEUX, P. Anatomie et connexions thalamiques chez le chien. *J. de. Neurol. 29, 525.* (1929).

[520] GRASTYÁN, E., LYSSAK, K., AND KEKESI, F. Facilitation and inhibition of conditioned alimentary and defensive reflexes by stimulation of the hypothalamus and reticular formation. *Acta physiol. Acad. Sci. Hungar., IX, 1-3, 133.* (1956).

[521] GREVING, K. Beiträge zur anatomie des zwischenhirns und seiner funktion. *Ztschr. ges. Neurol. u. Psychiatr., 99, 230.* (1925).

[522] GRINKER, R., AND SEROTA, H. Studies on cortico-hypothalamic relations in the cat and man. *J. Neurophysiol., 1, 6, 573.* (1938).

[523] GRÜNTHAL, E. Der zellenaufbau des hypothalamus beim hunde. *Ztschr. ges. Neurol. u. Psychiatr., 120, 157.* (1929).

[524] GUZMAN, F., AND DEL POZO, E. „jump reflex textquotedbl in hypothalamic cat. *J. Neurophysiol., 16, 4, 376.* (1953).

[525] HANBERY, J., AJMONE-MARSAN, C., AND DILWORD, M. Pathways of non-specific thalamocortical projection system. *EEG a. clin. Neurophysiol., 6, 1, 103.* (1954).

[526] HANBERY, J., AND JASPER, H. Independence of diffuse thalamocortical projection system shown by specific nuclear destruction. *Fed. Proc., 11, 64, 1952; J. Neurophysiol., 16, 252.* (1953).

[527] HESS, W. Das zwischenhirn. *Syndrome, Lokalisation, Funktionen. Basel.* (1949).

[528] HESS, W. The diencephalic sleep center. *Brain mechanisms and consciousness, Oxford.* (1954).

[529] HESS, W., AND AKERT, K. Experimental data on role of hypothalamus in mechanism of emotional behavior. *Arch. Neurol. a. Psychiatr., 73, 2, 127.* (1955).

[530] HORNET, F. Vergleichende anatomische untersuchungen über des corpus geniculatum mediale. *Arb. a.d. Neurol. Inst. d. Wien. Univ., 35, 76.* (1933).

[531] INGRAM, W., HANNETT, F., AND RANSON, S. The topography of the nuclei of the diencephalon of the cat. *J. comp. Neurol., 55, 339.* (1932).

[532] INGRAM, W., KNOTT, J., AND CHILES, W. Behavioral and electrocortical effects of diencephalic stimulation in unanesthetized unrestrained cats. *XIX Internat. Physiol. Congress. Abstracts, 487.* (1953).

[533] INGRAM, W., KNOTT, J., WHEATLEY, M., AND SUMMERS, T. Physiological relationship between hypothalamus and cerebral cortex. *EEG clin. Neurophysiol. 3, 37.* (1951).

[534] JASPER, H. Functional properties of the thalamic reticular system. *Brain mechanisms and consciousness, Oxford, 374.* (1954).

[535] JASPER, H., AND AJMONE-MARSAN, C. Thalamocortical integrating mechanisms. *Res. Publ. Ass. Nerv. a. Ment. Dis., 30, 493.* (1952).

[536] JASPER, H., AND AJMONE-MARSAN, C. A stereotaxic atlas of the diencephalon of the cat. *The Nation. Research. Council Ottawa, Canada.* (1954).

[537] JASPER, H., HUNTER, J., AND KNICHTON, R. Experimental studies of thalamocortical systems. *Trans. Amer. Neural. Ass., 73, 210.* (1948).

[538] JEWELL, P. The occurrence of vesiculated neurones in the hypothalamus of the dog. *J. Physiol., 121, 167.* (1953).

[539] JIMÉNEZ-CASTELLANOS, J. Thalamus of the cat in horsley-clarke coordinates. *J. comp. Neurol., 91, 307.* (1949).

[540] JIMÉNEZ-CASTELLANOS, J. Aportaciones morfológicas a la topografia esterotàxica del cuerpo geniculado medial del gato. *Arch. espan. Morf., 10, 35, 129.* (1953).

[541] KABAT, H., ANSON, B., MAGOUN, H., AND RANSON, S. Stimulation of the hypothalamus with special reference to its effect on gastrointestinal motility. *Amer. J. Physiol., 112, 214.* (1935).

[542] KAKHANA, M. On the regulatory functions of the hypothalamus and on the method of their being, immediately, affected. *Diss. M.* (1947).

[543] KLOSOVSKIY, B. The question of the structure of the connections of the cortex and the subcortical formations and the functional part of the latter. *Scientific conference of the department of clinical and medico-biological sciences AMS, USSR. Theses. M., 45.* (1956).

[544] KNOCHE, H. Ueber das vorkommen eigenartiger nervenfasern (nodulus-fasern) in hypophyse und zwischenhirn von hund und mensch. *Acta anat., 18, 3, 208.* (1953).

[545] KNOTT, J., AND SHIPTON. A method for accurate placement of electrodes in the hypothalamus of the dog. *EEG a. clin. Neurophysiol., VIII, 1, 136.* (1956).

[546] KOGAN, A. Electrophysiological investigations of the central mechanisms of some most complex reflexes. *M.* (1949).

[547] KOGAN, A. Materials to the determination of the topography of the nutritional center. *Bulletin of experimental biology and medicine, XXVIII, 3 (9), 190.* (1949).

[548] KRIAZHEV, V. The character of the higher nervous activity of hypophysecto-mized animals. *Soviet neurology, psychiatry psychhygiene, 1, 9, 550.* (1932).

[549] KUREPINA, M. Phylogenesis and ontogenesis of the optic thalamus. *In the book: In Memory of the Acad. A.N. Severtsov. M.-L., II, 1, 375.* (1940).

[550] LAGUEUR, G. Neurosecretory pathways between the hypothalamic paraventricular nucleus and the neurohypophysis. *J. comp. Neurol., 101, 3, 543.* (1954).

[551] LAGUTINA, N., AND ROZHANSKIY, N. On the location of the subcortical nutritional centers. *Physiological Journal USSR, XXXV, 5, 587.* (1949).

[552] LARSSON, S. On the hypothalamic organization of the nervous mechanism regulating food intake. *Acta physiol. Scand., 32, Suppl. 115.* (1954).

[553] LEVIN, G. On the development of the pulvinar of the optic thalamus. *Problems of morphology of the nervous system. L., 65.* (1956).

[554] LI CHAN LUH. The facilitatory effect of stimulation of an unspecific thalamic nucleus on cortical sensory neuronal responses. *J. Physiol., 131, 1, 115.* (1956).

[555] LISITSA, F. The influence of stimuli of the internal organs on the potentials of the cerebral cortex, hypothalamus and optic thalamus. *Bulletin of experimental biology and medicine, 12, 261.* (1941).

[556] MAGOUN, H. The ascending reticular system and wakefulness. *Brain mechanisms and consciousness. Oxford, 1.* (1954).

[557] MAGOUN, H., AND MCKINLEY, W. The termination of ascending trigeminal and spinal tracts in the thalamus of the cat. *Amer. J. Physiol., 137, 409.* (1942).

[558] MAGOUN, H., AND RANSON, S. The supraoptic decussations in the cat. *J. comp. Neurol., 76, 93.* (1942).

[559] MCCRUM, W. A study of diencephalon mechanisms in temperature regulation. *J. comp. Neurol., 98, 233.* (1953).

[560] MINKOWSKI, M. Ueber den verlauf der endigung und der zentralen repräsentation von gekreurten imd ungekreurten sehnervenfasern bei einigem säugetiere und beim menschen. *Schweiz. Arch. Neural. u. Psychiatr., 6, 201; 7, 268.* (1920).

[561] MINKOWSKI, M. Zur frage der endigung und der representation von gekreurten und ungekreurten sehnervenfasern im corpus geniculatum externum. *Psychiatr., Bl. 38, 514.* (1934).

[562] MOGILNITSKIY, B. The question of the connection of the hypophysis with the midbrain. *Medico-biological Journal, 11.* (1924).

[563] MONAKHOV, K. The cytoarchitecture of the hypothalamus. *Medico-biological Journal, 59.* (1926).

[564] MONAKOW, C. Experimentelle und pathologisch-anatomische untersuchungen über die haubenregion, den sehhügel und die regio subthalamica. *Arch. f. Psychiatr., 27, 1.* (1895).

[565] MORGAN, L. Symptoms and fiber degeneration following experimental lesions in the subthalamic nucleus of luys in the dog. *J. comp. Neurol., 44, 379.* (1927).

[566] MORGAN, L., AND JANSON, C. Experimental lesions in the tuber cinereum of the dog. *Arch. Neural. a. Psychiatr., 24, 4, 696.* (1930).

[567] MORRISON, R., AND DEMPSEY, E. A study of thalamocortical relations. *Amer. J. Physiol., 135, 281.* (1942).

[568] MOUNTCASTLE, V., AND HENNEMAN, F. Pattern of tactile representation in thalamus of cat. *J. Neurophysiol., 12, 85.* (1949).

[569] NARIKASHVILI, S. The influence of stimuli of subcortical formations on the electric activity of the cortex of the hemispheres. *Works of the Institute of physiology ASSSSR, Tbilisi, 9, 133.* (1953).

[570] NARIKASHVILI, S. Primary responsive reaction and "spontaneous" electric activity of the cortex of the hemispheres of the cerebrum. *Physiological Journal USSR, XLIII, 7, 642.* (1957).

[571] NASHOLD, B., HANBERY, J., AND OLSZEWSKI, J. Observations on the diffuse thalamic projections. *EEG a. clin. Neurophysiol., 7, 609.* (1955).

[572] NAUTA, W., AND WHITLOCK, D. An anatomical analysis of the nonspecific thalamic projection system. *Brain mechanisms and consciousness. Oxford, 81.* (1954).

[573] NEIDING, M. Ueber die kerne des diencephalon bei einigen säugetieren. *Berlin.* (1911).

[574] NICOLESCO, J., AND NICOLESCO, M. Quelques données sur les centres végétatifs de la région infundibulo-tubérienne et de la frontière diencephalo-télencéphalique. *Rev. Neural., 11, 3, 289.* (1929).

[575] NIEMER, W., AND JIMENEZ-CASTELLANOS, J. Cortico-thalamic connections in the cat as revealed by „physiological neuronography. textquotedbl *J. comp. Neurol., 93, 101.* (1950).

[576] O'LEARY, J. A structural analysis of the lateral geniculate nucleus of the cat. *J. comp. Anat., 73, 405.* (1940).

[577] OLSZEWSKY, J. The thalamus of the macaca mulatta. *An atlas for use with the stereotaxic instrument. Basel.* (1952).

[578] PAPEZ, J. The thalamus of a dog without a hemisphere. *Anat. rec., 67, 66.* (1937).

[579] PAPEZ, J. Subthalamo-tegmental tract. *Anat. rec., 94, 524.* (1946).

[580] PAPEZ, J. Central reticular path to infralaminar and reticular nuclei of thalamus for activating eeg related to consciousness. *EEG a. clin. Neurophysiol., 6, 1, 103.* (1954).

[581] PIKE, E., KLENKE, D., AND BASKERVILL, M. Some motor effects of experimental lesions of the region of the corpora quadrigemina in cats. *Bull. Neurol. Inst. New York, 5, 304.* (1936).

[582] PINES, L. On the subcortical optical center and its connections. *Problems of physiological optic, 6, 194.* (1918).

[583] PRIBYTKOV, G. The course of the fibers of the optic thalamus and on the place of their ending in the subcortical centers. *Diss. M.* (1895).

[584] PRIGONIKOV, I., AND PINES, L. The optic ducts. *In the book: Questions on the Morphology of the Cerebral Cortex. M., 51.* (1936).

[585] PROBST, M. Experimentelle untersuchungen über die anatomie und physiologic des sehhügels. *Mschr. Psychiatr. u. Neural., VII, 387.* (1900).

[586] RANSON, S., KABAT, H., AND MAGOUN, H. Autonomic responses to electrical stimulation of hypothalamus, preoptic region and septum. *Arch. Neural. a. psychiatr., 33, 3, 467.* (1935).

[587] RIOCH, D. A note of the centre median nucleus of luys. *J. Anat., 65, 111, 324.* (1931).

[588] RIOCH, D. Studies of the diencephalon of carnivora. *J. comp. Neurol., 49, 1, 1, 1930; 53, 2, 319.* (1931).

[589] ROBINER, I. The localization of samatic sensitivity in the cortex and the optic thalamus of the rabbit and the cat. *Diss. M.* (1950).

[590] ROSE, J. The thalamus of the sheep: cellular and fibrous structure and comparison with pig, rabbit and cat. *J. comp. Neurol., 77, 469.* (1942).

[591] ROSE, J. The cortical connections of the reticular complex of the thalamus. *Res. Publ. Ass. Nerv. a. Ment. Dis., 30, 454.* (1952).

[592] ROSE, J., AND MOUNTCASTLE, V. The thalamic tactile region in rabbit and cat. *J. comp. Neurol., 97, 441.* (1952).

[593] ROSE, J., AND WOOLSEY, C. The orbitofrontal cortex and its connections with the mediodorsal nucleus in rabbit, sheep and cat. *Res. Publ. Ass. Nerv. a. Ment. Dis., 27, 210.* (1948).

[594] ROSE, J., AND WOOLSEY, C. Structure and relations of limbic cortex and anterior thalamic nuclei in rabbit and cat. *J. comp. Neurol., 89, 279.* (1948).

[595] ROSE, J., AND WOOLSEY, C. Organization of the mammalian thalamus and its relationships to the cerebral cortex. *EEG a. clin. Neurophysiol., 1, 391.* (1949).

[596] ROUSSY, G., AND MOSINGER, M. L'hypothalamus chez l'homme et chez le chien. *Rev. Neurol., 63, 1, 1.* (1935).

[597] RUSSEL, G. A schematic presentation of thalamic morphology and connections. *Texas Rep. Biol. a. Med., 13, 4, 989.* (1955).

[598] SACHS, E. Eine vergleichende anatomische studie des thalamus opticus der säugetiere. *Arb. a.d. Neural. Inst. d. Wien. Univ., 17, 280.* (1909).

[599] SAKOVICH, M. The influence of the gray substance of the floor of the third ventricle and the optic thalamus on the body temperature. *Diss. St. P.* (1897).

[600] SANO, T. Beitrag zur vergleichenden anatomie der substantia nigra, des c. luysii und der zona incerta. *Mschr. Psychiatr. u. Neurol., 27, 110.* (1910).

[601] SAWYER, C., EVERETT, I., AND GREEN, I. The rabbit diencephalon in stereotaxic coordinates. *J. comp. Neurol., 101, 3, 801.* (1954).

[602] SCHWABAUER, B. The question of regulation of hydrosaline metabolism and blood sugar. *Medicobiological Journal, 69.* (1927).

[603] SHIMAMOTO, T., AND VERZEANO, M. Relations between caudate and diffusely projecting thalamic nuclei. *J. Neurophysiol., 17, 3, 278.* (1954).

[604] STARZL, T., AND MAGOUN, H. Organization of the diffuse thalamic projection system. *J. Neurophysiol., 14, 2, 133.* (1951).

[605] STEFANTSOV, B. The aftereffects of cutting through the cervical sympathetic nerves in dogs with a unilateral destruction of the region of the intermediate brain. *Transact. of the Acad. of Science, USSR, LXXXIX, 2, 369.* (1953).

[606] STIGLIANI, R., AND MONACI, M. Studio e documentazione delle neuricrinia nel systema ipotalamo-ipofisario con le più recenti metodiche. *Arch. „De Vecchi textquotedbl (Firenze), 17, 655.* (1952).

[607] SZAKÁCS, F., ENDRÖCZI, E., AND CSEKE, J. Wirkung der reizung der area hypothalamica posterior auf den bedingten ernährungsreflex am hund. *Acta physiol. Acad. Sci. Hungar., Suppl., IX, 49.* (1956).

[608] THOMPSON, W., AND BACH, L. Some functional connections between hypothalamus and medulla. *J. Neurophysiol., 13, 6, 455.* (1956).

[609] THUMA, B. Studies on the diencephalon of the cat. *The cytoarchitecture of the corpus geniculatum laterale. J. comp. Neurol., 46, 173.* (1928).

[610] TISHANKIN, V. The changes of the higher nervous activity as a result of the destruction of the subcortical formation. *In the book: The Problems of Higher Nervous Activity. Ed. by P.K. Anokhin, M., 281.* (1949).

[611] VALKENBURG, C. Caudal connections of the corpus mammillare. *Verslag. kon. Acad. v. Wetensch, 1118.* (1912).

[612] VASILYEV, M. To the problem of the cortex and the subcortex. *Works of the physiological laboratories of the Acad. of I.P. Pavlov, XVI, M.-L., Information I, 268; information II, 286; information IV, 316.* (1949).

[613] WALLER, W. Thalamic connections of the frontal cortex of the cat. *J. comp. Neurol., 73, 1, 117.* (1940).

[614] WALLER, W., AND BARRIS, R. Relationship of thalamic nuclei to the cerebral cortex in the cat. *J. comp. Neurol., 67, 317.* (1937).

[615] WALLS, G. The lateral geniculate nucleus and visual histophysiology. *Univ. California Publ. Physiol., 9, 1.* (1953).

[616] WEAVER, T. Anatomical relations of the commissures of meynert and gudden in the cat. *J. comp. Neurol., 66, 334.* (1937).

[617] WHEATLEY, M. The hypothalamus and affective behaviour in cat. *A study of the effects of experimental lesions, with anatomical correlations. Arch. Neurol. a. Psychiatr., 52, 296.* (1944).

[618] ZELIONYI, G., POLTYREV, S., AND ZAMALIN, N. To the question on the role of the subcortical ganglia in the formation of associations. *Work IV of All-Union convention of physiologists. Kharkov, 89.* (1930).

[619] ZVORYKIN, V. The medial geniculate body and hearing acuity. *Archive of anatomy, histology and embryology, 31, I, 22.* (1954).

Subcortical Nuclei

[620] AKERT, K., AND ANDERSON, B. Experimenteller beitrag zur physiologie des nucleus caudatus. *Acta physiol. Scand., 22, 281.* (1951).

[621] ANDERSEN, P., JANSEN, J., AND KAADA, B. Electrical stimulation of the amygdaloid nuclear complex in unanesthetized cats. *Acta psychiatr. et neurol. Scand., 29, 1, 55.* (1954).

[622] BAKLAVADZHIAN, O. Clinic of injury to the internal capsule in dogs. *In the book: Questions on the higher nervous activity and compensatory adaptations. Erevan, II, 139.* (1957).

[623] CHANG, H. Choreiform movements in a dog suffering from corticostriatal disease. *J. Neurophysiol., 8, 2, 89.* (1945).

[624] CHERKES, V. The changes of motor reflexes in the stimulation of the striated body. *Questions on Physiology, 7, 38.* (1954).

[625] DUSSER DE BARENNE, J. Kat, bij wie de greete hersenen (neopallium) geheel weggenomen zijn. *Ned. Tijdschr. Geneesk., 1, 848.* (1918).

[626] EDINGER, J. Corpus striatum and the basal forebrain bundle. *J. Neurol. a. Ment. dis., 14, 674.* (1887).

[627] FERRO, F., LUSSO, A., AND TERZUOLO, C. Contributo sperimentalle alla fisiologia del corp striato (nucleo caudato). *Minerva med., 2, 59-60, 255.* (1953).

[628] FOX, C. Certain basal telencephal centers in the cat. *J. comp. Neurol., 72, 1.* (1940).

[629] FOX, C. The stria terminalis, longitudinal association bundle and commissural fornix in the cat. *J. comp. Neurol., 79, 277.* (1943).

[630] FOX, C., AND SCHMITZ, J. The substantia nigra and the entopeduncular nucleus in the cat. *J. comp. Neurol., 80, 323.* (1944).

[631] FREY, E. Vergleichende, normale und pathologische anatomie des extrapyramidalen systems. *Schweiz. Arch. Neural. u. Psychiatr., 61, 1-2, 45.* (1950).

[632] GLEES, P. The anatomical basis of cortico-striate connections. *J. Anat., 78, 47.* (1944).

[633] GLOOR, P. Electrophysiological studies on the connections of the amygdaloid nucleus in the cat. *Part I. The neuronal organization of the amygdaloid projection system. EEG a. clin. Neurophysiol., 7, 2, 223.* (1955).

[634] GRASTYÁN, E., LISSAK, K., AND MOLNAR, L. The functional relation between gyrus cinguli and caudate nucleus in the cat. *Acta physiol. Hungar., 4, 3-4, 261.* (1953).

[635] GRINSTEIN, A. Materials on the study of the conducting tracts of the corporis striati. *M.* (1910).

[636] GRÜNTHAL, E. Comparative anatomic studies on cell structure of globus pallidus and nucleus basalis in mammals and man. *J. Psychol. a. Neurol., 44, 403.* (1932).

[637] GUREVICH, M. The cytoarchitecture of the neostriati in mammals. *Journal of Neuropathology and Psychiatry, 6, 105, 1930; see also: Journal for Anat., 93, 723.* (1930).

[638] HANDLEY, C., AND HODES, R. Effects of lesions on subcortically evoked movement in cat. *J. Neurophysiol., 16, 6, 587.* (1953).

[639] HARMAN, P. Volumes of basal ganglia and cortex in mammals. *Proc. Sox. Exper. Biol. a. Med., 54, 3, 297.* (1943).

[640] HOLMES, G. The nervous system of the dog without a forebrain. *J. Physiol., 27, 1.* (1901-1902).

[641] KLOSOVSKIY, B., AND VOLZHINA, N. On the functional character of the caudal bodies. *Questions of neurosurgery, I, 8.* (1956).

[642] KOGAN, A. On the usage of electroencephalography in the investigation of the subcortical region. *Rostov on the Don.* (1936).

[643] KOIKEGAMI, S., FUSE, S., YOKOYAMA, WATANABE, T., AND WATANABE, H. Contributions to the comparative anatomy of the amygdaloid nuclei of mammals with some experiments of their destruction or stimulation. *Fol. Psychiatr. et Neural. Japonica, 8, 336.* (1955).

[644] KOVALEVSKIY, P. The relation of the lenticular body to the cerebral cortex of man and animals. *Medical survey, XVIII, 903.* (1882).

[645] KUKUYEV, L. The development of the striopallidum in the onto- and phylogene-his. *Neuropathology and Psychiatry, XVI, 5, 38.* (1947).

[646] LANGLEY, I., AND GRÜNBAUM, A. On the degeneration resulting from removal of the cerebral cortex and corpora striata in dog. *J. Physiol., 11, 606.* (1890).

[647] LEBEDEV, I. The structure of the striated body of the brain of mammals. *Kiev.* (1872).

[648] LEONTOVICH, T. The delicate structure of the subcortical ganglia. *Journal of Neuropathology and Psychiatry named for S.S. Korsakov, 31, 2, 168.* (1954).

[649] LIDDEL, E., AND PHILIPPS, C. Experimental lesions in the basal ganglia of the cat. *Brain, 63, 264.* (1940).

[650] MARCHI, M. Sulla fine struttura dei corpori striati e dei thalami ottici. *Rivista sperim. di freniatr., 12, 285.* (1887).

[651] MARIENESCO, G. Les connexions du corps strié avec de lobe frontale. *C. r. Soc. biol., 2, 77.* (1895).

[652] METTLER, F. Relation between pyramidal and extrapyramidal functions. *In the book: The Diseases of the Basal Ganglia. Baltimore, 150.* (1942).

[653] MEZHERA, A. The location of the subcortical pain center. *Thes. X conference of physiologists of the South of BSFSB; Rostov on the Don, 37.* (1951).

[654] MINOR, D. The question on the significance of the corpori striati. *Diss. M.* (1882).

[655] MORGAN, L. The corpus striatum. *Arch. Neurol. a. Psychiatr., 18, 495.* (1927).

[656] MUSKENS, L. The central connections of the vestibular nuclei with the corpus striatum and their significance for ocular movement and for locomotion. *Brain, 45, 454.* (1922).

[657] NIESSI VON MAYENDORD, E. Die schweifkernbahen (projektionsvortrag). *Dtsch. Ztschr. Nervenheilk, 95, 122.* (1926).

[658] OLEFIRENKO, P., MUKHO, T., AND KALASHNIKOVA, Z. The functional condition of the hemispheres in the experimental injury of the subcortex and the cortex of the cerebrum. *In the book: Yaroslav State Medical Institute, Theses of lectures.* (1952).

[659] POLTYREV, S. The role of the cortex and the subcortical ganglia in the formation of conditioned reflexes. *Collected works of the Leningrad Veterinary Institute, 30.* (1933).

[660] RANSON, S., AND RANSON, S. Efferent fibers of the corpus striatum. *In the book: The Diseases of the Basal Ganglia. Baltimore 69.* (1942).

[661] RIESE, W. Beiträge zur faseranatomie der stammganglien. *J. Psychol. u. Neurol. 31, 81.* (1924).

[662] ROSEGAY, H. An experimental investigation of the connections between the corpus striatum and substantia nigra in the cat. *J. comp. Neurol., 80, 293.* (1944).

[663] RUSSEL, C. Functional interpretation of the mechanism of extrapyramidal function proposed by papez. *Diseases nerv. system., 14, 7, 221.* (1953).

[664] SCHÜLLER, A. Experimente am nucleus caudatus des hundes. *Jahrb. f. Psych. u. Neurol., 22, 90.* (1902).

[665] SHAIKEVICH, M. Physiological investigations of nuclei lenticularis. *Diss. St. P.* (1903).

[666] SHIMAMOTO, T., AND VERZEANO, M. Relation between caudate and diffusely projecting thalamic nuclei. *J. Neurophysiol., 17, 3, 278.* (1954).

[667] SHTIDA, V. The significance of nuclei caudati. *Experimental-critical investigation. Diss. St. P.* (1903).

[668] SPIEGEL, E. Die kerne im vorderhirn der sauger. *Arb. a.d. Neural. Inst. a.d. Wien. Univ., 22, 419.* (1919).

[669] TARASEVICH, I. The study of the fiber cords closely connected with the thalamus opticus and nuclei lenticularis. *Works of the Neural. Instit. of Vienna University., 9, 251.* (1902).

[670] TERZUOLO, C., AND STOUPEL, N. Donneées nouvelles sur les connexions et la physiologie du noyau caudé. *Brux. méd., 33, 411.* (1952).

[671] VASILYEV, M. The problem of the cortex and subcortex, information iii; the importance of the formations of the forebrain for the processes of higher nervous activity. *Works of the physiological laboratories named for I.P. Pavlov. M., XVI, 249.* (1949).

[672] VERHAART, W. Fiber analysis of the basal ganglia. *J. comp. Neurol., 93, 3, 425.* (1950).

[673] VON BONIN, G., AND SHARIFF, G. Extrapyramidal nuclei among mammals. *A quantitative study. J. comp. Neurol., 94, 3.* (1951).

[674] VON MONAKOW, C. Experimentelle und pathologisch-anatomische sowie entwicklungsgeschichtliche untersuchungen über die beziehungen des corpus striatum und des lilsenkerns zu den übrigen hirnteilen. *Schweiz. Arch. Neural. u. Psychiat., 16, 225.* (1925).

[675] VRIES, E. Bemerkungen zur ontogonie and vergleichenden anatomic des claustrums. *Folia Neuro-biol., 4, 481.* (1910).

[676] VRIES, E. Das corpus striatum der säugetiere. *Anat. Anz., 37, 385.* (1910).

[677] WILSON, S. An experimental research into the anatomy and physiology of the corpus striatum.

Brain, 36, 427. (1914).

[678] ZHUKOVSKIY, M. On the influence of the cerebral cortex and the subcortical ganglia on breathing. *Diss. St. P.* (1898).

Cerebral Cortex

[679] ABULADZE, K., AND ROSENTHAL, I. Conditioned reflectory activity of the dog after a partial destruction of cortical zones. *Works of physiological laboratories named for I.P. Pavlov. M., XIII.* (1948).

[680] ABULADZE, K., ZELIKIN, I., AND ROSENTHAL, I. The reactions of the dog after the removal of the entire cortex of the right hemisphere and the motor region of the left hemisphere. *Archive of Biological Sciences, 61, 3, 94.* (1941).

[681] ADRIANOV, O., AND MERING, T. Materials on the morphology and physiology of the cortical ends of the analysors of the dog. *VIII All-Union convention of physiologists, biochemists and pharmacologits. Theses of lectures. M., 9.* (1955).

[682] AIRAPETIANTS, E. New data on the physiology of the lateral and medial analysors. *Journal of Higher Nervous Activity. V, 5, 644.* (1955).

[683] AKELAITIS, A. Studies on the corpus callosum. *The higher visual functions in each homonymous field following complete section of the corpus callosum. Arch. Neurol. a. Psychiatr., 45, 788.* (1941).

[684] ALIEN, W. Relationship of conditioned olfactory-foreleg response to motor centers of brain. *Amer. J. Physiol., 121, 657.* (1938).

[685] AMASSIAN, V. Cortical representation of visceral afferents. *J. Neurophysiol. 14, 433.* (1951).

[686] ANOKHIN, P. The problem of localization from the point of view of systematized concepts on nervous functions. *Neuropathology and Psychiatr., IX, 6, 31.* (1940).

[687] ANOKHIN, P. The problem of localization of conditioned reflectory activity in the central nervous system. *In the book: Problems of the Higher Nervous Activity, Ed. by P.K. Anokhin. M.* (1949).

[688] ANOKHIN, P. Higher nervous activity and the reticular formation. *Scientific conference of the departments of clinical medicine and medico-biological sciences AMS, USSR. Theses of lectures, 5.* (1956).

[689] ANTHONY, R. Leçons sur le cerveau (cours d'anatomie comparée du museum). *Paris.* (1928).

[690] ANTONINI, A. La corticcia cerebrale nei mammiferi domestici. *Monit. Zool. ital.* (1892).

[691] ASRATIAN, E. Some observations on dogs without the cerebral cortex. *Physiological Journal USSR, XXIV, 1-2, 36.* (1938).

[692] ASRATIAN, E. The question of the anatomo-histological basis of conditioned reflectory activity in higher animals. *In the book: E.A. Asratian. Physiology of the central nervous system. M., 147.* (1953).

[693] BARD, P., AND RIOCH, D. A study of four cats deprived of neocortex and additional portions of the forebrain. *Johns Hopkins Hosp. Bull., 60, 73.* (1937).

[694] BAYANDUROV, B., AND MARKIN, V. Anatomo-physiological changes in whelps after removal of both hemispheres of the cerebrum. *Works of the chair of normal physiology of the Tomsk Medical Institute. Tomsk, 4, 106.* (1944).

[695] BELENKOV, N. Conditioned reflexes in cats without the cerebral cortex. *Bulletin of experimental biology and medicine. XXIX, 2, 100; 3, 182.* (1950).

[696] BERITASHVILI, I. Morphological and physiological bases of temporary connections in the cerebral cortex. *Works of the Institute of Physiology, named for I.S. Beritashvili. Tbilisi, 10, 3.* (1956).

[697] BREMER, F. Interaction dans l'aire auditive du chat, des influx transmis par le corps calleux et des influx sensoriels specifiques. *Rév. neurol., 87, 162.* (1952).

[698] BREMER, F. Some problems in neurophysiology. *London.* (1953).

[699] BREMER, F., AND TERZUOLO, C. Transfert interhémisp'erique d'informations sensorielles par le corps calleux. *J. physiol. (Paris), 47, 1, 105.* (1955).

[700] BRODMANN, K. Vergleichende lokalisationslehre der grosshirnrinde. *Leipzig.* (1909).

[701] BROMILEY, R. Conditioned responses in a dog after removal of neocortex. *J. comp. a. physiol. psychol., 41, 2, 102.* (1948).

[702] BURNS, B., AND GRAFSTEIN, B. The function and structure of some neurones in the cat's cerebral cortex. *J. Physiol., 118, 412.* (1952).

[703] BYKOV, K. The dog with a severed corpus callosum. *Physiological Journal USSR, VII.* (1924).

[704] CAMPBELL, A. Histological studies on the localization of cerebral function. *Cambridge.* (1905).

[705] CHERNYSHEV, A., AND GRIGOROVSKIY, I. The connections between the cerebrum and the cerebellum of the dog. *Archive of anatomy and histology, 10, 1, 134.* (1931).

[706] CLAES, E. Etude des centres oculomoteurs corticaux chez le chat non anesthésié. *Arch. int. Physiol., 48, 238.* (1939).

[707] CULLER, E., AND METTLER, F. Conditioned behavior in a decorticate dog. *J. comp. Psychol., 18, 291.* (1934).

[708] DEMOOR, I. Les centres sensivomoteurs et les centres d'association chez le chien. *Bruxelles.* (1899).

[709] DESHIN, A. The question of the evolution of the cortex. *The development of the central region of the cortex (islet of Reyle) and its tegment in man, Primates and Carnivora. Journal of Anthropology, 1-2, 68.* (1934).

[710] DUSSER DE BARENNE, J. „corticalization textquotedbl of function and functional localization in the cerebral cortex. *Arch. Neurol. a. Psychiatr., 30, 884.* (1933).

[711] ELLENBERGER, H. Ueber die furchen und windungen der grosshirnoberfläche des hundes. *Arch. f. wissensch. u. prakt. Tierheilk, 15.* (1899).

[712] FABRE, P. La brèche fonctionnelle des cellules corticales, condition de l'extiorisation de leur pulsation electrique. *C.r. Soc. biol., 143, 5-6.* (1949).

[713] FILIMONOV, I. The variants of cerebral fissures of the dog. *J. of Psychol. and Neurol., 3 , 32.* (1928).

[714] FILIMONOV, I. The fissure and gyri of the cerebral cortex in mammals. *Atlas of the cerebrum in man and in animals. M., 9.* (1937).

[715] FILIMONOV, I. A comparative anatomy of the cerebral cortex in mammals. *M.* (1949).

[716] FURSIKOV, D., AND YUMAN, M. Conditioned reflexes in the dog without one hemisphere. *Archive of biological sciences, XXV, 4-5, 147.* (1925).

[717] GANTT, W. The origin and development of behavior disorders in dogs. *Psychosom. med. Monogr.* (1943).

[718] GERVER, A. The emergence of efferent fibers from the so called sensory spheres of the cerebral cortex. *Journal of Neuropathology and Psychiatry, VI, 2, 21.* (1937).

[719] GIBBS, E., AND GIBBS, F. A purring center in the cat's brain. *J. comp. Neurol., 64, 209.* (1936).

[720] GIRDEN, E., METTLER, F., FINCH, G., AND CULLER, E. Conditioned responses in a decorticate dog to acoustic, thermal and tactile stimulation. *J. comp. Psychol., 21, 367.* (1936).

[721] GIURGEA, C. Elaborarea reflexului conditionat prin excitarea directa a scartei cerebrale. *Editura Academici Republicii Populare Romane.* (1953).

[722] GOLTZ, F. Zur physiologie der grosshirnrinde. *Neurol. Cbl., 5, 260.* (1886).

[723] GOLTZ, F. Der hund ohne grosshirn. *Pflüg. Arch., 51, 570.* (1892).

[724] GRUENSTEIN, A. Fasciculus subcallasus. *Journal of Neuropathology and Psychiatry named for S.S. Korsakov, 10, 504.* (1910).

[725] GUREVICH, M., AND BYKHOVSKAYA, G. The architectonics of the cerebral cortex (isocortex) of the dog. *Medico-biological Journal, 58.* (1927).

[726] GUREVICH, M., KHACHATURIAN, A., AND KHACHATUROV, A. The method of composing cytoarchitectural maps and the measuring of the areas. *To the cytoarchitecture of the cerebral cortex in phelides. In the book: The Higher Nervous Activity. M., 1, 159.* (1929).

[727] GUTNER, I. The question of the ontogenesis and structure of the cerebral cortex. *Announcement 2. Postembryonic ontogenesis of the cortex in the piglet, rabbit, mouse, and cat. Bulletin of experimental biology and medicine, 21, 3, 52.* (1946).

[728] HATAI, S. Observations on the developing neurons of the cerebral cortex of foetal cats. *J. comp. Neurol., 12, 199.* (1902).

[729] HITZIG, E. Alte und neue untersuchungen aber das gehirn. *Arch. f. Psychiatr., 34, 1, 1901; 35, 275, 585, 1902; 36, 1.* (1903).

[730] HÖNIG, H. Vergleichend-anatomische untersuchungen über den hirnfurchungstypus der caniden. *Berlin.* (1912).

[731] IVANOV-SMOLENSKIY, A. Outlines of pathophysiology of higher nervous activity. *M.* (1949).

[732] KELLOG, W. Locomotor and other disturbances following hemidecortication in the dog. *J. comp. a. physiol. psychol., 42, 6, 506.* (1949).

[733] KHACHATURIAN, A. The brain of the dog and of the cat. *In the book: Atlas of the Cerebrum of Man and Animals. M., 33.* (1937).

[734] KING, W. Observations on the role of the cerebral cortex in the control of the postural reflex. *Amer. J. Physiol., 80, 311.* (1927).

[735] KLATT, B. Studien zum domestikationsproblem. *Untersuchungen am Hirn. Leipzig.* (1921).

[736] KLEIN, E., LANGLEY, J., AND SCHÄFER, E. On the cortical areas removed from the brain of a dog and from the brain of a monkey. *J. Physiol., 4, 231.* (1883-4).

[737] KLEMPIN. Über die architektonik der grosshirnrinde des hundes. *J. Psychol. u. Neurol., 26, 5-6, 229.* (1921).

[738] KONONOVA, E. Methods of investigation of the architectonic structure of the cerebral cortex. *In the book: Cytoarchitecture of the Human Cerebral Cortex. M., 221.* (1949).

[739] KÖPPEN, M., AND LÖVENSTEIN, S. Studien über den zellenbau der grosshirnrinde bei den ungulaten und carnivoren und über die bedeutung einiger furchen. *Mschr. Psychiatr. u. Neural., 18, 480.* (1906).

[740] KORNMÜLLER, A. Die bioelektrischen erscheinungen der hirnrindefelder. *Leipzig.* (1937).

[741] LARENTE DE NO, R. Cerebral cortex: architecture, intracortical connections, motor projections. *In the book: J. Fulton. physiology of the Nervous System.* (1943).

[742] LAUGHTON, N. Studies on the occurrence of extensor rigidity in mammals as a result of cortical injury. *Amer. J. Physiol., 85, 78.* (1928).

[743] LEBEDINSKAYA, S., AND ROSENTHAL, I. The influence on conditioned reflexes after the removal of the cerebral cortex in the dog. *Works of the physiological laboratories named for I.P. Pavlov. M., VIII, 463.* (1938).

[744] LEWIS, B. On the comparative structure of the cortex cerebri. *Brain, 1, 79.* (1878).

[745] LINDBERG, A. The influence of the operative longitudinal cut through the corpus callosum, on motorism. *In the book: The Problems of Motorism in Neurology and Psychiatry. State Med. Publ. of the Ukranian SSR.* (1937).

[746] LOEB, I. Die elementaren störungen einfacher functionen nach oberflgchlicher umschriebener verletzung des grosshirns. *Neurol. Cbl., 4, 471.* (1885).

[747] LUCIANI UND SEPPILLI. Die functionslocalisation auf der grosshirnrinde. *Leipzig.* (1886).

[748] MACLEAN, P., AND PRIBRAM, K. Neuronographic analysis of medial and basal cerebral cortex. I. Cat. *J. Neurophysiol., 16, 312.* (1953).

[749] MAGOUN, H., AND RANSON, S. The behavior of cats following bilateral removal of the rostral portion of the cerebral hemispheres. *J. Neurophysiol., 1, I, 39.* (1938).

[750] METTLER, F. Effects of total removal of the cerebral cortex. *Arch. Neural. a. Psychiatr., 34, 1238.* (1935).

[751] MEYNERT, AND TH. Die windungen der conväxen oberfläche des vorderhirnes bei menschen, affen und raubtieren. *Arch. f. Psychiatr. u. Nervenkrankh., VII, 2, 257.* (1877).

[752] MIKLUKHO-MAKLAI, N. Notes on the gyri of the brain of the dingo. *Collected works. M.-L., III, 224.* (1952).

[753] MIVART, S. Notes on the cerebral convolutions of the carnivora. *J. Linnean soc. zool., XIX, 108, 1.* (1884).

[754] MONAKOW, C. Die localisation im grosshirn. *Wiesbaden.* (1914).

[755] MORAWSKY, J. Gehirnuntersuchungen bei katzen und hundefamilien mit berücksichtigung des geschlechts und der entwicklung. *Jahrb. f. Psych. u. Neural., 33, 306.* (1912).

[756] MORIN, G., GASTAUT, H., AND DUPLAY, I. Liberation des réflexes pasturaux en extension chez le chien décortiqué. *Rev. neurol., 79/3, 207.* (1947).

[757] MOSIDZE, V. A few data on the conditioned reflexes before and after a partial cut through the corpus callosum, in the dog. *Autoreferat of dissertation. L.* (1955).

[758] MUNK, H. Ueber die funktionen der grosshirnrinde. *Berlin.* (1890).

[759] MURATOV, V. Secondary degeneration after cutting through the stem. *Neurol. Cbl., 714.* (1895).

[760] NERRE, W., AND STEPHAN, H. Zur postnatalen morphogenese des hirnes verschiedener haushundrassen. *Gegenbaurs morphologisches Jahrbuch, 96, 210.* (1955).

[761] ORBELI, L. The question on the localization of conditioned reflexes in the central nervous system. *Works of the Society of Russian Physicians. St. P., 75, 291.* (1908).

[762] PANKRATOV, M. The formation of conditioned reflexes in the cat without the cerebral hemispheres. *Reports from the Institute Lesgaft, 21, 1-2.* (1939).

[763] PANSCH, A. Ueber gleichwertige regionen am grosshirn der carnivoren und der primaten. *Cbl. med. Wissensch., VIII, 38, 641.* (1875).

[764] PAVLOV, I. Pavlovskiye sredy. *M.-L., I, II, III.* (1949).

[765] PAVLOV, I. Lectures on the work of the cerebral hemispheres. *Complete collection of works. M.-L., IV.* (1951).

[766] PAVLOV, I. Twenty years of experience in the study of higher nervous activity (behaviour) in animals. *Conditioned reflexes. Complete collection of works. M.-L., III.* (1951).

[767] POLJAK, S. An experimental study of the association, callosal and projection fibers of the cerebral cortex of the cat. *J. comp. Neurol., 44, 197.* (1927).

[768] POPOV, N. Investigations on the physiology of the cerebral cortex in animals. *M.* (1953).

[769] PRESS, Y. The functional role of the nondecussated optic, auditory and motor conducting tracts. *In the book: Clinical Syndrome in the Disruption of Higher Functions of the Cerebrum and Their Anatomo-Physiological Bases. Kharkov, 70.* (1941).

[770] PRESSMAN, Y. The physiology of the relationship of the cortex of each hemisphere of the cerebrum to the ipsi- and contralateral receptors. *Physiological Journal USSR, XXXI, 4, 329.* (1939).

[771] RADEMAKER, G. Das stehen. *Berlin.* (1931).

[772] RAFIKI, M. The changes of the animals reactions after the extirpation of the cerebral cortex. *Physiological Journal USSR, XXI, 5-6, 703.* (1936).

[773] REDLICH, E. Zur vergleichenden anatomic der associationssysteme des gehirns der säugetiere. *Leipzig u. Wien.* (1903).

[774] RHEINGANSUWE, V. Das postnatale oberflächenwachstum der cytoarchitektonischen gebiete der grosshirnrinde des hundes. *Dtsch. Nation. Bibliogr., 17, 1229.* (1955).

[775] RIESE, W. Structure and function of the cerebral cortex in the newborn cat(felis domestica). *Confinia neurol., 7, 1/2, 55.* (1946).

[776] RINK, F. Furchen an der äusseren fläche des carnivorengehirns. *Zool. Jahrb., Abt. Morphol., 12.* (1899).

[777] ROITBAK, A. Bioelectrical phenomena in the cerebral cortex. *Tbilisi.* (1955).

[778] ROSE, M. Ler allocortex bei tier und mensch. *J. Psychol. u. Neurol., 34, 1.* (1927).

[779] ROSENTHAL, I. Summary of five years of work on the correlation of the analytical structure and function of the cortex of the hemispheres. *Archive of biological sciences, 61, 3, 38.* (1941).

[780] ROTHMANN, H. Zusammenfassender bericht über den rothmannschen grosshirnlosen hund nach klinischer und anatomischer untersuchung. *Ztschr. f.d. ges. Neurol. u. Psychiatr., 87, 247.* (1923).

[781] ROZHANSKIY, N. The problem of structure in the investigation of the central nervous system. *Physiological Journal USSR, XVII, 6, 1181.* (1934).

[782] ROZINA, E. The commissure of the endbrain in the individual development of man and in the comparative anatomical series of mammals. *Diss. M.* (1951).

[783] RUCH, F., PATTON, H., AND AMASSIAN, V. Topographical and functional determinants of cortical localization pattern. *Res. Publ. Assoc. Nerv. a. Ment. Dis., 30, 403.* (1952).

[784] RUDANOVSKIY, P. 'tudes photographiques sur la système nerveux de l'homme et de quelques animaux superieures d'après les coupes de tissu nerveux congélé, contenant xx planches et 203 figures photographiques. *Paris.* (1868).

[785] RÜDINGER, N. licher die hirne verschiedener hunderassen. *Sitzungsber. d. Wissensch. zu München.* (1894).

[786] RUSSEL, I. Further researches on eye movements. *J. Physiol., 17, 5, 378.* (1894-1895).

[787] SAGER, O. Cercetari asupra unor mecaniscercetari fiziol si neurol. *Studii si ceretari fiziol. Neurol., 6, 3-4, 561.* (1955).

[788] SARKISSOW, S. The postnatal development of separate cytoarchitectural areas in the dog. *Journal of Psychology and Neurol., 39, 486.* (1929).

[789] SARKISSOW, S. The correlation of bioelectric currents to the architectonic areas and their boundaries. *Neuropathology and Psychiatry, VI, 2, 139.* (1937).

[790] SARKISSOW, S. Bioelectric phenomena of the cerebral cortex and issues of localization. *Proceedings of the Institute of the brain. M., III-IV, 433.* (1938).

[791] SARKISSOW, S. A few peculiarities in the structure of neuronal connections of the cerebral cortex. *M.* (1948).

[792] SARKISSOW, S., KHACHATURIAN, A., AND CHERNYSHEV, A. Neurological and morphological changes in the extirpation of the cerebral cortex in the dog. *Neuropathology and psychiatry, IX, 6, 89.* (1940).

[793] SCHALTENBRAND, G., AND COBB, S. Clinical and anatomical studies on two cats without neocortex. *Brain, 53, 449.* (1931).

[794] SHIPOV. The connections of the fornix. *Review of psychiatry, neurology and experimental psychology.* (1902).

[795] SHITOV, F., YAKOVLEVA, V., PRESSMAN, Y., AND GLAGOVESHCHENSKAYA, V. The morphological foundations of conditioned reflectory activity. *Works of the session of the Brain Institute named for V.M. Bekhterev (L.), XI, 193.* (1939).

[796] SHOLL, D. Dendritic organization in the neurons of the visual and motor cortices of the cat. *J. Anat., 87, 4, 387.* (1953).

[797] SMITH, E. On the homology of the cerebral sulci. *J. Anat. a. Physiol., 36, 309.* (1902).

[798] SMITH, W. The representation of respiratory movements in the cerebral cortex. *J. Neurophysiol., 1, 55.* (1938).

[799] SOLLER, V. Aportaciones al estudio de las vias anatomicas de conexion inter-hemisferica (un estidio, en el gato, de la proyeccion walleriana subcortical tras hemiferectomias). *Arch. espanol. morfol, 10, 35, 229.* (1953).

[800] STRACK, D. Die äussere morphologie des grosshirns zwergwüchsiger und kurzköpfiger haushunde, ein beitrag zur entstehung des furdhungstyps. *Gaz. med. portug., 7, 210.* (1954).

[801] SUKHANOV, S. Materials on the question of the bead-shaped appearance of the protoplasmic processes of the nerve cells of the cerebral cortex. *Diss. St. P.* (1903).

[802] TEN-CATE, I. Akustische und optische reaktionen der katzen nach teilweisen und totalen extirpationen des neopalliums. *Arch. neerl. Physiol., 19, 191.* (1934).

[803] TROSHIN, G. The conjunctive systems of the hemispheres. *Diss. St. P.* (1903).

[804] URMANCHEYEVA, T. The influence of the removal of some sections of the cerebral cortex on the electric activity of different formations of the cerebrum of the cat. *Collection of theses and referats of the Rostov State Medical Institute. Rostov on the Don, 76.* (1954).

[805] VICTOROV, K. A case of the removal of one hemisphere in the dog. *Scientific notes of the University of Kazan. Kazan, 101, 4, 17.* (1941).

[806] VOGT, O. licher fasersysteme in den mittleren und caudalen balkenabschnitt. *Neurol. Cbl., 14, 208.* (1895).

[807] VOLKMER, D. Cytoarchitektonische studien an hirnen verschieder grosser hunde (königspudel und zwergpudel). *Kiel. Diss., 13, 6.* (1955).

[808] VON VALKENBURG, C. Der ursprung der fasern im corpus callosum und psalterium. *Verlag. d. kön. Acad. v. Weter, 1337.* (1911).

[809] VORONIN, L. Analysis and synthesis of the complex stimuli through the normal and injured hemispheres of the canine cerebrum. *M.* (1948).

[810] VUL, I., VLASOVA, B., AND NIKA, G. The forming of functions of some analysors in the early ontogenesis. *VIII All-Union congress of physiologists, biochemists and pharmacologists. Theses of lectures. M., 152.* (1955).

[811] WALBERG, F., AND BRODAL, A. Pyramidal tract fibers from temporal and occipital lobes. *Brain, 76, 3, 491.* (1953).

[812] WILDER, B. The outer cerebral fissures of the mammalia especially carnivora and the limits of their homology. *Proc. Ass. Amer. Anat.* (1873).

[813] YAKUBOVICH, N. Notes on the most delicate structure of the cerebrum and the spinal cord. *Medico-military Journal, 70, 2, 35.* (1857).

[814] YANISHEVSKIY, A. The commissurial systems of the cerebral cortex (corpus callosum, anterior commissure and lyre of david). *Diss. Kazan.* (1902).

[815] ZELENYI, G. The results of the removal of the cerebral hemispheres. *Medico-biological Journal, 1-2, 3.* (1930).

[816] ZELIKIN, I. The brain of the dog with only one hemisphere. *(To the question on the connections of the cerebral cortex.) Works of the Physiological Institute named for I.P. Pavlov. M.-L., 3, 107.* (1949).

[817] ZHUKOVA, G., LEONTOVICH, T., AND SAVICH, K. The differentiation of the neurons of the cerebrum in mammals. *Archive of Anatomy, Histology and Embryology, 31, 1, 3.* (1954).

[818] ZURABASHVILI, A. Synapses. *Tbilisi.* (1947).

Occipital Region (Optic Analysor)

[819] AGADZHANIANTS, K. The cortical center of vision. *Diss. St. P.* (1904).

[820] ALOUF, I. Die vergleichende cytoarchitektonik der area striata. *J. Psychol. u. Neurol., 38, 5.* (1929).

[821] BARRIS, R. A pupillo-constrictor area in the cerebral cortex of the cat and its relationship to the pretectal area. *J. comp. Neurol., 63, 353.* (1936).

[822] BAUMGARTNER, G. Verschiedene reaktionsweisen einzelner kortikaler neurone des optischen cortex der katze. *Boll. Soc. ital. biol. sperim., 30, 8-11, 1155.* (1954).

[823] BEKHTEREV, V. The localization of the visual center of the cortex on the internal surface of the occipital lobe in dogs. *Revue of psychiatry, neurology and experimental psychology, 8, 449.* (1911).

[824] BERITOV, I., AND CHICHINADZE, N. The question of the localization of cortical processes on visual stimulation. *VII Caucasian congress of physiologists, biochemists and pharmacologists. Rostov on the Don, 137.* (1937).

[825] BISHOP, C., AND CLARE, M. Radiation path from geniculate to optic cortex in cat. *J. Neurophysiol., 14, 497.* (1953).

[826] CHANG, H. Functional organization of central visual pathways. *Res. Publ. Ass. Nerv. a. Ment. Dis., Baltimore.* (1951).

[827] CLARK LE GROS, W. The visual centers of the brain and their connections. *Physiol. Review, 22, 205.* (1942).

[828] DANILLO, S. The relationship of the occipital lobes of newborn and young animals to the movements of the eyes. *The Physician, IX, 48, 955.* (1888).

[829] DONALD, M., MILES, R., AND RATOOSH, P. Absence of color vision in cat. *J. Neurophysiol., 17, 3, 289.* (1954).

[830] DUROV, V. The question of the discrimination of colors in dogs. *Works of the practical laboratory on zoo-psychology. M., I, 11.* (1928).

[831] ENTIN, T. Investigation of synapses in the optic region of the cerebral cortex. *Archive of anatomy, histology and embryology, XXXI, 4, 25.* (1954).

[832] ENTIN, T. The development of neurons and connections in the optic region of the cerebral cortex of the cat. *In the book: Problems of morphology of the nervous system. L., 59.* (1956).

[833] FROLOV, U. The physiology of vision. *Works of the Petrograd Society of Naturalists. Petrogr., 49, 1.* (1918).

[834] GHISELL, E. The relationship between the superior colliculus and the striate areas in brightness discrimination. *J. genet. Psychol., 52, 151.* (1938).

[835] GUNIN, V. The changes of the higher nervous activity in the extirpations of the cortical end of the optic analysor. *Journal of higher nervous activity. Ia, 6, 872.* (1956).

[836] GUNTER, R. The discrimination between lights of different wave lengths in the cat. *J. comp. a physiol. Psychol., 47, 2, 169.* (1954).

[837] HITZIG, E. Ueber das cortical sehen des hundes. *Arch. f. Psychiatr., 33, 707.* (1900).

[838] IMAMURA, S. Ueber die corticalen störungen des sehactes und die bedeutung des balkens. *Arch. ges. Physiol., 100, 495.* (1903).

[839] INGVAR, D., AND HUNTER, J. Influence of visual cortex on light impulses in the brain of the unanesthetized cat. *Acta physiol. Scand., 33, 2-3, 194.* (1955).

[840] KALBERLACH. Über die augenregion und die vordere grenze der sehsphäre munk's. *Arch f. Psychiatr., 37, 1014.* (1903).

[841] KEMPTON, G., WING, G., AND SMITH, K. The role of the optic cortex in the dog in the determination of the functional properties of conditioned reactions to light. *J. exper. Psychol., 31, 6, 478.* (1942).

[842] KOGAN, A., AND IVANNIKOVA, T. Optic conditioned reflexes in cats with a removed - at an early age - occipital lobes of the cerebral hemispheres. *Bulletin of experimental biology and medicine, 39, 3, 6.* (1955).

[843] KONONOVA, E. Anatomy and physiology of occipital lobes. *M.* (1926).

[844] KRIAZHEV, V., AND TSINDA, N. The disruption of the functions of the optic analyser in the bilateral removal of the occipital lobes of the cerebral hemispheres of the dog. *Journal of higher nervous activity, V, I, 110.* (1955).

[845] KUDRIN, A. Conditioned reflexes in the dog after the removal of the posterior half of the large hemispheres. *Diss. St. P.* (1910).

[846] KURZWEILL, F. Beiträge zur lokalisation der sehsphäre des hundes. *Arch. ges. Physiol., 129, 607.* (1909).

[847] LANNEGRACE. Influence des lésions corticales sur la vue. *Arch. méd. exper. et d'anat. pathol., 1, 87, Jan.* (1889).

[848] LEONTOVICH, A. The color discrimination in the dog. *Works of the III All-Union congress of physiologists. L., 207.* (1928).

[849] MARQUIS, D. Effects of removal of the visual cortex in mammals with observations on the retention of light discrimination in dogs. *Res. Publ. Ass. Nerv. Ment. Dis., 13, 558.* (1934).

[850] MARQUIS, D., AND HILGARD, E. Conditioned lid responses to light in dogs after removal of the visual cortex. *J. comp. Psychol., 22, 157.* (1936).

[851] MERING, T. The influence of the conditioned reflectory activity on the optic stimuli in dogs after injury to the temporal lobes. *Journal of higher nervous activity, IV, 3, 448.* (1954).

[852] MINKOWSKI, M. Zur physiologic der sehsphäre. *Pflüg. Arch. ges. Physiol., 141, 171.* (1911).

[853] MONAKOW, C. Experimentelle und pathologisch-anatomische untersuchungen über die optischen centren und bahnen. *Arch. f. Psychiatr., 20, 714.* (1889).

[854] NAGEL, W. Der farbensinn des hundes. *Zbl. f. Physiol., 21, 7, 205.* (1907).

[855] ORBELI, L. Condjtioned reflexes from the eyes of the dog. *Diss. St. P.* (1908).

[856] ORBELI, L. The question of color discrimination in dogs. *Questions of scientific medicine, I, 5-6, 513.* (1913).

[857] PAVLOVSKIY, A. The structure of the chiasm of optic nerves in man and some vertebrate animals. *Diss.* (1869).

[858] PINES, L., AND PRIGONNIKOV, I. The connections of the subcortical optic center. *Works of the session of the Institute V.M. Bekhterev, L., XI, 66.* (1939).

[859] POLJAK, S. Die verbindungen der area striata. *Ztschr. f. d. ges. Neurol. u. Psychiatr., 100, 545.* (1926).

[860] POLJAK, S. The vertebrate visual system. *Chicago.* (1957).

[861] POYEMNYI, F. The correlation of the optic cortex and the external geniculate body in the phylogenesis in mammals. *Diss. M.* (1940).

[862] PROBST, M. Ueher den verlauf der zentralen sehfasern (binten-sehhügelfasern) und deren endigung im zwischen- und mittelhirne und über die associations. *Arch. f. Psychiatr., 35, 9, 22.* (1902).

[863] ROSENZWEIG, B. The influence of the removal of the cortex of one hemisphere on the optic conditioned reflexes. *In the book: Higher Nervous Activity. M., 64.* (1929).

[864] SAMOILOV, A., AND FEOFILAKTOVA, A. The color discrimination in the dog. *Cbl. for Physiol., XXI, 5, 133.* (1907).

[865] SCHOLL, D. The organization of the visual cortex in the cat. *J. Anat., 89, 1, 33.* (1955).

[866] SHENGER-KRESTOVNIKOVA, N. The question on the differentiation of optic stimuli, and on the limits of differentiation in the optic analysor of the dog. *News from the Petrograd Scientific Institute Lesgaft, III, 1.* (1921).

[867] SHKOLNIK-YARROS, E. The morphology of the optic analyser. *Journal of higher nervous activity, 4, 2, 289.* (1954).

[868] SMITH, K. Visual discrimination in the cat. V. *The postoperative effects of removal of the striate cortex upon intensity discrimination. J. genet. Psychol., 51, 329.* (1937).

[869] SMITH, K., AND BOJAR, S. The nature of optokinetic reactions and their significance in the experimental analysis of the neural mechanisms of visual functions. *Psychol. Bull., 35, 193.* (1938).

[870] SPERRY, R., AND MINER, N. Pattern perception following insertion of mica plates into visual cortex. *J. compar. a. physiol. Psychol., 48, 6, 463.* (1955).

[871] STONE, C. Notes on light discrimination in the dog. *J. comp. Psychol., 1, 413.* (1921).

[872] TALBOT, S., AND MARSHALL, W. Physiological studies on neural mechanisms of visual localization and discrimination. *Amer. J. Ophth., 24, 1255.* (1941).

[873] TEN CATE, I. Bedingte reflexe bei hunden nach beiderseitiger extirpation der regio occipitalis der grosshirnrinde. *Arch. Neerl. d. Physiol. de l'homme et des animaux, 19, 191, 1934; 20, 467, 1935; 21, 219, 1938; 24, 153.* (1940).

[874] TOROPOV, P. Conditioned reflexes from the eye after the removal of the occipital lobes of the large hemispheres in dogs. *Diss. St. P.* (1908).

[875] TROSHIN, G. The conjunctive systems of the hemispheres. *Diss. St. P.* (1903).

[876] TSCHERMAK, A.   Über die lokalisation der sehsphäre des hundes. *Zbl. f. Physiol. 19, 335.* (1905).

[877] TSELERITSKIY, K. Experimental investigations on the functions of the cerebral cortex of the occipital lobe in higher animals. *Diss. St. P.* (1890).

[878] WING, G., AND SMITH, K. The role of optic cortex in the dog in the determination of the functional properties of conditioned reactions to light. *J. exper. Psychol., 31, 6, 478.* (1942).

[879] YUVCHENKO, A. Synapses of the cortex of the occipital lobe of the canine cerebrum. *Autoreferat of dissertation. Minsk.* (1955).

[880] ZVORYKIN, V., AND SHKOLNIK-YARROS, E. Figures on the relationship of the peripheric part of the optic analysor and the cerebral ends of the analysors in a series of mammals. *Archive of anatomy, histology and embryology, 30, 5, 43.* (1953).

Temporal Region (Auditory Analysor)

[881] ADES, H. Functional relationships between the middle and posterior ectosylvian areas in the cat. *Amer. J. Physiol., 159, 561.* (1949).

[882] ADES, H., AND BROOKHART, I. The central auditory pathway. *J. Neurophysiol., 13, 3, 189.* (1950).

[883] ALLEN, W. Effect of destroying three localized cerebral cortical areas for sound on conditioned differential responses of the dog's foreleg. *Amer. J. physiol., 144, 3, 415.* (1945).

[884] ANDREYEV, L. The characteristic of functional disturbances of the auditory analyser in the dog after partial destruction of the cochlea. *Works of II All-Uhion congress of physiologists. L., 138.* (1926).

[885] ANDREYEV, L. The high boundary of the acoustic area in the dog. *Russian Physiological Journal, XI, 3, 233.* (1928).

[886] ANDREYEV, L. The ability to distinguish tones of high frequencies in dogs. *Physiological Journal, 17, 6, 1248.* (1934).

[887] ANDREYEV, L. Some new data characterizing the activity of the auditory analysor. *In the book: Seventh Conference on Problems of Higher Nerve Activity, 3.* (1940).

[888] BABKIN, B. The characteristic of the acoustic analysor in the dog. *Works of the Society of Russian Physicians in St. P., 77, 197.* (1910).

[889] BABKIN, B. Further investigations of the normal and injured acoustic analysor in the dog. *Works of the Society of Russian Physicians in St. P., St. p., 78, 249.* (1910-1911).

[890] BREMER, F., BONNET, V., AND TERZUOLO, C. Etude electrophysiologique des aires auditives corticales du chat. *Arch. int. Physiol., 62, 3, 390.* (1955).

[891] BREMER, F., AND DOW, R. Cerebral acoustic area of the cat. *J. Neurophysiol., 2, 4, 308.* (1939).

[892] BROGDEN, W., GIRDEN, E., METTLER, F., AND CULLER, E. Acoustic value of the several components of the auditory system in cats. *Amer. J. Physiol., 116, 252.* (1936).

[893] BURMAKIN, V. Process of generalization of the conditioned acoustic reflex in the dog. *Diss. St. P.* (1909).

[894] CULLER, E. Acoustic value of the components of the auditory system in cats. *Amer. J. Physiol., 116, 33.* (1936).

[895] DELL, M., AND DELL, P. Etude critique des connexions attribuées la region temporale et de leur specificité. *Rév. neurol., 88, 5, 365.* (1953).

[896] DELL, P., BONVALLET, AND M. Projections sensorielles au niveau de la region temporale. *Les grandes activités du lobe temporal. Paris, 57.* (1955).

[897] DOWNMANN, C., AND WOOLSEY, C. Inter-relations within the auditory cortex. *J. Physiol., 123, 43.* (1954).

[898] EIYASON, M. Investigations of the auditory capacity of the dog under normal conditions and after a partial bilateral removal of the cortical center of hearing. *Diss. St. P.* (1908).

[899] GERSHUNI, G. Electrophysiological analysis of the activity of the auditory system. *Information I and II. Physiological Journal USSR, 29, 369, 380.* (1940).

[900] HIND, J. An electrophysiological determination of tonotopic organisation in auditory cortex of cat. *J. Neurophysiol., 16, 5, 475.* (1953).

[901] HUNTER, W. The function of the cerebral cortex in audition. *J. comp. Psychol. 32, 117.* (1941).

[902] IVANOV-SMOLENSKIY, A. About sound projection in the cerebral cortex. *Collected volumes, dedicated to the 75th anniversary of acad. I.P. Pavlov. L., 387.* (1924).

[903] IVANOV-SMOLENSKIY, A. The analysis of the successive acoustic conditioned stimulus. *Works of physiological laboratories named for I.P. Pavlov. M., II, 1, 47.* (1927).

[904] JOHNSON, H. Audition and habit formation in the dog. *Behav. Monogr., 2, 8, 78.* (1913).

[905] KALISCHER, O. Zur funktion des schlafenlappens des grosshirns. *Eine neue Hörprüfungsmethode bei Hunden, zugleich ein Beitrag zur Dressur als physiologische Untersuchungsmethode. Sitzungsber. d. Preuss. Acad. d. Wissensch., 1, X, 204.* (1907).

[906] KRYTER, K., AND ADES, H. Studies on the function of the higber acoustic nervous centers in the cat. *Amer. J. Psychol., 56, 501.* (1943).

[907] KRYZHANOVSKIY, I. Conditioned sound reflexes after removal of the temporal regions of the large hemispheres in the dog. *Diss. St. P.* (1910).

[908] KUDRIN, A. Conditioned reflexes in the dog after removal of the posterior halves of the large hemispheres. *Diss. St. P.* (1910).

[909] LARIONOV, V. Auditory tracts. *Neurological Herald.* (1898).

[910] LARIONOV, V. The cortical centers of hearing. *Diss. St. P.* (1898).

[911] LILLY, J. Equipotential maps of the posterior ectosylvian area and acoustic i and ii of the cat during responses and spontaneous activity. *Fed. Proc., 10, 84.* (1951).

[912] LILLY, J., AND CHERRY, R. New criterion for the division of the acoustic cortex into functional areas. *Fed. Proc., 11, 94.* (1952).

[913] MAKOVSKIY, I. Sound reflexes after removal of temporal regions of the large hemispheres in the dog. *Diss. St. P.* (1908).

[914] MERING, T. Conditioned reflexes in the dog after removal of the nucleus of the auditory analysor. *Journal of higher nerve activity, II, 6, 894.* (1952).

[915] MERING, T. The question of the topography of the auditory tract in the dog. *Archive of anatomy, histology and embryology, XXX, 5, 61.* (1953).

[916] MERING, T. The working of conditioned reflexes upon the successive complex stimuli in dogs with different types of nervous systems. *Journal of higher nerve activity, V, 5, 608.* (1955).

[917] METTLER, F. Connections of the auditory cortex of the cat. *J. comp. Neurol., 55, 139.* (1932).

[918] METTLER, F., FINCH, G., GIRDEN, E., AND CULLER, E. Acoustic value of the several components of the auditory pathway. *Brain, 57, 475.* (1934).

[919] MEYER, D., AND WOOLSEY, C. Effects of localized cortical destruction on auditory discriminative conditioning in cat. *J. Neurophysiol., XV, 2, 149.* (1952).

[920] NARIKASHVILI, S. Responsive bioelectric potentials of various regions of the auditory cortex of the large hemispheres in the cat and their changes depending on the strength and frequency of sound stimuli. *Works of the Institute of Physiology named for I.S. Beritashvili. Tbilisi, X, 73.* (1956).

[921] NEFF, W. Neural medhanisms of hearing: some experimental studies of the auditory nervous system. *Laryngoscope, LXI, 4, 289.* (1951).

[922] NEFF, W., ARNOTT, G., AND FISCHER, I. Function of the auditory cortex; the localization of sound in space. *Amer. J. Physiol., 163, 3, 738.* (1950).

[923] PERI, E., AND CASBY. Localization of cerebral electrical activity; the acoustic cortex of cat. *J. Neurophysiol., 17, 429.* (1954).

[924] ROSE, J. The cellular structure of the auditory region of the cat. *J. comp. Neurol., 91, 409.* (1949).

[925] ROSE, J., AND WOOLSEY, C. The relation of thalamic connections, cellular structure and evokable electrical activity in the auditory region of the cat. *J. comp. Neurol., 91, 441.* (1949).

[926] ROTHMANN, M. Ueber die ergebnisse der hörprüfung an dressierten hunden. *Arch. f. Anat. u. Physiol. Physiol. Abt., I-II, 103.* (1908).

[927] RÜDIGER, W., GRASTYÁN, E., AND MADARÁSZ, I. Ueber die beziehungen von effekten der elektrischen reizung der kortikalen hörsphäre zur bedingtreflextorischen tätigkeit beim hunde. *Acta physiol. Acad. Sci. Hungar., IX, 1-3, 163.* (1956).

[928] SKIPIN, G. Materials on the question of the formation of the conditioned reflex and differentiation to the successive complex stimulus. *Works of the physiological laboratories named for I.P. Pavlov, IX, 49.* (1940).

[929] STOLL, I., AJMONE-MARSAN, C., AND JASPER, H. Electrophysiological studies of subcortical connections of anterior temporal region in cat. *J. Neurophysiol., 14, 4, 305.* (1951).

[930] SWIFT, B. Demonstration eines hundes, dem beide schläfenlappen exstirpiert sind. *Berl. Gesellschaft f. Psychiat. u. Nervenheilk, Mai, 9.* (1910).

[931] TUNTURI, A. The audio frequency localization in the acoustic cortex of the dog. *Amer. J. Physiol., 141, 397.* (1944).

[932] TUNTURI, A. A study on the pathway from the medial geniculate body to the acoustic cortex in the dog. *Amer. J. Physiol., 147, 2, 311.* (1946).

[933] TUNTURI, A. Physiological determination of the boundary of the acoustic area in the cerebral cortex of the dog. *Amer. J. Physiol., 160, 2) 395.* (1950).

[934] TUNTURI, A. Effect of lesions of the auditory and adjacent cortex on conditioned reflexes. *Amer. J. Physiol., 181, 2, 225.* (1955).

[935] USIYEVICH, M. Physiological investigation of the auditory capacity of the dog. *News Military-Medical Academy, XXIV, 484, 1911; XXV, 872.* (1912).

[936] VOSKRESENSKIY, L. Materials on the physiology of the normal and injured auditory analysor. *Works of the physiological laboratories named for I.P. Pavlov. M., X, 183.* (1941).

[937] WOOLARD, H., AND HARPMAN, J. The cortical projection of the medial geniculate body. *J. Neurol. a. Psychiat., 2, 35.* (1939).

[938] WOOLSEY, C., AND WALZL, E. Topical projection of nerve fibers from local regions of the cochlea to the cerebral cortex of the cat. *Johns Hopkins Hosp. Bull., 71, 315.* (1942).

[939] ZELENYI, G. Materials on the question of the reaction of the dog to acoustic stimulations, diss. *St. Petersburg.* (1907).

[940] ZIMKINA, A., AND ZIMKIN, H. On the disruption of the balance between stimulation and inhibition. *Physiological Journal USSR, XVIII, 3, 433.* (1935).

Postcoronal Area (Cutaneous Analysor)

[941] AMASSIAN, V. Cortical representation of visceral afferents. *J. Neurophysiol. 14, 6, 433.* (1951).

[942] AMASSIAN, V. Studies on organization of a somesthetic association area, including a single unit analysis. *J. Neurophysiol., 17, 1, 39.* (1954).

[943] ARKHANGELSKIY, V. The physiology of the cutaneous analyser. *Archive biological sciences, XXII, 45.* (1922).

[944] BAILEY, P., AND BREMER, F. A sensory cortical representation of the vagus nerve. *J. Neurophysiol., 1, 405.* (1938).

[945] BYKHOVSKAYA, G. Conditioned reflexes to tactile stimulus after extirpation of gyrus coronarius. *Works of III All-Union congress of physiologists. L., 57.* (1928).

[946] CAROL, H. The functional organization of the sensory cortex of cat. *J. Neuropath. exper. Neurol., 1, 320.* (1942).

[947] DUSSER DE BARENNE, J., AND MCGULLOCH, W. The direct functional interrelation of sensory cortex and optic thalamus. *J. Neurophysiol., 1, 117.* (1938).

[948] HAMUY, T., BROMILY, P., AND WOOLSEY, C. Somatic afferent areas i and ii of the dog's cerebral cortex. *Amer. J. Physiol., 163, 719.* (1950).

[949] HARD, P. Studies on the cortical representation of somatic sensibility. *Bull. N.Y. Harv. Lect., 33, 143.* (1938).

[950] HAYES, G., AND WOOLSEY, C. The pattern of organization within the primary tactile area of the cerebral cortex of the cat. *Fed. Proc., 3, 18.* (1944).

[951] KASHERININOVA, N. Materials on the study of conditioned salivary reflexes on the mechanical stimulus of the skin in the dog. *Diss. St. P.* (1908).

[952] KUPALOV, P. Functional mosaic in the cutaneous part of the cerebral cortex and its influence on the limitation of sleep. *Russian Physiological Journal. IX, 1, 147.* (1926).

[953] MARSHALL, W. Observations on subcortical somatic sensory mechanisms of cats under nembutal anesthesia. *J. Neurophysiol., 4, 25.* (1941).

[954] MARSHALL, W., WOOLSEY, C., AND BARD, P. Observations on cortical somatic sensory mechanisms of cat and monkey. *J. Neurophysiol., 4, 1.* (1941).

[955] MICKLE, W., AND ADES, H. A composite sensory projection area in the cerebral cortex of the cat. *Amer. J. Physiol., 170, 628.* (1952).

[956] MOUNTCASTLE, V., COVIAN, M., AND HARRISON, C. The central representation of some forms of deep sensibility. *Res. Publ. Ass. Nerv. a. Ment. Dis., 30, 339.* (1952).

[957] PANKRATOV, M. Reflexes from the skin of the cat. *Seventh conference on the problems of higher nerve activity. L., 42.* (1940).

[958] POLTYREV, S., AND ALEKSEYEV, V. The possibility of forming conditioned reflexes in dogs from the surface of the body opposite the hemisphere with the removed cortex. *Collected works of the Leningrad Veterinary Institute. L., 79.* (1934).

[959] POPOV, N., AND PALATNIK, S. The changes of cutaneous sensitivity and muscular stimulation in dogs and in the monkey with the unilaterally excluded cerebral cortex. *Bulletin All-Union Institute of Experimental Medicine, 9-10, 26.* (1935).

[960] ROSENTHAL, I. The ipsilateral cortical representation for the tactile sensitivity in the dog. *Physiological Journal USSR, XXXV, 6,667.* (1949).

[961] SCHERRER, I., AND OECONOMOS, D. Responses evoquées corticales somesthesiques des mammiferes adulte et nouveau-né. *Les grandes activités du lobe temporal. Paris.* (1955).

[962] SHISHLO, A. The temperature center in the cerebral cortex and the somniferous reflexes. *Diss. St. P.* (1910).

[963] VOSKRESENSKIY, L. Materials on the physiology of the cutaneous analysor. *Works of physiological laboratories named for I.P. Pavlov. M., X, 178.* (1941).

[964] WOOLSEY, C. "second" somatic receiving areas in the cerebral cortex of cat, dog and monkey. *Fed. Proc., 2, 55.* (1943).

[965] WOOLSEY, C. Patterns of sensory representation in the cerebral cortex. *Fed. Proc., 6, 437.* (1947).

[966] ZHURAVLEV, I. Materials on the question of the negative induction and influence of a partial extirpation of the cutaneous analysor in the dog. *Works of physiological laboratories named for I.P. Pavlov. M., IX, 89.* (1940).

[967] ZUBEK, I. Studies in somesthesis. *II. Role of somatic sensory areas I and II in roughness discrimination in cat. J. Neurophysiol., 15, 5, 401.* (1952).

Precoronal Region (Motor Analyser)

[968] ADRIANOV, O. The question about the morpho-physiological peculiarities of the cortical nuclear zone of the canine motor analysor. *Journal of higher nervous activity, II, 3, 358.* (1952).

[969] ADRIANOV, O. The changes of tonic reflexes in the dog without a cortical nuclear zone of the motor analysor. *Journal of Neuropathology and Psychiatry named for S.S. Korsakov, 53, 5, 328.* (1953).

[970] ADRIANOV, O. The question of the participation of the nuclear zone of the motor analysor in the visual functions of the dog. *Journal of higher nervous activity, III, 3, 428.* (1953).

[971] ALLEN, W. Effect of prefrontal brain lesions on correct conditioned differential responses in dogs. *Amer. J. Physiol., 159, 3, 525.* (1949).

[972] ANOKHIN, P., AND ARTEMYEV, E. The study of the dynamics of higher nervous activity. *Information IV. Physiological Journal USSR, XVI, 2.* (1933).

[973] ANOKHIN, P., AND CHERNEVSKIY, A. The study of the dynamics of higher nervous activity. *Information VII. Physiological Journal USSR, XVIII, 3, 421.* (1935).

[974] ARKHANGELSKIY, V. The physiology of the motor analysor. *Archive of biological sciences, XXII, 45.* (1922).

[975] ASRATIAN, E. The defensive motor conditioned reflex in the dog without the motor region of the cortex of the large hemispheres. *Transact. of the Acad. of Sc. of USSR, I, 2-3, 159.* (1935).

[976] BARI, A. The excitability of the cerebral cortex in newborn animals. *Diss. St. P.* (1898).

[977] BARTLEY, H., AND NEWMAN, E. Studies on the dog's cortex. *I. The sensory motor area. Amer. J. Physiol., 99, 1, 1.* (1931).

[978] BELITSKIY, U. The cerebral centers of accommodation. *Diss. St. P.* (1903).

[979] BELITSKIY, U. The influence of the cortical center of salivation on the activity of salivary glands. *Review of psychiatry, neurology and experimental psychology, XI, 1, 34.* (1906).

[980] BETZ, V. Anatomical information on two cerebral centers. *Cbl. med. Wissensch., 12, 578, 594, 1874 and also in the book: Betz, V.A.: Anatomical and Histological Research. M., 223.* (1950).

[981] BOHM, E., AND PETERSEN, I. Differences in sensitivity to dial of motor effects elicited by stimulation of fore- and hindlimb areas of the cat's motor cortex. *In a book: In honour of S. Ramon y Cajal, 143, Stockholm.* (1953).

[982] BONIN, G. Studies of the size of the cells in the central cortex. *II. The motor area of man, cebus and cat. J. comp. Neurol., 69, 381.* (1938).

[983] BOROVSKIY, M. Cytological and cytoarchitectonic investigations in postembryonal development of the motor zone of the cerebral cortex in the cat. *Arch. Bio. Science, 47, 2, 115.* (1937).

[984] BRODMANN, K. Der riesenpyramidentypus und sein verhalten zu den furchen bei den karnivoren. *J. Psychol. u. Neurol., 7, 1-2, 108.* (1905).

[985] BULYGIN, I. The cortical regulation of the movements of the stomach and the cortical reception of impulses from it after the removal of the premotor zone. *Bulletin of experimental biology and medicine, 11, 2, 173.* (1941).

[986] BURMISTROVA, T. Data on the influence of chronic stimulation of the motor zone of the cerebral cortex on the functional condition of the neuromuscular complex. *Information I. Bulletin of experimental biology and medicine, 7, 47.* (1950).

[987] BYKHOVSKAYA, G. The question of the homology between s. coronalis of the canine and s. centralis of primates. *Higher nervous activity. M., I, 49.* (1929).

[988] BYKHOVSKAYA, G., AND ROBINSON, I. Materials on the question of the change of the cerebral cortex after the severing of the pyramids. *Higher nervous activity. M., I, 149.* (1929).

[989] CHERNIGOVSKIY, V. The physiological characteristic of the interoceptive analysor. *Journal of higher nervous activity, 6, 1, 53.* (1956).

[990] CLARK, C. The mode of representation in the motor cortex. *Brain, 71, 3, 320.* (1948).

[991] DUSSER DE BARENNE, J. The disturbances after laminar thermocoagulation of the motor cerebral cortex. *Brain, 57, 517.* (1934).

[992] FEODOROV, V. Physiological peculiarities of the motor analysor of the dog. *M.* (1955).

[993] FRANK, F., AND PIETRES, A. Les dégénérations secondaires de la moelle eponière consecutives a l'ablation du gyrus sigmoide chez le chien. *Progr. méd., 8, 145.* (1880).

[994] FRANZ, S. Variations in distribution of the motor centers. *Neurol. Cbl., 35, 379.* (1916).

[995] FRITSCH, G., AND HITZIG, E. Über die elektrische erregbarkeit des grosshirns. *Arch. Anat., Physiol. u. Wissensch. Med., 111, 300.* (1870).

[996] GARDNER, E., AND HADDAD, B. Pathways to the cerebral cortex for afferent fibers from the hindleg of the cat. *Amer. J. Physiol., 172, 475.* (1953).

[997] GARDNER, E., AND NOER, R. Projection of afferent fibers from muscles and joints to the cerebral cortex of the cat. *Amer. J. Physiol., 168, 2, 437.* (1952).

[998] GAROL, H. The "motor" cortex of the cat. *J. Neuropath. Exper. Neurol., 1, 139.* (1942).

[999] GLIKI, V. The question of the electric excitability of the cerebrum. *Diss. M.* (1876).

[1000] GRIGHEL, E., CHIVU, V., AND STERIADE, M. Cercetari asupra functiunicāli piramidale. *Studii cerset. fiziol. neurol., 5, 1-2, 155.* (1954).

[1001] HITZIG, E. Untersuchungen über das gehirn. *Berlin.* (1874).

[1002] HOLMES, G., AND MAY, W. Rage on the exact origin of the pyramidal tracts in man and other mammals. *Brain, 32, 1.* (1909).

[1003] HUBER, E. A phylogenetic aspect of the motor cortex of mammals. *Quart. Review of Biol., 9, 55.* (1934).

[1004] HUGELIN, A., BONVALET, M., AND DELL, P. Topographie des projections cortico-matrices au niveau du télencéphale, du diencéphal du tronic cerebral et du cervelet chez le chat. *Rév. neural., 89, 5, 419.* (1953).

[1005] IVANOV, E. The centers of the cerebral cortex and the subcortical ganglia for the movements of the vocal cords and for the manifestation of voice. *Diss. St. P.* (1899).

[1006] KAPLAN, L. The development of the gigantic pyramid cells in the motor region of the cerebral cortex in a series of mammals. *Archive of anatomy, histology and embryology, 2, 18.* (1952).

[1007] KAPLAN, L. The place of ending of the fibers entering into the motor part of the cerebral cortex. *Archive of anatomy, histology and embryology, XXXIII, 4, 38.* (1956).

[1008] KARIVA, K. Experimentelle untersuchung über die corticalen extrapyramidalen fasern aus dem sog. *motorischen Rindezentrum (area 4 u. 6) der Katze. Fol. anat. jap., 14, 241.* (1936).

[1009] KASYANOV, V. The changes of the conditioned reflectory activity of the dog after the extirpation of the motor zone of the cortex of the large hemispheres. *Scientific reports of the Moscow State Pedagogical Instituted named for V.I. Lenin. M., LXXXIV, 2, 3.* (1955).

[1010] KONORSKIY, U., AND MILLER, S. Conditioned reflexes of the motor analysor. *Works of physiological laboratories named for I.P. Pavlov. M., VI, 1, 119.* (1936).

[1011] KRASNOGORSKIY, N. The process of retention and the localization of the cutaneous and motor analysor in the cortex of the large hemispheres in the dog. *Diss. St. P.* (1911).

[1012] KUKUYEV, L. The question of the evolution of the nucleus of the motor analysor and the subcortical ganglia. *Journal of higher nervous activity, III, 5, 766.* (1953).

[1013] KUVATOV, G., AND MUTLI, A. The changes of auditory conditioned reflexes in the hypothermia of the motor region of the large hemispheres in the dog. *In the book: Problems of Physiology and Pathology of the Sense Organs. M., 147.* (1936).

[1014] LANCE, J., AND MANNING, R. Origin of the pyramidal tract in the cat. *J. Physiol. 12, 2, 385.* (1954).

[1015] LISITSA, F., AND PENTSIK, A. Cervical reflexes in the injury of the cerebral cortex in the dog. *Medical works. 2, 119.* (1934).

[1016] LONGO, V., AND FERRARI, E. Rilievi sperimentali sulla rappresentazione motoria omolaterale nella corteccia cerebrale del cane utili per l'interpretazione fisiopatologica degli effetti dell emisferectomia nella fronastenia cerebropatica. *Acta neurol., 10, 5, 667.* (1955).

[1017] MAGOUN, H., AND RANSON, S. Corticofugal pathways for masticatorion lapping and other motor functions in cat. *Arch. Neurol. a. Psychiatr., 30, 292.* (1933).

[1018] MCKIBBEN, P., AND WHEELIS, D. Experiments on the motor cortex of the cat. *J. comp. Neurol., 56, 373.* (1932).

[1019] MICKLE, W., AND ADES, H. Cortical projection of postural impulses. *Fed. Proc., 10, 92.* (1951).

[1020] MINKOWSKI, M. Experimentelle und anatomische untersuchungen zur lehre von der atetose. *Zugleich ein Beitrag zur Kenntnis der anatomischen Verbindungen der Regio sigmoido-coronalis (Area gigantopyramidalis) bei der Katze. Ztschr. ges. Neurol. u. Psychiatr., 102, 650.* (1926).

[1021] MORIN, G., BONNET, V., AND ZWIRN, P. Comparaison des modifications du tonus consécutives à la décortication motrice unilatérale, à l'ablation d'un hémisphère cerebral au la section d'une pyramide bulbaire chez le chien. *J. Physiol. (Paris), 41, 2, 242.* (1949).

[1022] MORIN, G., POURSINES, J., AND MAFFRÉ, S. Sur l'origine de la voie pyramidale documents obtenus par le methode de dégénérescences descendentes chez le chien. *J. Physiol. (Paris), 43, 75.* (1951).

[1023] MURATOV, V. Secondary palingeneses in focal afflictions of the motor sphere of the cerebral cortex. *Diss. M.* (1893).

[1024] ORSHANSKIY, I. Materials on the physiology of the brain. *Psychomotor centers. Diss. St. P.* (1877).

[1025] PANETH, I. Ueber lage, ausdehnung und bedeutung der absoluten motorischen felder auf der hirnoberfläche des hundes. *Arch. ges. Physiol., 37, 523.* (1885).

[1026] PASTERNATSKIY, I. The question of the psychomotor centers of the brain. *Diss. Warsaw.* (1876).

[1027] PHILLIPS, C. Cortical motor threshold and the thresholds and distribution of excited betz cells in the cat. *Quart J. exper. Physiol., 41, 1, 70.* (1956).

[1028] PHILLIPS, C. Intracellular records from betz cells in the cat. *Quart. J. exper. Physiol., 41, 1, 58.* (1956).

[1029] PROTOPOPOV, V. The conjunctive-motor reaction to sound stimuli. *Diss. St. P.* (1909).

[1030] REDLICH, E. Ueber die anatomischen folgeerscheinungen ausgedehnter extirpationen der matorischen rindencentren bei der katze. *Neural. Cbl., 16, 818.* (1897).

[1031] ROSENTHAL, I. Conditioned motor nutritional reflex in dogs, either without the motor or without the cutaneous analysor. *Physiological Journal USSR, XXIV, 345.* (1938).

[1032] SANDMEYER, W. Sekundäre degeneration nach exstirpation motorischen zentren. *Ztschr. f. Biol., XXVIII, 177.* (1891).

[1033] SHUMILINA, A. Morphophysiological analysis of the localization of motor stimulation. *In the coll.: Problems of Higher Nervous Activity. M., 299.* (1949).

[1034] SHUMILINA, A. The participation of the pyramidal and extrapyramidal systems in the motor activity of the deafferentiated extremity. *In the coll.: Problems of Higher Nervous Activity, Ed. by P.K. Anokhin. M., 196.* (1949).

[1035] SHUSTIN, N. The localization of the vocal part of the motor analysor. *Physiological Journal USSR, XXXVII, 5, 562.* (1951).

[1036] SIMPSON, S. Secondary degeneration following unilateral lesions of the cerebral motor cortex. *Intern. Mschr. f. Anat. u. Physiol., 304.* (1902).

[1037] SKIPIN, G. The mechanism of the formation of the conditioned nutritional reflexes. *M.* (1947).

[1038] SMITH, W. The extent and structure of the electrically excitable cerebral cortex in the frontal lobe of the dog. *J. comp. Neurol., 62, 431.* (1935).

[1039] TARKHANOV, I. The psychomotor centers and their development in man and animals. *St. P.* (1879).

[1040] TOWER, S. The dissociation of cortical excitation from cortical inhibition by pyramid section and the syndrome of that lesion in the cat. *Brain, 58, 238.* (1935).

[1041] TOWER, S. Extrapyramidal action from the cat's cerebral cortex: motor and inhibitory. *Brain, 59, 408.* (1936).

[1042] TRAPEZNIKOV, A. The central innervation of deglutition. *Diss. St. P.* (1897).

[1043] VVEDENSKIY, N. The correlations between the psychomotor centers. *Complete works. L., III, 158.* (1952).

[1044] WOOLSEY, C. Postural relations of the frontal and motor cortex of the dog. *Brain, 56, 353.* (1933).

[1045] ZALMANZON, A. Conditioned defensive reflexes in the local poisoning of the motor centers of the cerebral cortex with strychnine and cocaine. *Higher nervous activity. M., I, 39.* (1929).

[1046] ZHUKOV, N. The influence of the removal of motor centers of the cerebral cortex upon the excitability of the adjacent cortical regions. *Diss. St. P.* (1895).

[1047] ZHUKOVA, G. The question of the development of the cortical end of the motor analysor. *Archive of anatomy, histology and embryology, 30, 1, 32.* (1953).

[1048] ZURABASHVILI, A. The question of the stratified synapsoarchitectonic of the motor cortex. *Information of A.S. of the Georgian SSR. Tbilisi, 10, 367.* (1949).

Frontal Region

[1049] AFANASYEV, N. Materials on the study of the functions of the frontal lobes. *Diss. St. P.* (1913).

[1050] BABKIN, B. Materials on the physiology of the frontal lobes of the large hemispheres in the dog. *News Mil.-Med. Acad., XIX, 1-2, 16.* (1909).

[1051] BEKHTEREV, V. The study of the functions of the pre-frontal and other regions of the cerebral cortex with the help of conjunctive motor reflexes. *Review of psychiatry, neurology and experimental psychology, 4, 5, 6, 336; 7, 8, 9, 353.* (1914-1915).

[1052] BIANCHI, L. The mechanism of the brain and the function of the frontal lobes. *Edinburgh.* (1922).

[1053] BRADFORT, F. Ablations of frontal cortex in cats with special reference to enhancement of the scratch reflex. *J. Neurophysiol., 2, 192.* (1939).

[1054] BREGADZE, A. Individual behaviour of the cat without the frontal lobes of the large hemispheres. *Works of the Institute of Physiology named for I.S. Beritashvili. Tbilisi, 7.* (1947).

[1055] BRUTKOWSKI, S. Wplyw usuwania okolic czolowych na ślinowe odruchy warunkowe u psów. acta physiol. *polon., 5, 4, 503.* (1954).

[1056] COLE, S. The comparative anatomy of the frontal lobe and its bearing upon the pathology of insanity. *Ment. Sci., LVII, 52.* (1911).

[1057] DELMAS-MARSALET, P. Le syndrome frontal de déséquilibre chez le chien. *C. r. Soc. biol., 110, 966.* (1932).

[1058] DEMIDOV, V. Conditioned (salivary) reflexes in the dog without the anterior halves of both hemispheres. *Diss. St. P.* (1908).

[1059] EBERSTALLER, O. Das stirnhirn. *Wien-Leipzig.* (1890).

[1060] FELICIANGELI, G. Experimenteller beitrag zur kenntnis der funktion des stirn-lappens des hundehirns. *Folia neuro-biol., IV, 5, 449.* (1910).

[1061] FRANZ, S. On the functions of the cerebrum. The frontal lobes. *Neurol. Cbl. 28, 805.* (1909).

[1062] ICHISHIMA, S. Über die kortikalen extrapyramidalen fasern aus der. *Area 8 der Grosshirnrinde der Katze. Ztschr. f. mikr.-anat. Forsch., 40, 541.* (1936).

[1063] KALISCHER, O. Über die bedeutung des stirnteils des grosshirns für die fresston-dressur. *Sitzungs. physiol. Gesellschaft. Berlin, XXXV, 70.* (1910).

[1064] KURAYEV, C. Examination of dogs with injured anterior lobes of the hemispheres during a late postoperative period. *Diss. St. P.* (1912).

[1065] LANGWORTHY, O. The area frontalis of the cerebral cortex of the cat, its minute structure and physiological evidence of its control of the postural reflex. *Johns Hopkins Hosp. Bull., 42, 20.* (1928).

[1066] LAWICKA, B. The effect of the prefrontal lobectomy on the vocal conditioned reflexes in dogs. *Acta biol. exp., 17, 2, 317.* (1957).

[1067] MORIN, G., DONNET, V., AND MAFFRÉ, S. Mouvements de manège et troubles de la vision par lésions de l'écorce frontale chez le chien. *Soc. Biol., 145, 17/18, 1344.* (1951).

[1068] PEACOCK, S., AND HODES, R. Influence of the forebrain on somatomotor activity. II. Facilitation. *J. comp. Neurol., 94, 3, 409.* (1951).

[1069] SAGER, O., BROSTEANU, R., NESTIANU, V., AND FLOREA-CIOCOIV, V. Les connexions du tractus optique avec le lobe frontale, comm. *Acad. Rep. Popul. Rom., 5, 1199.* (1955).

[1070] SATURNOV, N. Further investigations of conditioned reflexes in dogs without anterior halves of both hemispheres. *Diss. St. P.* (1911).

[1071] SCHEWIOR. The frontal lobe of the dog. *J. comp. Neurol., 62, 421.* (1935).

[1072] SHUMILINA, A. Functional significance of the frontal region of the cerebral cortex in the conditioned reflectory activity of the dog. *In the book: Problems of Higher Nervous Activity, Ed. by P.K. Anokhin. M., 561.* (1949).

[1073] SHUSTIN, N. Traced conditioned reflexes in the dog after the removal of the frontal lobes. *Works of the Institute of Physiology named for I.P. Pavlov. M.-L., II, 76.* (1953).

[1074] SHUSTIN, N., AND GILINSKIY, E. The disruption of the cortical activity caused by the removal of the frontal lobes. *Works of the I.P. Pavlov Institute Institute of Physiology. M.-L., V, 461.* (1956).

[1075] SIEBENS, A., AND WOOLSEY, C. Cortical autonomic center for the eyes on the mesial surface of the frontal lobe in cat. *Fed. Proc., 5, 95.* (1946).

[1076] SPECKMAN, T., AND BABKIN, B. Changes in behaviour following frontal lobectomy in dogs and cats. *Arch. Neurol. a. Psychiatr., 63, 433.* (1950).

[1077] STEPIEN, I. Wplyw usuwania platow czolowych na zachowanie kotow. *Acta physiol. polon., 5, 109.* (1954).

[1078] STRATFORD, J. Cortico-thalamic connections from gyrus proreus and first and second somatic sensory areas of the cat. *J. comp. Neurol., 100, 1, 1.* (1954).

[1079] SVETUKHINA, B. Cytoarchitecture of the cortex of the anterior part of the hemisphere in a series of carnivora. *Diss. M.* (1956).

[1080] TARABRINA, M. The influence of early lobotomy on higher nervous activity in animals. *Collection of student scientific papers of the Rostov State University. Rostov on the Don, 2, 26.* (1953).

[1081] TIKHOMIROV, N. Test of strictly objective investigation of the functions of the large hemispheres in the dog. *Diss. St. P.* (1906).

[1082] TOWER, S., AND HINIS, M. Dissociation of the pyramidal and extrapyramidal function of the frontal lobe. *Science, 82, 376.* (1935).

[1083] USIYEVICH, M., KUDRIASHOVA, K., AND SO-VIETOV, A. The influence of the exclusion of the frontal lobes of the cerebrum (lobotomy) upon the higher nervous activity in the dog. *Bulletin of experimental biology and medicine, XXVIII, Information 1; 1, 11; Information 2; 9, 3, 183.* (1949).

[1084] VALSHONOK, O., AND SVETNIK, Z. Conducting tracts of the frontal lobe. *Medical works, 2.* (1934).

[1085] VARGHA, M., BEUTZIK, M., AND KOZAA, M. Leikotomie beim hunde für experimentelle zwecke. *Acta neurochir. (Wien), 3, 248.* (1953).

[1086] WILLIAM, C., HARLEY, S., AND CLAIBORN, L. An experimental study of the function of the frontal lobes in dogs. *Arch. Neurol. a. Psychiatr., XXVII, 961.* (1932).

[1087] ZHUKOVSKIY, M. The anatomical connections of the frontal lobes. *Neurological Herald, V, 4.* (1897).

[1088] ZHUKOVSKIY, M. The functions of the frontal lobes. *Review of psychiatry, neurology and experimental psychology, V, 4, 905.* (1897).

Parietal, Limbic Regions, Archicortex, Paleocortex and Intermediate Cortex and Other Cortical Regions

[1089] ADEY, W. An experimental study of the hippocampal connections of the cingulate cortex in the rabbit. *Brain, 74, 233.* (1951).

[1090] ADLER, A. Zur topik der corticalen geschmacksphäre. *Ztschr. f.d. ges. Neurol. u. Psychiatr., 152, 25-33.* (1935).

[1091] ALLEN, W. Effect of ablating the pyriform-amygdaloid areas and hippocampi on positive and negative olfactory conditioned reflexes and on conditioned olfactory differentiation. *Amer. J. Physiol., 132, 81.* (1941).

[1092] ANAND, B., AND DUA, S. Effect of electrical stimulation of the limbic system (visceral brain) on gastric secretion and motility. *Indian J. Med. Research, 44, 1, 125.* (1956).

[1093] ANAND, B., AND DUA, S. Electrical stimulation of the limbic system of brain (visceral brain) in the waking animals. *Indian J. Med. Research., 44, 1, 107.* (1956).

[1094] ANDERSSON, S., AND GERNAND, B. Cortical projection of vestibular nerve in cat. *Acta oto-laryngol., Suppl., 116, 10.* (1954).

[1095] ARONSON, L. Conduction of labyrinthine impulses to the cortex. *J. Nerv. a. Ment. Dis., 78, 250.* (1933).

[1096] BABAYAN, S. Efferent tracts of the parietal region in the dog. *Diss. M.* (1957).

[1097] BABKIN, B., AND KITE, W. Gastric motor effects of acute removal of cinguiate gyrus and section on brain stem. *J. Neurophysiol., 13, 335.* (1950).

[1098] BARI, A. The question of the cortical centers of salivation. *Neurological Herald, VII, 4, 1.* (1899).

[1099] BARRAQUER-BORDAS, L. Fisiologia y clinica del sistema limbico. *Madrid, Paz Montalvo.* (1954).

[1100] BELITSKIY, U. The question of the cortical gustatory center. *Revue of psychiatry and neurology, 12, 728.* (1908).

[1101] BLINKOV, S. The limbic area. *In the book: Cytoarchitecture of the Cerebral Cortex in Man. M., 390.* (1949).

[1102] BĂLĂCEANA-STOLNICI, C. Relatiile aparatului vestibular cu scoarta cerebrală. *Nota I. Reflexele labirintice neconditionate la pisici decorticate si hemide-corticate. Nota II. Reflexele vestibulare labirintice neconditionate după leziuni partiale ale scoartei cerebrale la pisici. Bul. stiint Acad. Rep. Popul. Rom. Soc. med., 5, 2, 247.* (1953).

[1103] BUNICHI, H. Über die projection der labyrinth'gren erregung in die regio hypothalamica im potentialbild. *Ztschr. f. Neurol. u. Psychiatr., 169, 5, 606.* (1940).

[1104] CERLETTI, U. Über einen neunen befund im bulbus olfactorius des hundes. *Vortrag, gehalten auf dem psych. Kongress zu Perugia, Mai 3.* (1911).

[1105] CHERNYSHEV, A. The superior limbic region of terrestrial carnivora. *Works of the Brain Institute. M., III-IV, 393.* (1938).

[1106] CHERNYSHEV, A., AND BLINKOV, S. Some peculiarities of the architecture of the cortex of the superior limbic region of the brain. *Neuropathology, psychiatry and psychphygiene, 12, 4, 45.* (1935).

[1107] CLARK, G., CHOW, K., GILLASPY, C., AND KLOTZ, D. Stimulation of anterior limbic region in dogs. *J. Neurophysiol., 12, 459.* (1949).

[1108] FULTON, J. Cortical representation of somatic sensation with comment on the limbic system. *Iuprensa med., 19, 11, 627.* (1955).

[1109] GEREBTZOFF, M. Recherches sur la projection corticale du labyrinthe. *I. Des effets de la stimulation labyrinthique sur l'activité electrique de l'ecorce cerebrale. Arch. int. Physiol., 50, 59.* (1940).

[1110] GORSHKOV, Y. The centers of taste and olfaction in the cerebral cortex. *Diss. St. P.* (1901).

[1111] GORSHKOV, Y. The central conductors of gustatory sensations. *Neurological Herald, X, I, 11.* (1902).

[1112] GORSHKOV, Y. The question of the central conductors of olfactory sensations. *Neurological Herald, X, I, 1.* (1902).

[1113] HESS, H., AKERT, K., AND MCDONALD, D. Functions of the orbital gyri of cats. *Brain, 75, 11, 244.* (1952).

[1114] KAADA, B. Somato-motor, autonomic and electrocorticographic responses to electrical stimulation of "rhinencephalic" and other structures in primates, cat and dog. *Acta physiol. Scand., Suppl. 24, 1.* (1951).

[1115] KARR, D. An investigation of olfactory centrifugal fiber system. *J. Neurophysiol., 18, 4, 362.* (1955).

[1116] KASTANIAN, E. Theory on the conducting tracts in the olfactory centers. *Diss. Rostov on the Don.* (1902).

[1117] KASYANOV, V. The physiological significance of the limbic area in the canine brain. *In the book: Problems of Higher Nervous Activity. Ed. by P.K. Anokhin. Information 1 and 2. M., 223 and 246.* (1949).

[1118] KEMPINSKY, W. Cortical projection of vestibular and facial nerves in cat. *J. Neurophysiol., 14, 203.* (1951).

[1119] KENNARD, M. Effect of bilateral ablation of cingulate area on behavior of cats. *J. Neurophysiol., 18, 3, 159.* (1955).

[1120] KREMER, W. Autonomic and somatic reactions induced by stimulation of the cingular gyrus in dogs. *J. Neurophysiol., 10, 5, 371.* (1947).

[1121] LANGUTINA, N., ROZHANSKIY, N., AND URMANICHEYEVA, T. Materials on the characteristic of the "archeocortex" of the cerebrum. *Physiological Journal USSR, XLII, 7, 533.* (1956).

[1122] LISITSA, F. Efferent tracts of the parietal lobe. *Soviet psychoneurology. 2, 77.* (1936).

[1123] LUCIANI, L. On the sensorial localisation in the cortex cerebri. *Brain, 7, 145.* (1884).

[1124] MACLEAN, P. The limbic system and its hippocampal formation. *Studies in animals and their possible application to man. J. Neurophysiol., 17, 29.* (1954).

[1125] MICKLE, W., AND ADES, H. Rostral projection pathway of the vestibular system. *Amer. J. Physiol., 176, 2, 243.* (1954).

[1126] OSIPOV, V. The physiological significance of the horns of ammon. *Arch. Anat. and Physiol., Dept. of Physiol., Suppl., 1.* (1900).

[1127] OVSIANNIKOV, F. The most delicate structure of the lobi olfactorii in mammals. *Selected works. M., 47.* (1955).

[1128] PONIATOVSKIY, A. The theory of the central cerebral tracts of olfactory sensations. *Diss. M.* (1895).

[1129] POPOV, N., AND BAYANDUROV, B. The physiology of the central end of the space analysor in the dog. *Report of the Azerbaidzhan State University, 3, 248.* (1923-1924).

[1130] PRIBRAM, K., AND KRUGER, L. Functions of the "olfactory brain. " *Ann. N.Y. Acad. Sci., 58, 2, 109.* (1954).

[1131] REDLICH, E. Zur vergleichenden anatomie der associations-systeme des gehirns der säugetiere. *I. Das Cingulum. Arb. a.d. Neurol. Inst. d. Wien. Univ., 10, 1.* (1903).

[1132] ROSE, I., AND WOOLSEY, C. Structure and relation of limbic cortex and anterior thalamic nuclei in rabbit and cat. *J. comp. Neurol., 89, 279.* (1948).

[1133] ROSE, M. Der allocortex bei tier und mensch. *J. Psychol. u. Neurol., 34, 1-2, 1.* (1926-1927).

[1134] ROSE, M. Gyrus limbicus anterior und regio retrosplenialis (cortex holoprotoptychos quinquestratificatus). *Vergleichende Architectonik bei Tier und Mensch. J. Psychol. u. Neurol., 35, 3-4, 65.* (1927-1928).

[1135] ROTHFIELD, L., AND HARMAN, P. On the relation of the hippocampal fornix system to the control of rage responses in cat. *J. comp. Neurol., 101, 2, 265.* (1954).

[1136] RUWALDT, M., AND SNIDER, R. Projections of vestibular areas of cerebellum to the cerebrum. *J. comp. Neurol., 104, 3, 387.* (1956).

[1137] SAVICH, K. The pathway of the radicles of the olfactory tract and their relationship to the formation of the archeocortex. *Archive of anatomy, histology and embryology, 31, 2, 3.* (1954).

[1138] SCHREINER, L., AND KLING, A. Rhinencephalon and behavior. *Amer. J. Physiol., 184, 3, 486.* (1956).

[1139] SLOAN, N., AND JASPER, H. Studies of the regulatory functions of the limbic cortex. *EEG a. clin. Neurophysiol., 2, 317.* (1950).

[1140] SMITH, W. The results of ablation of the cingular region of the cerebral cortex. *Proc. Am. Soc. Exp. Biol., 3, 42.* (1944).

[1141] SMITH, W. The functional significance of the rostral cingular cortex as revealed by its responses to electrical excitation. *J. Neurophysiol., 8, 4, 241.* (1945).

[1142] SPIEGEL, E. Cortical centers of the labyrinth. *J. Nerv. a. Ment. Dis., 75, 504.* (1932).

[1143] SPIRTOV. Demonstration of the cortical center of salivation. *Review of psychiatry, neurology and experimental psychology, 57.* (1909).

[1144] TELIATNIK, F. The nervous elements of the olfactory bulb. *Neurological Herald, III, 3.* (1895).

[1145] WALZL, E., AND MOUNTCASTLE, V. Projection of vestibular nerve to cerebral cortex of the cat. *Amer. J. Physiol., 159, 595.* (1949).

[1146] WARD, A. The cingular gyrus: area 24. *J. Neurophysiol., 11, 1, 13.* (1948).

[1147] WOOLSEY, C., DICK, F., AND FRANTZ, R. Electrical responses in gyrus cinguli evoked by electrical stimulation of ipsilateral mammillary body in cat and monkey. *Fed. Proc., 5, 116.* (1946).

[1148] ZAMBRZHITSKIY, I. Cytoarchitecture and neural structure of the limbic area in some mammals. *Archive of anatomy, histology and embryology, XXXIII, 4, 41.* (1956).

[1149] ZAVADSKIY, I. Gyrus pyriformis and the olfaction of the dog. *Archive of biological sciences, XV, 3 and 4, 221.* (1910).

SYMBOLS

a, processus acominis
aa, area acustica
aki, cornu Ammonis et area cornu Ammonis
am, nucleus amygdalae
an, sulcus ansatus
and, nucleus anterodorsalis
anm, nucleus anteromedialis
anv, nucleus anteroventralis
ap, area postrema
are, fibrae arcuatae externae
area, fibrae arcuatae externae anteriores
arep, fibrae arcuatae externae posteriores
ari, fibrae arcuatae internae
aS, aquaeductus Sylvii
asp, ramus ascendens sulci splenialis
bb, "bigeminal body"
bcbp, brachium corporis bigemini posterioris
BO, bulbus olfactorius
c, central group of cells of the anterior horn of the spinal cord
C, gyrus cinguli
CA, cornu Ammonis et area cornu Ammonis
ca, cornu anterius
caa, commissura anteriores alba medullae spinalis, commissura alba anterior medullae spinalis
caa, commissura alba anterior
CAB, cornu Ammonis et area cornu Ammonis
cag, commissurae anteriores grisea, commissura grisea anterior
CAi, cornu Ammonis inferius
cal, calamus scriptorius
cal, area regio entorhinalis
can, commissura anterior
CAP, cornu Ammonis et area cornu Ammonis
CAs, cornu Ammonis superius
cba, corpus bigeminum anterius
cbp, corpus bigeminum posterius
cc, canalis centralis
ccba, commissura corporis bigemini anterioris
ccbp, commissura corporis bigemini posterioris
ccgm, capsula corporis geniculatum medians
ccl, corpus callosum
ce, capsula externa
cer, cerebellum
cex, capsula extrema
cf, columna fornicis
cgl, corpus geniculatum laterale
cgm, corpus geniculatum mediale
ch, chiasma nervorum opticorum
ci, capsula interna
cl, cornu lateralia

cL, corpus Luysi
cl, cornu lateralis
cla, columnae anteriores
cll, columnae laterales
cll, columna lateralis
clp, columnae posteriores
clp, columna posterior
cls, claustrum
cm, commissura grisea media s. commissura mollis
cm, commissura grisea media
cmd, centrum medianum Luysi
cml, nucleus lateralis corporis mamillaris
cmm, nucleus medians corporis mamillaris
cmp, commissura posterior
cmp, commissura posterior
cnl, nucleus centralis lateralis
cnl, nucleus centralis lateralis thalami optici
cnm, nucleus centralis medialis
cnm, nucleus centralis medialis thalami optici
Cor, gyrus coronalis
cor, sulcus coronalis
cp, corna posteriores
cp, cornu posterius
cpg, commissura grisea posterior
cpg, commissura grisea posterior
cps, area regio entorhinalis
cr, sulcus cruciatus
ctr, corpus trapezoides
ctr, corpus trapezoides
cu, culmen
D, regio diagonalis
D_1, areae regio diagonalis
D_2, areae regio diagonalis
de, declive
dF, decussatio Foreli
dF, decussatio Foreli
dg, sulcus diagonalis
dlm, decussatio lemniscorum
dlm, decussatio lemniscorum medialium
dM, decussatio Meynerti
dM, decussatio Meynerti s. decussatio tectospinalis
dpy, decussatio pyramidum
dpy, decussatio pyramidum
dW, decussatio pedunculorum cerebelli anteriorum s. decussatio Wernekinki
E, regio entorhinalis
ea, area regio entorhinalis
Ecl, gyrus ectolateralis
ecl, sulcus ectolateralis
egn, sulcus ectogenualis
Enl, gyrus entolateralis

enl, sulcus entolateralis s. fissura confinis

ep, area regio entorhinalis

EP, epiphysis

epr, area regio entorhinalis

eprl, area regio entorhinalis

epria, area regio entorhinalis

epriam, area regio entorhinalis

eprle, area regio entorhinalis

epro, area regio entorhinalis

Es, gyrus ectosylvius

es, sulcus ectosylvius

Esa, gyrus ectosylvius anterior

esa, sulcus ectosylvius anterior

Esm, gyrus ectosylvius medius

esm, sulcus ectosylvius medius

Esp, gyrus ectosylvius posterior

esp, sulcus ectosylvius posterior

et, eminentia tares

et, eminentia teres

eta, area regio entorhinalis

etl, area regio entorhinalis

etp, area regio entorhinalis

f, fornix

F-L$_2$, subarea frontolimbica

F$_1$, area frontalis prima

F$_2$, area frontalis secunda

F$_3$, area frontalis tertia

F$_4$, area frontalis quarta

fa, nucleus filiformis anterior

fc, funiculus cuneatus

fct, fasciculus centralis tegmenti

FD, fascia dentata

FDi, fascia dentata inferior

FDs, fascia dentata superior

fg, funiculus gracilis

fhp, fasciculus habenulo-peduncularis

fin, fossa interpeduncularis

fl, flocculus

flc, fissura longitudinalis cerebri

flp, fasciculus longitudinalis posterior

flp, Fasciculus longitudinalis posterior s. medians

fM, foramen Monroi

fma, fissura mediana anterior

fmt, fasciculus mamillothalamicus s. fasciculus Vicq d'Azyr

foc, fibrae olivocerebellares

fp, filiformis principalis

fp, nucleus filiformis principalis

fpm, fissura paramediana

fpr, fissura prima

frM, tractus habenulo-peduncularis s. fasciculus retroflexus Maynerti

frM, fasciculus retroflexus Maynerti

frs, fasciculus rubrospinalis

fs, fissura secunda

fscd, Fasciculus spinocerebellaris dorsalis

fscd, fasciculus spinocerebellaris dorsalis Flechsigi

fscv, Fasciculus spinocerebellaris ventralis

fscv, fasciculus spinocerebellaris ventralis Gowersi

fsl, tractus s. fasciculus solitarius

fsp, fasciculus striopeduncularis

fsp, fasciculus striopeduncularis

fsth, fasciculus spinotactalis

fsth, fasciculus spinothalamicus

fts, fasciculus tectospinalis

fts, Fasciculus tectospinalis s. praedorsalis

fvc, fibrae vestibule-cerebellares

fvc, fasciculus vestibulo-cerebellaris

G, gyrus genualis

gc, substantia grisea centralis

gen, genu corporis callosi

gen, genu corporis callosi

gi, gangl. interpedunculare

gi, ganglion interpedunculare

gn, sulcus genualis

GVII, genu nervi facialis

H$_1$, fasciculus thalamicus

h^1, cornu Ammonis et area cornu Ammonis

H$_1$, fasciculus thalamicus Foreli

h^1, h^2, ..., (cm. CA)

H$_2$, fasciculus lecticularis

h^2, cornu Ammonis et area cornu Ammonis

H$_2$, fasciculus lenticularis Foreli

hip, fissura hippocampi s. sulcus cornu AMMonis

hp, nucleus tractus habenulo-peduncularis

hpa, nucleus hypothalamicus anterior

hpf, nucleus perifornicalis

hpl, area hypothalamica lateralis

hpl, area hypothalamica lateralis

hpmd, nucleus hypothalamicus dorsomedialis

hpmv, nucleus hypothalamicus ventromedialis

hpp, nucleus hypothalamicus posterior

hpr, area praeoptica

hpr, area praeoptica hypothalami

hprl, area praeoptica lateralis

hprl, area praeoptica hypothalami lateralis

hprm, area praeoptica medians

hprm, area praeoptica hypothalami medialis

hps, ramus horizontalis posterior sulci splenialis

hyp, hypophysis

I$_1$, I$_2$, area insularis prima, secunda

iam, nucleus interanteromedialis

iam, nucleus interantoromedians

iam, nucleus interanteromedialis thalami optici

II, nervus opticus

III, n. oculomotorius

imd, nucleus intermediodorsalis

imd, nucleus intermediodorsalis thalami optici

in, infundibulum

ipr, sulcus interprorealis s. sulcus intraorbitalis

IV, nervus trochlearis

IX, nervus glossopharyngeus

l, sulcus lateralis

L$_1$, L$_2$, area limbica prima, secunda

lc, lobulus centralis
li, lingula
ll, lemniscus lateralis
lm, lemniscus medians
lmd, lamina medullaris
lmi, sulcus lateromedialis inferior
lms, sulcus lateromedialis superior
lmt, nucleus limitans
lp, sulcus limitans posterior
lpm, lobulus paramedianus
lqd, lobulus quadrangularis
lsm, lobulus semilunaris
lta, pars anterior
lta, pars anterior nucleus lateralis thalami optici
lti, pars intermedia nucleus lateralis
lti, pars intermedia nucleus lateralis thalami optici
ltp, pars posterior nucleus lateralis
ltp, pars posterior nucleus lateralis thalami optici
M, inner group of cells of the anterior horn of the spinal cord
md, nucleus medians dorsalis
mo, medulla oblongata
na, nucleus album
nap, nucleus commissura posterioris
narc, nucleus arcuatus medullae oblongatae
narc, nucleus arcuatus
nB, nucleus angularis Bechterevi
nc, nucleus funiculi cuneati
nC, nucleus interstitialis Cajali
nc_1, nucleus nervi cervicalis primus
nca, nucleus interstitialis commissurae anterioris
nca, nucleus interstitialis commissurae anterioris
ncd, corpus nuclei caudati
ncd, nucleus caudatus
nce, cuneiform fasciculus
nce, nucleus externus funiculi cuneati
ncp, nucleus commissurae posterioris
ncr, nucleus centralis formatio reticularis
nct, nucleus centralis tegmenti
nD, nucleus Deitersi
ndn, nucleus dentatus
nDr, nucleus Darkschewitschi
nDr, nucleus Darkschewitschi
ndv, nucleus radicis descendentis nervus vestibularis
ndv, nucleus radicis descendentis nervi vestibularis
neb, nucleus emboliformis
nfs, nucleus fastigii
ng, nucleus funiculi gracilis
ngb, nucleus globosus
ngc, nucleus gigantocellularis formatio reticularis
nh, habenula s. nucleus habenulae
nh, nucleus habenulae
nhl, nucleus lateralis habenulae
nhm, nucleus medialis habenulae
NIII, nucleus nervi oculomotorii
nIIIE, nucleus Edinger-Westphali
nIIIm, nucleus motorius nervi oculomotorii

nIIIP, nucleus Perlia
nin, nucleus intercalates
nin, nucleus intercalatus
nIV, nucleus nervi trochlearis
nll, nuclei lemniscus lateralis
nll, nucleus lemniscus lateralis
nlt, nucleus lateralis
nlt, nucleus lateralis medullae oblongatae s. nucleus lateralis reticularis
nod, nodulus
nod, nodulus
npar, nucleus paraventricularis
npc, nucleus pontis caudalis
npd, nucleus peripeduncularis
npo, nucleus pontis oralis
npp, nuclei proprii pontis
nr, nucleus ruber
nR, nucleus sublingualis
nR, nucleus Rolleri
nr, nucleus ruber
nret, nucleus reticularis
nret, nucleus reticularis thalami optici
nsl, nucleus tractus solitarius
nsp, nucleus supraopticus diffusus
nsp, nucleus supraopticus diffuses
nst, nucleus interstitialis striae terminalis
nst, nucleus interstitialis stria terminalis
ntr, nucleus triangularis
ntr, nucleus triangularis
nVa, nucleus radicis ascendentis (s. mesencephalicus) nerve trigemini
nVd, nucleus radicis descendentis n. trigemini
nVd, nucleus radicis descendentis nervi trigemini
nvest, nuclei nervi vestibularis
nVI, nucleus nervi abducentis
nVII, nucleus nervi facialis
nVIIIcv, nucleus s. ganglion ventralis nervi cochlearis
nVm, nucleus motorius nervi trigemini
nVs, nucleus sensibilis nervi trigemini
nXa, nucleus motorius n. vagi s. nucleus ambiguus
nXa, nucleus ambiguus nervi vagi
nXd, nucleus dorsalis nervi vagi
nXId, nucleus dorsalis n. accessorii
nXId, nucleus dorsalis nervus accessorii
nXId, nucleus dorsalis nervi accessorii
nXII, nucleus hypoglossi
nXII, nucleus nervi hypogiossi
nXIv, nucleus ventralis nervus accessorii
o, oliva
O_1, O_2, area occipitalis prima, secunda
oe, pallidum externum
oi, oliva inferior
oid, oliva inferior accessoria dorsalis
oin, sulcus occipitalis inferior
oiv, oliva inferior accessoria ventralis
oiv, oliva inferior accessoria ventralis
Ol, gyrus olfactorius lateralis

Om, gyrus olfactoris medialis
OP, area occipito-parietalis
Or, gyrus orbitalis
or, sulcus orbitalis
os, oliva superior
osl, oliva superior lateralis
osl, oliva superior lateralis
osm, oliva superior medialis
ot, sulcus occipito-temporalis
P, area parietalis
p, sulcus posticus
Pas, parasubiculum
pas, ramus praeascendens sulci uplenialis
pc, pedunculi cerebri
Pc_1, Pc_2, Pc_3, Pc_4, area postcoronalis: prima, secunda, tertia, quarta
pci, pedunculi inferior s. pedunculi cerebelli ad medullam oblongatum
pci, pedunculi cerebelli inferior s. pedunculi cerebelli ad medullam oblongatum
pcm, s. pedunculi cerebelli medius
pcm, pedunculi cerebelli medius, s. pedunculi cerebelli ad pontem
pcn, nucleus paracentralis
pcs, pedunculi cerebelli superior
pcs, pedunculi cerebelli superiores
pcs, pedunculum cerebelli superior
pcs, pedunculi cerebelli superior s. pedunculi cerebelli ad corpora quadrigemina
pcs4, Pci4, subarea quarta superior et inferior
pe, pallidum externum
pen, nucleus paracentralis
per, systema periventricularis
per, massa periventricularis
pev, sulcus praectolateralis verticalis
pfl, paraflocculus
pi, pallidum internum
Pi, gyrus piriformis
pi, pallidum internum
Pl_1, Pl_2, area parainsularis prima et secunda
pl, sulcus postlateralis
pm, pedunculi corporae mamillariae
Pm, regio periamygdalaris
pm, pedunculi corporae mamillariae
Pm, Pmm, Pml^1, Pml^2, areae regio periamygdalaris
post, nucleus posterior thalami optici
pp, pes pedunculi
Pp, regio praepiriformis
pp, pes pedunculi cerebri
Pp, Pp^1, Pp^2, Pp_o^1, Pp_o, Pp^{oo}, Pple, Ppl1, Ppla, areae et subareae regio praepiriformis
Pr, prorea s. gyrus proreus
pr, sulcus proreus
pra, nuclei paraventriculares anterior
pra, nucleus paraventricularis anterior
Prc_2, L2, subarea praecoronalis limbica
Prci, Prc2, areae praecoronalis prima et secunda

prcr, sulcus praecruciatus
prf, nucleus parafascicularis
prf, nucleus parafascicularis thalami optici
prp, nuclei paraventriculares posterior
prp, nucleus paraventricularis posterior
prs, sulcus praesylvius
Prspl, gyrus praesplenialis
prt, area praetectalis
prt, area praetectalis
Psb, regio praesubicularis
Psb, Psb^1, Psb^2, areae regio praesubicularis
pscr, sulcus postcruciatus
Pspl, gyrus postsplenialis
pssp, sulcus praesuprasplenialis
pt, nucleus parataenialis
Pt_1, Pt_2, Pt_3, area peritectalis prima, secunda et tertia
pul, pulvinar thalami optici
put, putamen
pV, pons Varolii
py, Fasciculus corticospinalis s. pyramidalis
py, fasciculus pyramidalis
py, pyramis, fasciculus pyramidalis
pyr, pyramis vermis cerebelli
r, raphe
R, gyrus rectus
r, raphe
Rb, regio retrobulbaris
rc, radix nervi cervicalis
rdv, radix descendens nervi vestibularis
rest, corpus restiforme
ret, formatio reticularis
reu, nucleus reuniens thalami
rha, sulcus rhinalis anterior
rhm, nucleus rhomboidalis
rhp, sulcus rhinalis posterior
RIII, radix nervi oculomotorii
ros, sulcus rostralis
rslp, sulcus retrosplenialis
rV, radix nervi trigemini
rV1, radix nervi abducentis
rVd, radix descendentis nervi trigemini
rVII, radix nervi facialis
rVIIIc, ramus cochlearis nervi acustici
rVIIIv, ramus vestibularis nervi acustici
rVm, nucleus motorius n. trigemini
rXII, radix nervi hypoglossi
S, gyrus Sylvii
s, sulcus Sylvii
Sa, gyrus Sylvii anterior
sa, striae acusticae
sam, stratum album medium
sam, stratum album medium corporis bigemini anterioris
sap, stratum album profundum
sap, stratum album profundum corporis bigemini anterioris
scc, sulcus corporis callosi
scg, nucleus suprageniculatus

scm, nucleus supramammillaris
scm, nucleus supramamillaris
Sg, gyrus sigmoideus
Sga, gyrus sigmoideus anterior
sgc, substantia gelatinosa centralis
sgm, stratum griseum medium
sgm, stratum griseum medium corporis bigemini anterioris
sgp, stratum griseum profundum
Sgp, gyrus sigmoideus posterior
sgp, stratum griseum profundum corporis bigemini anterioris
sgR, substantia gelatinosa Rolandi
sgs, stratum grisum superficiale
sgs, stratum griseum superficiale corporis bigemini anterioris
sip, sulcus intermedius posterior
siR, substantia innominata Reicherti
sla, sulci laterales anterior
sla, sulcus lateralis anterior
slfr, sulcus lateralis fossae rhomboideae
sln, sulcus basilaris s. sulcus longitudinalis
sln, sulcus longitudinalis
slp, sulci laterales posterior
slp, sulcus lateralis posterior
sma, sulcus medianus anterior
smd, nucleus submedium
smd, nucleus submedius thalami optici
smfr, sulcus medianus fossae rhomboideae
smp, sulcus medianus posterior
smt, stria medullaris thalami
sn, substantia nigra
snc, substantia nigra zona compacta
snr, substantia nigra zona reticularis
so, stratum opticum
so, stratum opticum corporis bigemini anterioris
Sp, gyrus Sylvii posterior
spa, substantia perforata anterior
Spl, gyrus splenialis
spl, sulcus splenialis
spn, splenium corporis callosi
spp, sulcus praepyramidalis
sprf, nucleus subparafascicularis thalami optici
spt, massa septii pellucidi
spt, septum pellucidum
Ss, gyrus suprasylvius
ss, sulcus suprasylvius
Ssa, gyrus suprasylvius anterior
ssa, sulcus suprasylvius anterior
ssc, stratum subcallosum
Ssm, gyrus suprasylvius medius

ssm, sulcus suprasylvius medius
Ssp, gyrus suprasylvius posterior
ssp, sulcus suprasylvius posterior
Sspl, gyrus suprasplenialis
sspl, sulcus suprasplenialis
st, stria terminalis
stc, stratum complexum pontis
stp, stratum profundum pontis
sts, stratum superficiale pontis
sub, subiculum
sz, stratum zonale
sz, stratum zonale corporis bigemini anterioris
T_1, T_2, T_3, T_4, areae temparales: prima, secunda, tertia, quarta
ta, taenia anterior
tac, tuberculum acusticum
tc, tuber cinereum
TE_1, TE_2, area temporoentorhinalis prima et secunda
tg, nucleus tangentialis
th, thalamus opticus
TO, tuberculum olfactorium
to, tractus opticus
TO^1, TO^2, area prima et secunda tuberculi olfactorii
Tpc, area temporopostcoronalis
tr, sulcus transsecans
trn, truncus corporis callosi
T^s_1, T^i_1, subarea temporalis prima superior et inferior
tt, taenia tecta
tub, tuber vermis cerebelli
uv, uvula
V, nervus trigeminum
v, ventral group of cells of the anterior horn of the spinal cord
vlII, ventriculus tertius
VIII, nervus statoacusticus
vlV, ventriculus quartus
vl, ventriculus lateralis
vm, vellum medullare anterius
vmp, velum medullare posterius
vna, pars anterior nucleus ventralis thalami opticii
vnar, pars arcuata nucleus ventralis
vne, pars externa nucleus ventralis
vnm, pars medialis nucleus ventralis
vs, fasciculus vestibulo-spinalis
X, nervus vagus
XI, nervus accessorius Willissii
XII, nervus hypoglossus
zin, zona incerta
zm, zona marginalis

INDEX

aquaeductus Sylvii, aS, 18, 62, 64, 66, 68, 70, 72

area acustica, aa, 9

area frontalis prima, F_1, 111, 115, 148, 172, 176–178

area frontalis quarta, F_4, 111, 115, 180, 182–184, 186

area frontalis secunda, F_2, 111, 115, 172, 176, 178–180

area frontalis tertia, F_3, 111, 115, 178, 180–182

area hypothalamica lateralis, hpl, 22, 76, 78, 80, 82, 84, 86, 88

area insularis prima, I_1, 106, 113, 114, 146–148, 150, 152, 154, 155

area insularis secunda, I_2, 106, 113, 148–150, 172, 176

area limbica prima, L_1, 116, 120, 126, 188–190, 196

area limbica secunda, L_2, 94, 111, 116, 170, 174, 188, 190, 191, 196

area occipitalis prima, O_1, 104, 106, 112, 118–120, 122, 188

area occipitalis secunda, O_2, 106, 112, 118, 120–123, 125, 126, 130, 142, 188

area occipto parietalis, OP, 105, 106, 112, 120, 123–126, 128, 188

area parainsularis prima, PI_1, 106, 113, 132, 144, 150–152

area parainsularis secunda, PI_2, 106, 113, 150, 152, 153, 166

area parietalis, P, 104, 106, 112, 123, 126, 127, 136, 138, 156, 188

area peritectalis prima, Pt_1, 116, 192, 194

area peritectalis secunda, Pt_2, 116, 192, 194

area peritectalis tertia, Pt_3, 116, 190, 194, 195

area postcoronalis prima, Pc_1, 105, 106, 111, 114, 126, 156–158, 160, 162, 166, 168, 170, 188

area postcoronalis quarta, Pc_4, 111, 114, 160, 164, 166, 169, 172

area postcoronalis secunda, Pc_2, 106, 111, 114, 156, 158–160, 162, 166, 168, 170

area postcoronalis tertia, Pc_3, 106, 111, 114, 158, 160–162, 164, 169, 170, 172

area postrema, ap, 9, 38, 40

area praecoronalis prima, Prc_1, 105, 111, 156, 160, 171, 172

area praecoronalis secunda, Prc_2, 105, 111, 172–174, 176, 178, 180

area praeoptica lateralis, hprl, 24, 90

area praeoptica medians, hprm, 90

area praeoptica, hpr, 24, 92

area praetectalis, prt, 20, 72, 74, 76

area temporalis prima, T_1, 105, 106, 113, 120, 130–132, 134, 136, 140–142

area temporalis quarta, T_4, 106, 113, 126, 130, 134, 136, 138, 142

area temporalis secunda, T_2, 106, 113, 130, 132–134, 137, 140, 142, 144, 150, 152

area temporalis tertia, T_3, 106, 113, 130, 132, 134–136, 142, 152, 166

area temporoentorhinalis prima, TE_1, 106, 130, 140, 142, 144

area temporoentorhinalis secunda, TE_2, 105, 106, 132, 140, 144, 145

area temporopostcoronalis, TPc, 105, 106, 111, 114, 134, 156, 158, 166, 167

brachium corporis bigemini posterioris, bcbp, 18

calamus scriptorius, cal, 9, 38

canalis centralis, cc, 5, 26, 30, 32, 34, 36

canalis nervus hypoglossi, 12

capsula externa, ce, 23, 80, 82, 84, 86, 88, 90, 92, 94

capsula extrema, cex, 80, 82, 88, 90, 92, 94

capsula interna, ci, 23, 78, 80, 82, 84, 86, 88, 90, 92

cavum septi pellucidi, 24

centrum medianum Luysi, cmd, 20

chiasma nervorum opticorum, ch, 86, 88, 90

claustrum, cls, 23, 78, 80, 82, 84, 86, 88, 90, 92, 94

columna fornicis, cf, 90

columnae anteriores, cla, 26

columnae fornicis, 20, 24

columnae laterales, cll, 26

columnae posteriores, clp, 26

commissura anterior, can, 20, 24, 90, 92, 94

commissura corporis bigemini anterioris, ccba, 66, 68, 70, 72

commissura corporis bigemini posterioris, ccbp, 18

commissura fornicis, 24

commissura grisea media s. commissura mollis, cm, 20

commissura grisea posterior, cpg, 26

commissura posterior, cmp, 19, 72

commissurae anteriores grisea, cag, et alba, caa, 26

contractile tonus, 19

corna posteriores, cp, 26

cornu Ammonis inferius, CAi, 78, 80

cornu Ammonis superius CAs, 78

cornu lateralis, cl, 26

corpus bigeminum anterius, cba, 18, 66, 68, 70, 72

corpus bigeminum posterius, cbp, 18

corpus callosum, ccl, 20, 23, 24, 78, 82, 86, 88, 90, 92, 94

corpus geniculatum laterale, cgl, 19, 72, 74, 76

corpus geniculatum mediale, cgm, 13, 18, 19, 68, 70, 74

corpus juxta restiforme, 17

corpus Luysi, cL, 19, 21, 74, 76, 78, 80, 82

corpus nuclei caudati, ncd, 24, 84, 86, 88, 90, 92, 94
corpus restiforme, rest, 5, 9, 38, 40, 42, 44, 46, 48, 50
corpus trapezoides, ctr, 48, 50, 52, 54
crura cerebelli ad pontem s. crura pontis, 9
culmen, cu, 15
cuneiform fasciculus (nce), 38

declive, de, 15
decussatio Foreli, dF, 8
decussatio lemniscorum, dlm, 5
decussatio Meynerti, dM, 8
decussatio pyramidum, dpy, 7, 9, 30

eminentia tares, et, 9
epithalamus, 19

fascia dentata inferior, FDi, 78, 80
fascia dentata superior, FDs, 78
fasciculus centralis tegmenti, fct, 14, 17, 52, 54, 56,
       58, 60, 62, 64, 66, 68, 70, 72
fasciculus colliculorubralis, 18
Fasciculus corticospinalis s. pyramidalis, py, 7
fasciculus lecticularis, H2, 19
fasciculus lecticularis, H_2, 19, 21, 74, 76, 78, 80
Fasciculus longitudinalis posterior s. medians, flp, 8
fasciculus longitudinalis posterior, flp, 30, 32, 34, 36,
       38, 40, 42, 44, 46, 48, 50, 52, 54, 56, 58,
       60, 62, 64, 66
fasciculus mamillothalamicus s.   fasciculus Vicq
       d'Azyr, fmt, 20, 80, 82, 84, 86, 88
fasciculus mamillothalamicus s.   fasciculus Vicq
       d'Azyri, fmt, 76
fasciculus pyramidalis, py, 9, 32, 34, 36, 38, 40, 42,
       44, 46, 48, 50, 52, 54, 56, 58
Fasciculus reticulospinalis, 8
fasciculus rubrospinalis, frs, 8, 30, 32, 34, 36, 38, 40,
       42, 44, 46, 48, 50, 52, 54, 56, 58, 60, 62, 64
fasciculus spinocerebellaris dorsalis Flechsigi, fscd, 30,
       32, 34, 36
Fasciculus spinocerebellaris dorsalis, fscd, 5
fasciculus spinocerebellaris ventralis Gowersi, fscv, 30,
       32, 34, 36, 38, 40, 42, 44, 46
Fasciculus spinocerebellaris ventralis, fscv, 7
fasciculus spinoreticularis, 7
fasciculus spinotactalis, fsth, 7
fasciculus spinothalamicus, fsth, 7, 30, 32, 34, 36, 38,
       40, 42, 44, 46, 48, 50, 52, 54, 56, 58, 60,
       62, 64, 66, 68, 70, 72, 74
fasciculus striopeduncularis, fsp, 66, 68, 70, 72, 74,
       76, 80
Fasciculus tectospinalis s. praedorsalis, fts, 8
fasciculus tectospinalis, fts, 30, 32, 34, 36, 38, 40, 42,
       44, 46, 48, 50, 52, 54, 56, 58, 60, 62, 64,
       66, 68
fasciculus thalamicus, H_1, 21, 78, 80
fasciculus uncinatus, 17
Fasciculus vestibulospinalis Lowentali, 8

fibrae arcuatae externae anteriores, area, 38, 40
fibrae arcuatae externae posteriores, arep, 5, 36
fibrae arcuatae internae, ari, 5
fibrae cerebello-olivares, 17
fibrae cortico-pontines, 17
fibrae cortico-pontino-cerebellares, 17
fibrae olivocerebellares, foc, 17, 34, 36, 38, 40
fibrae vestibule-cerebellares, fvc, 13, 50, 52
fissura longitudinalis cerebri, flc, 24
fissura mediana anterior, fma, 1, 9, 26
fissura paramediana, fpm, 15
flocculus, fl, 15
foramen Monroi, fM, 24, 90
formatio reticularis, ret, 5, 14, 26, 30, 34, 36, 38, 40,
       42, 44, 46, 48, 50, 52, 54, 56, 58, 62, 64,
       68, 70, 72
fornix, f, 24, 78, 80, 82, 86, 88, 90, 92
fossa interpeduncularis, fin, 18
fossa rhomboidea, 9
fossa Sylvii, 97
funiculus cuneatus, fc, 5, 9, 30, 32, 36
funiculus gracilis, 9
funiculus gracilis, fg, 5, 9, 30, 32, 36

gangl. interpedunculare, gi), 19
gangl. spinale s. intervertebrale, 5
genu corporis callosi, gen, 94
glandula pinealis s. epiphysis, 19

H_1, 19, 82, 84
habenula s. nucleus habenulae, nh, 19
hypophysis, hyp, 19, 22
hypothalamus, s. regio hypothalamica, 19

III, 88
infundibulum, in, 19, 22, 80

lamina quadric gemina, 18
lamina terminalis, 20
laminae medullares, 20
lemniscus lateralis, ll, 50, 52, 54, 56, 58, 60, 64, 66,
       70
lemniscus medians, lm, 5, 36, 38, 40, 42, 44, 46, 48,
       50, 52, 54, 56, 58, 60, 62, 64, 66, 68, 70
lingula, li, 15
lobulus centralis, lc, 15
lobulus quadrangularis, lqd, 15

m. ciliaris, 19
m. sphincter pupillae, 19
massa septii pellucidi, spt, 92
medulla oblongata, mo, 9

n. oculomotorius, III, 19
nervus abducens, VI, 13
nervus accessorius Willisii, XI, 12
nervus cochlearis, rVIIIc, 12, 13
nervus glossopharyngeus, IX, 12

nervus hypoglossus, XII, 9
nervus opticus, II, 92
nervus trigemini, nVm, 13, 56
nervus trigeminum, V, 13
nervus trigeminus, V, 56
nervus trochlearis, IV, 19
nervus vagus, X, 12
nervus vestibularis, rVIIIv, 12
nodulus, nod, 15
nuclei cornu posterioris, 26
nuclei lemniscus lateralis, nll, 13, 58
nuclei proprii pontis, npp, 14, 54, 56, 58, 60, 62, 64
nucleus amygdalae, am, 78, 80, 82, 84
nucleus anterodorsalis, and, 20, 84, 86, 88
nucleus anteromedialis, anm, 20, 84, 86, 88
nucleus anteroventralis, anv, 20, 84, 86, 88
nucleus arcuatus medullae oblongatae, narc, 42, 44
nucleus centralis formatio reticularis, ncr, 14
nucleus centralis formation reticularis, ncr, 40
nucleus centralis lateralis, cnl, 20, 76, 78, 80, 82, 84
nucleus centralis medialis, cnm, 20, 78, 80, 82, 84, 86
nucleus centralis tegmenti, nct, 14, 56, 58
nucleus commissura posterioris, nap, 19
nucleus commissurae posterioris, ncp, 72
nucleus Darkschewitschi, nDr, 19, 72
nucleus Deitersi, nD, 13, 44, 46, 48, 50, 52
nucleus dentatus, s. nucleus lateralis, ndn, 17
nucleus dorsalis nervus accessorii, nXId, 12, 30
nucleus emboliformis, neb, 17
nucleus externus funiculi cuneati s. nucleus Burdach,
    s. Monakowi, s. Bechterewi, nce, 36
nucleus fastigii s. tecti, s. nucleus medians, nfs, 17
nucleus filiformis anterior, fa, 22, 86, 88
nucleus filiformis principalis, fp, 22, 88
nucleus funiculi cuneati, nc, 5, 30, 32, 34, 36, 38
nucleus funiculi gracilis, ng, 5, 30, 32, 34, 36, 38
nucleus gigantocellularis formatio reticularis, ngc, 42,
    44, 46, 48, 50
nucleus gigantocellularis, ngc, 14
nucleus globosus, ngb, 17
nucleus habenulae, nh, 21
nucleus hypoglossi, nXII, 36
nucleus hypothalamicus anterior, hpa, 22, 86, 88
nucleus hypothalamicus dorsomedialis, hpmd, 22, 82,
    84
nucleus hypothalamicus posterior, hpp, 22, 76, 78, 80
nucleus hypothalamicus ventromedialis, hpmv, 22, 82,
    84
nucleus interanterodorsalis, 20
nucleus interanteromedialis, iam, 20, 88
nucleus interantoromedians, iam, 86
nucleus intercalates, nin, 38, 42
nucleus intermediodorsalis, imd, 20, 80, 82
nucleus interparataenialis, 20
nucleus interpositus, 17
nucleus interstitialis commissurae anterioris, nca, 24

nucleus interstitialis commissurae anterioris, nca s. \,
    90
nucleus interstitialis striae terminalis, nst, 90
nucleus lateralis, 20
nucleus lateralis corporis mamillaris, cml, 19, 22, 76,
    78
nucleus lateralis habenulae, nhl, 21, 74, 76, 78
nucleus lateralis medullae oblongatae, s. nucleus lat-
    eralis reticularis, nit, 14
nucleus lateralis, nlt, 32, 34, 36, 38, 40
nucleus lemnisci lateralis, nll, 56
nucleus lenticularis, 80
nucleus limitans, lmt, 20
nucleus medialis habenulae, nhm, 21, 74, 76, 78
nucleus medians corporis mamillaris, cmm, 19, 22, 76,
    78
nucleus medians dorsalis, md, 20, 76, 78, 80, 82, 84,
    86
nucleus motorius n. trigemini, rVm, 54
nucleus motorius n. vagi s. nucleus ambiguus, nXa,
    38, 40
nucleus n. cervicalis I, nc1, 30
nucleus nervi abducentis, nVI, 13, 50
nucleus nervus trochlearis, nIV, 64
nucleus paracentralis, pcn, 20, 80, 82, 84
nucleus parafascicularis, prf, 20, 74, 76, 78
nucleus parataenialis, pt, 20, 80, 82, 84, 86, 88
nucleus paraventricularis anterior, pra, 20, 80, 82, 84,
    86, 88
nucleus paraventricularis posterior, prp, 20, 78
nucleus peripeduncularis, npd, 74, 76
nucleus pontis caudalis, npc, 14
nucleus pontis oralis, npo, 14
nucleus posterior, post, 20
nucleus radicis descendentis n. trigemini, nVd, 13, 36,
    38, 40, 42, 44, 46, 48, 50
nucleus radicis descendentis nervus vestibularis, ndv,
    44
nucleus reticularis, nret, 20, 74, 76, 78, 80, 82, 84, 86,
    88, 90
nucleus reuniens thalami, reu, 20, 80, 82, 84, 86, 88
nucleus rhomboidalis, rhm, 20, 80, 82, 84
nucleus ruber, nr, 19, 68, 70, 72
nucleus sensibilis nervi trigemini, nVs, 13
nucleus sensorius nervi trigemini, nVs, 54, 56
nucleus sublingualis, nR, 40, 42, 44, 46
nucleus submedium, smd, 20, 84
nucleus suprageniculatus, scg, 20, 72, 74, 76
nucleus supramammillaris, scm, 22
nucleus supraopticus diffusus, nsp, 22, 86, 88
nucleus sympaticus lateralis Jacobsohni, 5
nucleus tangentialis, tg, 22, 86, 88, 90
nucleus tractus habenulopeduncularis, hp, 20, 74, 76,
    78
nucleus tractus solitarius, nsl, 12, 34, 36, 38, 40, 42,
    44
nucleus triangularis, ntr, 12, 42, 44, 46, 48, 50

nucleus ventralis, 20
nucleus ventralis nervus accessorii, nXlv, 12, 30
nXd, 36

oliva inferior accessoria dorsalis, oid, 38
oliva inferior accessoria ventralis, oiv, 38
oliva superior lateralis, osl, 13, 50, 52
olive inferior, oi, 14, 34, 36, 38, 42

pallidum externum, pe, 23, 80, 84, 86, 88, 92
pallidum internum, pi, 23, 80, 82, 84, 86
paraflocculus, pfl, 15
pars anterior nucleus ventralis, vna, 21, 82, 84, 86, 88
pars anterior, lta, 20, 80, 82, 84
pars arcuata nucleus ventralis, vnar, 21, 76, 78, 80, 82, 84
pars externa nucleus ventralis, vne, 21, 76, 78, 80, 82, 84, 86
pars intermedia nucleus lateralis, lti, 20, 78, 80, 82
pars medians nucleus ventralis, vnm, 21, 78, 80, 82, 84, 86
pars posterior nucleus lateralis, ltp, 20, 74, 76, 78, 80
Pe, 82
pedunculi cerebelli superior, pcs, 18
pedunculi cerebelli superiores, pcs, 9, 17, 52, 54, 56, 58
pedunculi cerebri, pc, 18
pedunculi corporae mamillariae, pm, 22, 70, 74
pedunculi inferior s. pedunculi cerebelli ad medullam oblongatum, pci, 17
pedunculum cerebelli superior, pcs, 19
pes pedunculi, pp, 18, 19, 60, 62, 66, 68, 70, 72, 74, 76, 78, 80, 82, 84
plexus chorioideus, 24
pons Varolii, pV, 9
processus acominis, a, 97
pulvinar, pul, 20, 72, 74, 76, 78
putamen, put, 23, 80, 82, 84, 86, 88, 90, 92, 94
pyramid, pyr, 15

radiatio thalami optici, 21
radix descendens nervi trigemini, rVd, 9, 13, 32, 36, 38, 40, 42, 44, 46, 48, 50, 52, 54
radix descendens nervi vestibularis, rdv, 44
raphe, r, 15, 36, 38, 40, 42, 44, 46, 48, 50
regio diagonalis, D, 90, 92
regio entorhinalis, E, 78, 80
regio periamygdalaris, Pm, 80, 82, 84, 86, 88
regio praepiriformis, Pp, 82, 84, 86, 88, 90, 92, 94
regio subthalamica s. subthalamus, 19
rXII, 36

s. pedunculi cerebelli medius, pcm, 9, 17, 52, 54, 58
stratum album medium, sam, 18
stratum album profundum, sap, 18
stratum complexum, stc, 14
stratum ganglionare, 17
stratum granulosum, 17

stratum griseum medium, sgm, 18
stratum griseum profundum, sgp, 18
stratum grisum superficiale, sgs, 18
stratum moleculare, 15
stratum opticum, so, 18
stratum profundum pontis, stp, 14, 54, 56, 58
stratum subcallosum, ssc, 88, 90, 92, 94
stratum superficial pontis, sts, 14, 54, 56, 58, 60, 62, 64
stratum zonale, sz, 18
stria medullaris thalami, smt, 19, 21, 76, 82, 84, 86, 88
stria terminalis, st, 20
subarea fronto-limbica, F-L_2, 111, 180, 182, 186, 187, 190
subarea postcoronalis quarta inferior, Pc^i_4, 164, 165
subarea postcoronalis quarta superior, Pc^s_4, 114, 162–164
subarea praecoronalis secunda limbica, Prc_2-L_2, 172, 174, 175, 180, 190
substantia gelatinosa centralis, 26
substantia gelatinosa Rolandi, sgR, 26, 30, 32
substantia grisea centralis, gc, 56, 58, 60, 62, 64, 66, 68, 70, 72
substantia innominata Reicherti, siR, 90, 92
substantia nigra zona compacta, snc, 68, 70
substantia nigra zona reticularis, snr, 68, 70
substantia nigra, sn, 19, 64, 66, 72
substantia perforata posterior, 18
sulci laterales anterior, sla, 1
sulci laterales posterior, slp, 1
sulcua ectosylvius medium, esm, 97
sulcus ansatus, an, 97
sulcus arcuatus secundus, 97
sulcus basilaris s. sulcus longitudinalis, sln, 9
sulcus coronalis, 97
sulcus ectosylvius anterior, esa, 97
sulcus ectosylvius posterior, esp, 97
sulcus ectosylvius, es, 97
sulcus intermedius posterior, sip, 9
sulcus lateralis anterior, sla, 9
sulcus lateralis fossae rhomboideae, slfr, 9
sulcus lateralis posterior, slp, 9, 26
sulcus limitans posterior, 97
sulcus medianus anterior, sma, 26
sulcus medianus fossae rhomboideae, smfr, 9
sulcus medianus posterior, smp, 1, 9, 26
sulcus suprasylvius anterior, ssa, 97
sulcus suprasylvius medium, ssm, 97
sulcus suprasylvius posterior, ssp, 97
sulcus suprasylvius, ss, 97
sulcus Sylvii, sulcus pseudosylvius, s, 97
systema periventricularis, per, 22, 74, 76, 78, 80, 82, 84

taenia tecta, tt, 94
tectum, 18

thalamus opticus, th, 19
to, 80, 82, 84
tractus habenulo-peduncularis s. fasciculus retroflexus
       Maynerti, frM, 21
trigonum hypoglossi, 9
tuber cinereum, tc, 19, 22, 80
tuber, tub, 15
tuberculum acusticum, tac, 13, 48, 50
tuberculum olfactorium, TO, 94

uvula, uv, 15

vellum medullare anterius, vm, 18
velum medullare posterius, vmp, 38, 40
ventriculus lateralis, vl, 78, 80, 86, 88, 90, 92, 94
ventriculus tertius, vIII, 19
vIII, 78, 80, 82, 84, 90

zona incerta, zin, 19, 21, 74, 76, 78, 80, 82, 84
zona marginalis, zm, 26

Lightning Source UK Ltd.
Milton Keynes UK
172976UK00001B/8/P